Principles of Research Methodology

Phyllis G. Supino • Jeffrey S. Borer
Editors

Principles of Research Methodology

A Guide for Clinical Investigators

Foreword by Stephen E. Epstein

Springer

Editors
Phyllis G. Supino
Professor of Medicine, College of Medicine
Professor of Public Health, School of Public Heath
Director of Clinical Epidemiology and Clinical Research
Division of Cardiovascular Medicine
State University of New York (SUNY) Downstate Medical Center
Brooklyn, NY, USA

Jeffrey S. Borer
Professor and Chair, Department of Medicine
Chief, Division of Cardiovascular Medicine
Director of The Howard Gilman Institute for Heart Valve Disease
Director of the Cardiovascular Translational Research Institute
SUNY Downstate Medical Center
Brooklyn, NY, USA

ISBN 978-1-4939-4292-3 ISBN 978-1-4614-3360-6 (eBook)
DOI 10.1007/978-1-4614-3360-6
Springer New York Heidelberg Dordrecht London

Printed on acid-free paper

Springer is part of Springer Science+Business Media (www.springer.com)

Foreword

This superb book on research philosophy and methodology that Drs. Phyllis Supino and Jeffrey Borer have written and edited came out of an experience common to most of us involved in training investigators beginning their research careers. How do you teach these investigators the mostly unwritten ways of an area as complex as medical research? How do you help the research neophyte develop into a creative and reliable researcher? For me and my associates in the Cardiology Branch of the NIH (of which Dr. Borer was one) in the 1970s and 1980s, the teaching process was mostly based on an apprenticeship model, with learning coming in the actual doing of the research. This time-honored approach led to the development, in many research centers, of a cadre of superb researchers—but it was hard to master and the results were necessarily inconsistent, with many young investigators going down wrong paths.

Drs. Supino and Borer's book represents a unique collaboration between an accomplished educator specializing in research methodology and a prominent physician-scientist. Drs. Supino and Borer began their collaboration more than 20 years ago at Cornell University Medical College, continuing their work together in what became the Howard Gilman Institute for Valvular Heart Diseases. The Institute, of which Dr. Borer is the Director, now is located at the State University of New York Downstate Medical Center. Working within the context of a research institute housed within a medical school, Dr. Borer soon discovered that most of the fellows coming into his program had no formal research training and scant knowledge of research methodology. Prior to joining the Institute, Dr. Supino had been conducting continuing education in research methodology for scientists and health professionals since late 1970's. When Dr. Supino joined the Institute in 1990, she applied her accumulated expertise in this field to develop a curriculum and lead a comprehensive course providing formal training in research methodology for Dr. Borer's fellows and others at the institution. This curriculum and course, developed in partnership with Dr. Borer, turned out to be our good fortune. During the ensuing 20+ years Drs. Supino and Borer gradually developed the pedagogical framework for writing what is one of the best books in the field.

This book provides in depth chapters containing information critical to creating good research—from the kind of mind-set that generates valuable research questions to study design, to exploring a variety of online data bases, to the elements making for compelling research grants and papers, and to the wonderfully informing chapter on the history of the application of ethics to medical research. There also is a valuable chapter on statistical considerations and a fascinating discussion on the origins and elements of hypothesis generation.

It's also important to emphasize that this superb text is not only for the new investigator, but for experienced investigators as well. This results from the fact that Drs. Supino, Borer, and their coauthors write their chapters in ways that are not only easily accessible to the new investigator, but at the same time are sufficiently sophisticated so that the seasoned investigator will profit.

As an example, I particularly enjoyed the first chapter, written by Dr. Supino, which provides some down to earth examples of, in essence, why there should be a clearly defined primary endpoint in clinical investigations. As I was reading her chapter, I realized I had forgotten the "why" of this requirement, and that I was just taking the requirement for granted—a situation that could make investigators vulnerable to dismissing its importance. In this regard, over the years I've found it not uncommon for investigators, who find that the efficacy of the intervention they're studying significantly improves one or another secondary endpoints but not the primary endpoint, to freely attack this "requirement" and argue they've proven the efficacy of their intervention. But Dr. Supino reminds us what good science is by providing an elegantly simple example of the marksman who boasts his skills after interpreting the results of his shooting a gun at a piece of paper hung on the side of a barn. The marksman, it turns out, does not prospectively define the "bull's eye". Rather, after multiple bullets are fired at the piece of paper, he inspects the bullet hole-riddled paper, sees the random bullet hole patterns, and then draws a circle (bull's eye) around a group of holes that by chance have fallen into a tight cluster. The post hoc definition of the bull's eye (i.e., now the "primary endpoint") speaks (unjustifiably) to the marksman's skill. By this simple anecdote, Dr. Supino makes the critical importance of prospectively defining the primary endpoint exquisitely clear.

A foreword is no place to provide extensive details of what a book contains. I'll therefore limit myself and just enthusiastically say this first chapter I read is representative of the high quality of the chapters to come. Drs. Supino and Borer have used the many years they have developed their course extraordinarily well—they and their outstanding coauthors have produced a book that is well written, beautifully edited, and contains wisdom and insight. It is a book, whether reading it in its entirety or perusing individual chapters, that presents the reader with a superb learning experience. The authors have certainly hit the bull's eye.

Washington, DC, USA Stephen E. Epstein, MD

Preface

This book has been written to aid medical students, physicians, and other health professionals as they probe the increasingly complex and varied medical/scientific literature for knowledge to improve patient care and search for guidance in the conduct of their own research. It also is intended for basic scientists involved in translational research who wish to better understand the unique challenges and demands of clinical research and, thus, become more successful members of interdisciplinary medical research teams.

The book is based largely on a lecture series on research methodology, with particular emphasis on issues affecting clinical research, that the editors designed and have offered for 21 years to more than 1,000 members of the academic medical communities of Weill Cornell Medical College and the State University of New York (SUNY) Downstate Medical Center, both located in New York City. The book spans the entire research process, beginning with the conception of the research problem to publication of findings.

The need for such a book has become increasingly clear to us during many years of conducting a program of training and research in cardiovascular diseases and in our general teaching of research methodology to students, trainees, and postgraduate clinical physicians and researchers. Though agreement on the fundamental principles of scientific research has existed for more than a century, the application of these principles has changed over time. The precision required in defining study populations and in detailing methodologies (and their deficiencies) is continually increasing. In addition, a bewildering arsenal of statistical tools has developed (and continues to grow) to identify and define the magnitude and consistency of relationships. Simultaneously, acceptable formats for communicating scientific data have changed in response to parallel changes in the world at large, and under the pressure of an "information explosion" which mandates succinctness and clarity.

Despite these demands, there are few books, if any, that comprehensively and concisely present these concepts in a manner that is relevant and comprehensible to a broad professional medical community. This text is designed to resolve this deficiency by combining theory and practical application to familiarize the reader with the logic of research design and hypothesis construction, the importance of research planning, the ethical basis of human subjects research, the basics of writing a clinical protocol, the logic and techniques of data generation and management, and the fundamentals and implications of various sampling techniques and alternative statistical methodologies. This book also aims to offer guidance for assembling and interpreting results, writing scientific papers, and publishing studies.

The book's 13 chapters emphasize the role and structure of the scientific hypothesis (reinforced throughout the various chapters) in informing methods and in guiding data interpretation. Chapter 1 describes the general characteristics of research and differentiates among various types of research; it also summarizes the steps typically utilized in the hypothesis-testing (hypothetico-deductive) method and underscores the importance of proper planning. Chapter 2 reviews the origins of clinical research problems and the types of questions that are commonly asked in clinical investigations; it also identifies the characteristics of well-conceived research problems and explains the role of the literature search in research problem development. Chapter 3 introduces the reader to various modes of logical inference utilized for hypothesis generation, describes the characteristics of well-designed research hypotheses, distinguishes among various types of hypotheses, and provides guidelines for constructing them. Chapter 4 takes the reader through classic epidemiological (observational) methods, including cohort, case–control, and cross-sectional designs, and describes their respective advantages and limitations. Chapter 5 discusses the meaning of internal and external validity in the context of studies that aim to examine the effects of purposively applied interventions, identifies the most important sources of bias in these types of studies, and presents a variety of alternative study designs that can be used to evaluate interventions, together with their respective strengths and weaknesses for controlling each of the identified biases. Chapter 6 defines and describes the purpose of the clinical trial and provides in-depth guidelines for writing the clinical protocol that governs its conduct. Chapter 7 describes methodologies used for data capture and management in clinical trials and reviews associated regulatory requirements. Chapter 8 explains the steps involved in designing, implementing, and evaluating questionnaires and interviews that seek to obtain self-reported information. Chapter 9 reviews the pros and cons of systematic reviews and meta-analyses for generating secondary data by synthesizing evidence from previously conducted studies, and discusses methods for locating, evaluating, and writing them. Chapter 10 describes the various methods by which subjects can be sampled and the implications of these methods for drawing conclusions from clinical research findings. Chapter 11 introduces the reader to fundamental statistical principles used in biomedical research and describes the basis of determination of sample size and definition of statistical power. Chapter 12 describes the ethical basis of human subjects research, identifies areas of greatest concern to institutional review boards, and outlines the basic responsibilities of investigators towards their subjects. Finally, Chapter 13 provides practical guidance on how to write a publishable scientific paper.

The authors of this book include prominent medical scientists and methodologists who have extensive personal experience in biomedical investigation and in teaching various key aspects of research methodology to medical students, physicians, and other health professionals. They have endeavored to integrate theory and examples to promote concept acquisition and to employ language that will be clear and useful for a general medical audience. We hope that this text will serve as a helpful resource for those individuals for whom performing or understanding the process of research is important.

Brooklyn, NY, USA

Phyllis G. Supino
Jeffrey S. Borer

Special Acknowledgments

We wish to give special thanks to the following individuals, who provided particular assistance to the editors and authors in the preparation of this book:

From our publishers, we especially thank Richard Lansing for his belief in the importance of our project as well as Kevin Wright, senior developmental editor, for his excellent pre-production work.

From SUNY Downstate Medical Center, we thank Ofek Hai DO for his efforts in the preparation of figures and tables; Rachel Reece BS for her assistance in helping us to secure permission for the reproduction of images; and Dany Bouraad BA, Jaclyn Wilkens BA, Daniel Santarsieri BS, and Romina Arias BA for their assistance in literature searching, proof reading, and other essential background work.

Finally, we thank our colleagues at Weill Cornell Medical College and SUNY Downstate Medical Center who participated in our teaching programs on which this book is largely based, and to our families for their unfailing support of this project.

Contents

Contributors

Jeffrey S. Borer, MD Department of Medicine, Division of Cardiovascular Diseases, Howard Gilman Institute for Valvular Heart Diseases, and Cardiovascular Translational Research Institute, State University of New York (SUNY) Downstate Medical Center, Brooklyn, NY, USA

Todd A. Durham, MS Axio Research, LLC, Seattle, WA, USA

Helen-Ann Brown Epstein, MLS, MS, AHIP Clinical Librarian, Samuel J. Wood Library and C.V. Starr Biomedical Information Center, Weill Cornell Medical College, New York, NY, USA

Peter L. Flom, PhD Peter Flom Consulting, LLC, New York, NY, USA

Joseph A. Franciosa, MD Department of Medicine, SUNY, Downstate Medical Center, Brooklyn, NY, USA

Eli A. Friedman, MD Department of Medicine, SUNY, Downstate Medical Center, Brooklyn, NY, USA

Mario Guralnik, PhD Synergy Research Inc, Irvine, CA, USA

Gary G. Koch, PhD Department of Biostatistics, University of North Carolina at Chapel Hill Gillings School of Global Public Health, Chapel Hill, NC, USA

Lisa M. LaVange, PhD Department of Biostatistics, University of North Carolina at Chapel Hill Gillings School of Global Public Health, Chapel Hill, NC, USA

Martin L. Lesser, PhD Biostatistics Unit, Departments of Molecular Medicine and Population Health, Feinstein Institute for Medical Research, Hofstra North Shore-LIJ School of Medicine, Manhasset, NY, USA

Lorenzo Paladino, MD Department of Emergency Medicine, SUNY Downstate Medical Center, Brooklyn, NY, USA

N. Philip Ross, BS, MS, PhD SUNY Downstate Medical Center, Bethesda, MD, USA

Richard H. Sinert, DO Department of Emergency Medicine, SUNY Downstate Medical Center, Brooklyn, NY, USA

Phyllis G. Supino, EdD Department of Medicine, College of Medicine, SUNY Downstate Medical Center, Brooklyn, NY, USA

Richard C. Zink, PhD JMP Life Sciences, SAS Institute, Inc, Cary, NC, USA

Overview of the Research Process

1

Phyllis G. Supino

The term "research" can be defined broadly as a process of solving problems and resolving previously unanswered questions. This is done by careful consideration or examination of a subject or occurrence. Although approach and specific objectives may vary, the ultimate goal of research always is to discover *new* knowledge. In biomedical research, this may include the description of a *new* phenomenon, the definition of a *new* relationship, the development of a *new* model, or the application of an existing principle or procedure to a *new* context. Increasingly, the methodology of research is acknowledged as an academic discipline of its own, whose specific rules and requirements for securing evidence, though applicable across disciplines, mandate special study. This chapter describes the characteristics of the research process and its relation to the scientific method, distinguishes among the various forms of research used in the biomedical sciences, outlines the principal steps involved in initiating a research project, and highlights the importance of planning.

P.G. Supino, EdD (✉)
Department of Medicine, College of Medicine,
SUNY Downstate Medical Center,
450 Clarkson Avenue, Box 1199, Brooklyn,
NY 11203, USA
e-mail: phyllissupino@aol.com

Characteristics of Research

No discussion of research methodology should begin without examining the characteristics of research and its relation to the scientific method. The reason for this starting point is that the term "research" has been used so loosely in common parlance and defined in so many different ways by scholars in various fields of inquiry [1] that its meaning is not always appreciated by those without a formal background. To understand more readily what research is, it is useful to begin by considering some examples of what it is *not*.

Leedy, in his book *Practical Research* [2], describes two young students: one whose teacher has sent him to the library to do "research" by gleaning a few facts about Christopher Columbus and another who completes a "research" paper on the Dark Lady in Shakespeare's sonnets by gathering facts, assembling a bibliography, and referencing statements without drawing conclusions or otherwise interpreting the collected data. Both students think that research has taken place when, in fact, all that has occurred has been information gathering and transport from one location to another. Leedy argues that these misconceptions are reinforced at every grade level and that most students facing the rigors of a graduate program lack clear understanding about the specific requirements of the research process and underestimate what is involved. In academic medical programs, it is not uncommon for a resident to comment, "I have a 2-week block available to

P.G. Supino and J.S. Borer (eds.), *Principles of Research Methodology: A Guide for Clinical Investigators*,
DOI 10.1007/978-1-4614-3360-6_1, © Phyllis G. Supino and Jeffrey S. Borer 2012

conduct a research project" and to expect to design, execute, and complete it in that time frame.

There is general consensus that information gathering, including reviewing and synthesizing the literature, is a critically important activity to be undertaken by an investigator. However, in and of itself, it is not research. The same can be said for data gathering activities aimed at personal edification or those undertaken to resolve organization-specific issues. So what, then, characterizes research?

Tuckman [3] has argued that in order for an activity to qualify as research, it should possess a minimum of five characteristics:

1. *It should be systematic.*
   While some important research findings have occurred serendipitously (e.g., Fleming's accidental discovery of penicillin, Pasteur's chance finding of microbial antibiosis), most arise out of purposeful, structured activity. Structure is engendered by a series of the rules for defining variables, constructing hypotheses, and developing research designs. Rules also exist for collecting, recording, and analyzing data, as well as for relating results to the problem statement or hypotheses. These rules are used to generate formal plans (or protocols) which guide the research effort, thereby optimizing the likelihood of achieving valid results.
2. *It should be logical.*
   Research employs logic that may be inductive, deductive, or abductive in nature. Inductive logic is employed to develop generalizations from repeated observations, abductive logic is used to form generalizations that serve as explanations for anomalous events, and deductive logic is used to generate specific assertions from known scientific principles or generalizations. Further elaboration of these distinctions is covered in Chap. 3. Logic is used both in the development of the research design and selection of statistics to ensure that valid inferences may be drawn from data (internal validity). Logic also is used to generalize from the results of the particular study to a broader context (external validity or extrapolability).
3. *It should be empirical.*
   Despite the deductive processes that may precede data collection, the findings of research must always be based on observation or experience and, thus, must relate to reality. It is the empirical quality of research that sets it apart from other logical disciplines, such as philosophy, which also attempts to explain reality. Recognition of this fact may pose a problem for physicians who, according to some researchers [4, 5], have a cognitive style that tends to be more deterministic than probabilistic, causing personal experience to be valued more than data. Under these circumstances, the importance of subordinating the hypothesis to data may not be fully appreciated. As part of the education of the physician scientist, he or she must learn that when confronted with data that do not support the study hypothesis, it is the hypothesis and *not* the data that must be discarded, unless it is abundantly clear that something untoward occurred during the performance of the study.
4. *It should be reductive.*
   As Tuckman [3] has noted, a fundamental purpose of research is to reduce "the confusion of individual events and objects to more understandable categories of concepts" (p. 11). One heuristic tool used by scientists for this purpose is the creation of abstractive constructs such as "intervening variables" (e.g., *resistance* and *solubility* in the physical sciences, *conditioning or reflex reserve* in the behavioral sciences) to explain how phenomena cause or otherwise interact with each other [6]. Another powerful tool available to the researcher for this purpose is a constellation of techniques for numerical and graphical data analysis (the specific methodology employed depending on the objectives and design of the study as well as the number of observations generated by the study). As Tuckman observes, whenever data are subjected to analysis, some information is lost, specifically the uniqueness of the individual observation. However, such losses are offset by gains in the capacity to

conceptualize general relationships based on the data. As a result, the investigator can explain and predict, rather than merely describe.

5. *It should be replicable and transmittable.* The fact that research procedures are documented makes it possible for others to conduct and attempt to replicate the investigation. The ability to replicate research results in the confirmation (or, in some unhappy cases, refutation) of conclusions. Confirmation of conclusions, in turn, results in the validation of research and confers upon research a respectability that generally is absent in other problem-solving processes. In addition, the fact that research is transmittable also enables the general body of knowledge to be extended by subsequent investigations based on the research. For this reason, researchers are encouraged to present their findings as soon as possible at local, national, and international scientific sessions and to publish them expeditiously as letters (communications) or full-length articles in peer-reviewed journals (to ensure their quality and validity).
6. *It should contribute to generalizable knowledge.* The Tuckman criteria speak to the structure and process of research, but not to its intended objectives. The Belmont Report [7], which codified the definition of human subjects research for the US Department of Health and Human Services, argues additionally that for an activity to be considered research, it must contribute to generalizable knowledge (the latter expressed in theories, principles, and statements of relationships). For knowledge to be generalizable, the *intent* of the activity must be to extrapolate findings from a sample (e.g., the study subjects) to a larger (reference) population to define some universal "truth," and be conducted by individuals with the requisite knowledge to draw such inferences [8]. Because research seeks generalizable knowledge, it differs from information gathering for diagnosis and management of individual patients. It also differs from formal evaluation procedures (e.g., review of data performed for clinical quality improvement [CQI] or formative and summative appraisals of educational programs) which, while employing many of the same rigorous and systematic methodologies as scientific research, principally aim to inform decision making about particular activities or policies rather than to advance more wide-ranging knowledge or theory. As Smith and Brandon [9] have noted, research "generalizes" whereas evaluation "particularizes."

Types of Research

There are multiple ways of classifying research, and the categorizations noted below are by no means exhaustive. Research can be classified according to its theoretical versus practical emphasis, the type of inferential processes used, its orientation with respect to data collection and analysis, its temporal characteristics, its analytic objective, the degree of control exercised by the investigator, or the characteristics of the measurements made during the investigation. These yield the following categorizations: basic versus applied versus translational, hypothesis testing versus hypothesis generating, retrospective versus prospective, longitudinal versus cross-sectional, descriptive versus analytic, experimental versus observational, and quantitative versus qualitative research.

Basic Versus Applied Versus Translational Research

Traditionally, research in medicine, as in other disciplines, has been classified as basic or applied, though the lines between the two can, and do, intersect. In basic research (alternatively termed "fundamental" or "pure" research), the investigation often is driven by scientific curiosity or interest in a conceptual problem; its objective is to expand knowledge by exploring ideas and questions and developing models and theories to explain phenomena. Basic research typically does not seek to provide immediate solutions to practical problems (indeed, it can progress for decades before leading to breakthroughs and paradigm shifts in practice), though it can yield unexpected applications (e.g., the discovery of the laser and its value for fiber-optic communications [10]), and it often provides the theoretical underpinnings of applied research. Applied research, in contrast, is conducted specifically to find solutions to practical problems in as rapid a time frame as possible. In medicine, applied research searches for explicit knowledge to improve the treatment of a specific disease or its sequelae. Examples of applied research include clinical trials of new drugs and devices in human subjects or evaluation of new uses for existing therapeutic interventions.

In recent years, "translational" or "translative" research has emerged as a paradigm alternative to the dichotomy between basic and applied research. Currently practiced in the natural, behavioral, and social sciences, and heavily reliant on multidisciplinary collaboration, translational research is a method of conceptualizing and conducting basic research to render its findings directly and more immediately applicable to the population under study. In medicine, this iterative approach is used to translate results of laboratory research more rapidly into clinical practice and vice versa ("bench to bedside and back" or T1 translation) and from clinical practice to the population at large ("to the community and beyond and back" or T2 translation) to enhance public knowledge. This is one of the major initiatives of the US National Institutes of Health (NIH) "Roadmap for Medical Research." Examples of T1 translation include the development of a technique for evaluating endothelium-dependent vasodilator responses as a diagnostic test in patients with atherosclerosis and the elucidation of the role of the p53 tumor suppressor gene in the regulation of apoptosis in the treatment of patients with cancer [11]. Examples of T2 translation would include the implementation, evaluation, and ultimate adoption of interventions that have been shown to be effective in clinical research for primary or secondary prevention in heart disease, stroke, and other disorders. (For an in-depth discussion of purpose, challenges, and techniques of translational research in clinical medicine and associated career opportunities, the reader is referred to the collective works of Schuster and Powers [12], Woolf [13], Robertson and Williams [14], and Goldblatt and Lee [15].)

Hypothesis-Generating Versus Hypothesis-Testing Research

Although some studies are undertaken to describe a phenomenon (e.g., incidence of a new disease or prevalence of an existing disorder in a new population), most research is performed to generate a hypothesis or to test a hypothesis. In hypothesis-generating research, the investigator begins with an observation (e.g., a newly discovered pattern, a rare event) and constructs an argument to explain it. Hypothesis-generating research typically is conducted when existing theory or knowledge is insufficient to explain particular phenomena. Popular "tools" for hypothesis generation in preclinical research include gene expression microarray studies; hypotheses for clinical or epidemiological research may be generated secondary to a project's initial purpose by mining existing datasets. In contrast, in hypothesis-testing research (sometimes called the "hypothetico-deductive" approach), the investigator begins with a general conjecture or hunch put forth to explain a prior observation or to clarify a gap in the existing knowledge base.

It is vitally important that the investigator keep these differences in mind when designing and drawing inferences from a study. To underscore what can happen when these distinctions are blurred, it is instructive to step back from scientific inquiry and mull over the following scenario:

A Texas cowboy fires his gun randomly at the side of a barn. Figure 1.1 (left panel) shows his results. He pours over his efforts, paints a target centered around his largest number of hits (Fig. 1.1, right panel), and claims to be a sharpshooter.

Do you agree that the Texan is a sharpshooter? Do you think that if he repeated his so-called

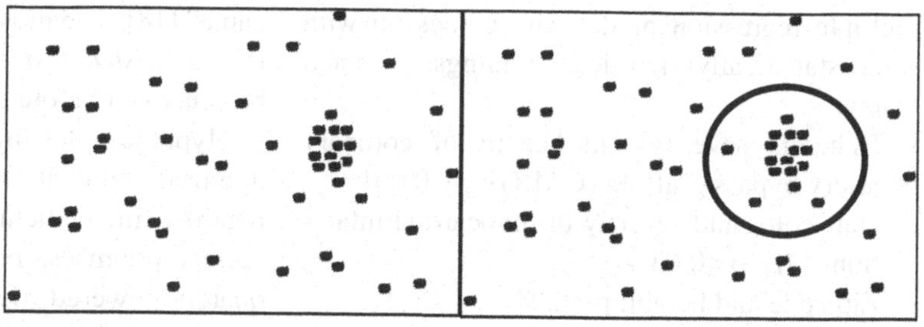

Fig. 1.1 The Texas sharpshooter fallacy

Fig. 1.2 Variables included in an exploratory dataset based on 95 patients with chronic coronary artery disease

- Age at study entry
- Incidence of sudden death
- Hair color
- Angina severity
- MI history
- Number of coronary vessels diseased
- Systolic blood pressure
- Income
- Sudden death
- Marital status
- Preop Ischemia severity
- CABG benefit
- Body mass index
- Family history of MI
- History of hypertension
- Height
- History of PTCA
- Beta blocker use
- Gender
- College education
- Zip code
- Number of children
- Exercise capacity
- Heart rate
- Eye color
- Smoking history
- Ethnicity
- IQ score
- ETOH consumption
- LV mass

target practice, he would again be able to get that many bullets in the circle? Note: the Texan defined his target only after he saw his results. He also ignored the bullets that were not in the cluster! This parable illustrates what epidemiologists call the "Texas Sharpshooter Fallacy" [16] to underscore the dangers of forming causal conclusions about cases of disease that happen to cluster in a population due to chance alone or to reasons other than the chosen cause. As per Atul Gawande, in his classic article in *The New Yorker*, of the myriad of cancer "clusters" studied by scientists in the United States, "not one has convincingly identified an underlying environmental cause" [17]. In a more general sense (and particularly germane to the activities of some biomedical researchers), the Texas Sharpshooter Fallacy is related to the "clustering illusion," which refers to the tendency of individuals to interpret patterns in randomness when none actually exists, often due to an underlying cognitive bias.

Consider a more clinical example: A resident inherits a dataset that contains information about 95 patients with chronic coronary artery disease. Figure 1.2 depicts the variables in that dataset.

He believes that he could satisfy his research elective if he could draw inferences about this study group, though he has no a priori idea about what relationships would be most reasonable to explore. He recruits a friend who happens to have a statistical package installed on his computer, enters all of the variables in the dataset into a multiple regression model, and comes up with some statistically significant findings, as noted below:

- Ischemia severity and benefit of coronary artery bypass grafting (CABG): $p<0.001$
- Hair color and severity of myocardial infarction (MI): $p<0.03$
- Zip code and height: $p<0.04$

He concludes that he has *confirmed the hypothesis* that there is a strong association between preoperative ischemia severity and benefit of coronary artery bypass grafting because not only was the obtained probability (p) value low, his hypothesis also makes clinical sense. He also decides that he would not report the other findings because, while also statistically significant, he cannot explain them. What methodological error has the resident made in drawing his conclusion?

The answer is that, analogous to the rifleman who defined his target only after the fact, the resident "confirmed" a hypothesis that did not exist before he examined patterns in his data. The fallacy would not have occurred if the resident had, in mind, a prior expectation of a particular association. It also would not have occurred had the resident used the data to generate a hypothesis and validated it, as he should have, with an independent group of observations if he wanted to draw such a definitive conclusion. This is an important distinction because the identification of an association between two or more variables may be the result of a chance difference in the distribution of these variables—and hypotheses identified this way are suggestive at best, not proven. What one cannot do is to use the same data to generate and test a hypothesis.

Moreover, the resident compounded his error by capitalizing on only one association that he found, ignoring all of the others. Working with hypotheses is like playing a game of cards. You cannot make up rules after seeing your hand, or change the rules midstream if you do not like the hand that you have been dealt. Similarly, if you gather your data first and draw conclusions based only on those you believe to be true, you have, in the words of the famed behavioral scientist, Fred Kerlinger, violated the rules of the "scientific game" [18]. The most important take-home point is *if you wish to test it*, a hypothesis always should be generated before data collection begins.

Hypothesis-testing studies (especially randomized clinical trials [RCTs]) are highly regarded in medicine because, when based on correct premises, properly designed, and adequately powered, they are likely to yield accurate conclusions [19]; in contrast, conclusions drawn from hypothesis-generating studies, even when well designed, are more tentative than those of hypothesis-testing studies due to the myriad of explanations (hypotheses) one can infer from the observation of a phenomenon.

For these reasons, hypothesis-generating studies are appropriately regarded as exploratory in nature. These differences notwithstanding, there is general consensus that hypothesis-testing and hypothesis-generating activities *both* are vital aspects of the research process. Indeed, the latter are the crucial initial steps for making discoveries in medicine. As Andersen [20] has correctly argued, without hypothesis-generating activities, there would be no hypotheses to test and the body of theory and knowledge would stagnate. The critical role of the hypothesis in the research process and the logical issues entailed in formulating and testing them are further discussed in Chap. 3.

Retrospective Versus Prospective Research

Research often is classified as retrospective or prospective. However, as pointed out by Catherine DeAngelis, former editor-in-chief of the Journal of the American Medical Association (JAMA), these terms "are among the most frequently misunderstood in research" [21] in part because they are used in different ways by different workers in the field and because some forms of research do not neatly fall within this dichotomy. Many methodologists [22, 23] consider research to be retrospective when data (typically recorded for purposes other than research) are generated prior to initiation of the study and to be prospective when data are collected starting with or subsequent to initiation of the study. Others, including

DeAngelis, prefer to distinguish retrospective from prospective research according to the investigator's and subject's orientation in the data acquisition process. According to the latter view, a study is retrospective if subjects are initially identified and classified on the basis of an outcome (e.g., a disease, mortality, or other event) and are followed backward in time to determine the relation of the outcome to exposure to one or more risk factors (genetic, biological, environmental, or behavioral); conversely, the study is prospective if it begins by identifying and classifying subjects on the basis of the exposure (even if the exposure preceded the investigation), with outcome (s) observed at a later point in time [21].

There are various types of retrospective studies. The simplest (and least credible from the standpoint of scientific evidence) is the "case study" (or "case report"), which typically provides instructive, albeit anecdotal, information about unusual symptoms not previously observed in a medical condition or new combinations of conditions within a single individual [24]. The "case series" (or "clinical series") is an uncontrolled study that furnishes information about exposures, outcomes, and other variables of interest among multiple similar cases. Though lack of control precludes evaluation of cause and effect, this type of study can provide useful information about unusual presentations or infrequently occurring diseases and can be used to generate hypotheses for testing, using more rigorous studies [24]. The most common type of retrospective research used to draw inferences about the relation of prior exposures to diseases (and the most rigorous of the various retrospective designs) is the case–control study. In this type of investigation, a group of individuals who are positive for a disease state (e.g., lung cancer) is compared with a group comprised of those who are negative for that disease state (e.g., free of lung cancer). By looking back at the medical record, we attempt to determine differences in risk factors (e.g., prior exposure to cigarette smoke or asbestos) that may account for the disease. Because of the temporal sequence and interval between the factor and the outcome variable and the availability of a comparison group (e.g., nondiseased subjects), the case–control study can be used to infer cause and effect associations, though various biases (discussed in depth in Chap. 4) may limit its value for this purpose.

The two most typical examples of prospective research in clinical medicine are observational cohort and experimental studies. In an observational cohort study, subjects within a defined group who share a common attribute of interest (e.g., newly diagnosed cardiac patients, new dialysis patients) who are free of some outcome of interest are identified on the basis of exposure to risk factors whose presence or absence is outside the control of the investigator. These individuals are followed over time until the occurrence of an outcome (or outcomes) that usually (but not always) is measured at a later date. In an experimental study, outcomes also are assessed at a later date, but subjects initially are differentiated according to their exposure to one or more interventions which have been purposively applied. (Further distinctions between observational and experimental studies are discussed below.)

Prospective research is less prevalent in the literature than retrospective research principally due to its relatively greater cost. In most prospective studies, the investigator must invest the time and resources to follow subjects and sometimes even apply an intervention if the study is experimental. Moreover, prospective studies usually require larger sample sizes. Why, then, would anyone choose a prospective design over a retrospective approach? One reason is that prospective studies (particularly RCTs and concurrent cohort studies, described below) potentially have more control over temporal sequence and extraneous factors, including selection and recall bias, although loss to follow-up can be problematic. Second, prospective designs are more appropriate than retrospective designs for rare exposures and relatively more common outcomes. Finally, if it is desired that the exposure be manipulated by the investigator, as in an experimental study, the relation between exposure and outcome can be evaluated only with a prospective design.

In many prospective studies (all RCTs, many cohort studies), the exposure takes place coincident with or following the initiation of the study.

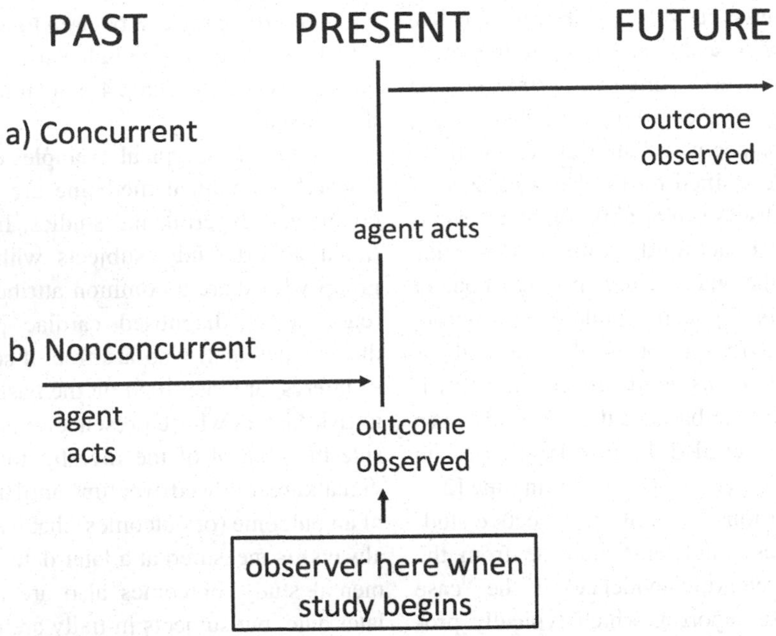

Fig. 1.3 Concurrent versus noncurrent "prospective" research (Reprinted with permission from [21])

This type of prospective research has been termed concurrent [25, 26] because the investigator moves along in parallel with the research process (i.e., from application or assessment of the exposure to ascertainment of the outcomes associated with the exposure). In other instances, the exposure and even the outcomes will have taken place in the past, i.e., before the investigator's involvement in the study. If the logic of the study is to follow subjects from exposure to outcome, the research may be termed a nonconcurrent prospective study [25, 26], a historical cohort study, or a retrospective cohort study (departing from the view of prospective research held by DeAngelis and others). These distinctions are shown in Fig. 1.3.

Longitudinal Versus Cross-Sectional Research

As noted above, prospective studies sample members of a defined group at a common starting point (e.g., exposure to a putative risk factor or intervention) and follow them forward in time until the occurrence of a specified outcome (e.g., a disease state or event), whereas retrospective studies begin with existing cases and look back in time at the history of the subject to identify relevant exposures or other instructive trends. Both are examples of longitudinal research because subjects are examined on multiple occasions that are separated in time.

Not all studies have defined temporal windows between putative risk factors and outcomes. One that does not is the cross-sectional (or prevalence) study. With this approach, several variables are measured at the same point in time to determine their frequency and/or possible association within a group of individuals who are selected without regard to exposure or disease status. They are usually based on data collected in the past for other purposes but can be based on information acquired de novo. When used with large representative samples (to permit valid generalizations), cross-sectional studies can provide useful information about the prevalence of risk factors, disease states, and health-related knowledge, attitudes, and behaviors in a specified population. Cross-sectional studies are prevalent in the literature principally because they are relatively quick, easy to conduct, and can be used to evaluate multiple associations. However, unlike the case–control study, where temporality between risk factor and outcome variables can be established (or at least inferred) in order to buttress a cause and effect relationship, cross-sectional studies are best suited for generating, rather than testing, such hypotheses [23].

Descriptive Versus Analytic Research

Research can be further subdivided into descriptive and analytical subtypes. In descriptive studies, the presence and distribution of characteristics (e.g., health events or problems) of a single group of subjects are examined and summarized (but are not intervened upon or otherwise modified) to determine who, how, and when they were affected and the magnitude of these effects. Descriptive studies can involve a single case or a large population. Though they are considered to be among the simplest types of investigation, they can yield fundamental information about an individual or group that is of importance when little is known about the subject in question. Modes of data collection for descriptive studies are primarily observational and include survey methods, objective assessments of physiological measures, and review of historical records. Methods of analysis include computation of descriptive statistics such measures of central tendency and dispersion (quantitative studies) and verbal descriptions and content analysis (qualitative studies) [27]. Because descriptive studies contain no reference groups, they cannot be used to test hypotheses about cause and effect; however, they can be useful for hypothesis generation, thus providing the foundation for future analytic studies. Descriptive studies may be either retrospective or prospective. Retrospective descriptive studies include the single case study and case series formats. Prospective descriptive studies include natural history investigations that follow individual subjects or groups over time to determine changes in parameters of interest.

While descriptive studies attempt to examine *what* types of problems exist in a population, analytic studies attempt to determine *how* or *why* these problems came to be. Thus, the ultimate goal of analytic studies is to test prestated hypotheses about risk factors or interventions versus outcomes to elucidate causality. Analytic studies can be performed with two or more equivalent or matched comparison groups, in which case inferences are drawn on the basis of analysis of intergroup differences ("comparative" research) or by comparisons within a single group in which assessments are made over time before and after imposition of an intervention or a naturally occurring event. Analytic research can be retrospective (e.g., case–control studies) or prospective (e.g., observational cohort or experimental studies). Correlational analysis of cross-sectional data is classified as analytic by some [28] but not all [22] workers in the field.

Observational Versus Experimental Research

In this dichotomy, research is differentiated by the amount of control that the investigator has over the factors in the study by which the outcome variables are compared. In observational studies, the investigator is passive with respect to the factors of interest as these usually are naturally occurring risk factors or exposures outside of the investigator's control. He or she can identify them and measure them but cannot allocate subjects to treatment groups or deliberately manipulate a treatment to systematically study its effect. The investigator's sole responsibility is to select a design which can validly assess the impact of the risk factor on the outcome variable. In contrast, in experimental studies, the input of interest not only is measured or observed but is purposively applied by the investigator, who manipulates events by arranging for the intervention to occur or, at the very least, arranges for random allocation of subjects to alternative treatment or control groups. As a consequence, most of the inherent differences that exist between comparison groups are minimized, if not eliminated, thereby providing greater capacity to determine cause and effect relationships between the intervention and the outcome. Unlike observational studies, which can either be prospective or retrospective, experimental studies, as noted earlier, always are prospective. Midway between observational and experimental studies is a methodology known as quasi-experimental research. With this approach, the investigator evaluates the impact of an intervention (e.g., a therapeutic agent, policy, program, etc.) which has been applied either to an entire population or to one or more subgroups on a nonrandom basis. Although he or she may have been directly involved in arranging the intervention, control is nonetheless suboptimal due to limitations in the quality of reference data; as such, inferences drawn from quasi-experimental studies, while stronger than those generated with purely observational data, are less robust than those drawn from true experimental investigations. Characteristics of the true experimental and quasi-experimental approaches are detailed more fully in Chap. 5.

Quantitative Versus Qualitative Research

Finally, research also can be differentiated according to whether the information sought is collected quantitatively or qualitatively. Quantitative research involves measurement of parameters (e.g., demographic, functional, geometric, or physiological characteristics; mortality, morbidity, and other outcome data; attitudes, knowledge, and behaviors) that have been obtained under standardized conditions by structured or semi-structured instrumentation and that may be subjected to formal statistical analysis. Typically, numerous subjects are studied and the investigator's contact with them is relatively brief and minimally interactive to avoid introduction of "bias." In contrast, qualitative research gathers information about how phenomena are experienced by individuals or groups of individuals (and the context of these experiences) based on open-ended (unstructured) interviews, questionnaires, observation, and focus group methodology. Fewer subjects are studied than with quantitative research, but the investigator's contact with them is longer and more interactive. As Portney and Watkins [29] have noted, quantitative methods can be used across "the continuum of research approaches" to describe, generate, and test hypotheses, whereas qualitative methods typically are used for descriptive or exploratory (hypothesis-generating) research. Quantitative and qualitative research each subsumes many different methodologies.

Steps in the Research Process

As mentioned earlier, research is structured by a series of methodological rules which govern the nature and order of procedures used in the investigation. It is, therefore, necessary that a plan be developed prior to the study which incorporates these procedures. This is true, irrespective of the type of research involved. The following is a brief listing of the steps, identified by DeAngelis [21], which comprise the research process in general and the hypothetico-deductive approach in particular:

In the first stages of the project, the investigator will:

1. Identify the problem area or question.
2. Optimally restate the question as a hypothesis.
3. Review the published literature and other information resources, including meeting abstracts and databases of funded resource summaries or blogs, to determine whether the hypothesis has been adequately evaluated or is in need of further study.

Prior to developing the research design, he/she will:

4. Identify all relevant study variables, knowledge of whose presence, absence, change, or interrelationship is the objective of the study.

In order to bring precision to the research, he/she will:

5. Construct operational definitions of all variables.
6. Develop a research design and analytic plan to test the hypothesis. The design will identify the nature and number of subjects from whom data will be obtained, the timing and sequence of measurements, and the presence or absence of comparison groups or other procedures for controlling bias. The analytic plan will define the statistical procedures to be performed on the data and must be prespecified to minimize the likelihood of reaching spurious conclusions.
7. If data collection instruments are available, they must be specified. If not, they must be constructed. (Data collection instruments include all tools used to collect relevant observations in the study such as physiological measurements questionnaires, interviews, and case report forms, to name a few.)
8. A data collection plan, containing provisions for accrual of subjects and for recording and management of data, must be designed.

Only after these important preparatory steps have been taken should the investigator proceed to:

9. Collect and process the data.
10. Conduct statistical analysis to describe the dataset and test hypotheses.
11. After the data are analyzed, conclusions are drawn and these are related to the problem statement and/or hypotheses.
12. Finally, the research report is written and, if accepted after peer review, is presented and/or published as a journal article.

The importance of following a research plan was addressed by Marks [30], who described a number of typical planning errors and their negative consequences. To cite one example, Marks detailed the experience of an investigator who failed to receive renewal of his multiyear research grant because he could not report the results of the data analysis to the granting agency. This occurred because he failed to develop a mechanism for the storage, handling, and analysis of data. Due to staffing changes and other factors, some of the data were lost, and what was located had not been recorded uniformly. As a result, years of hard work were wasted. In a second example, addressing scheduling problems, Marks describes the failure of an investigator, studying the effects of a drug developed for patients undergoing elective coronary artery bypass grafting, to complete his research project within his specified time frame. Though the investigator had the foresight to calculate his required sample size and to estimate patient accrual rates, he made the mistake of allowing only 4 months to study 30 points. Much to his chagrin, a poorly worded consent form submitted to his institutional review board (IRB) delayed him approximately 6 weeks and, by then, the number of nonemergency operations had dropped dramatically due to the winter holidays. After 4 months, only a quarter of his sample had been accrued—and no data analysis had been performed.

Other common problems associated with poor planning include inability to implement or complete a study (due to disregard of organizational, political, or ethical factors), loss of statistical power to confirm hypotheses (due to inadequate attention to patient accrual factors, attrition of subjects, or excess variability in the study population), ambiguity of findings (due to lack of operational definitions or nonuniformity of data collection procedures), and unsound conclusions brought about by weak research designs, among others.

Marks' vignettes about the adverse consequences of poor research planning depict errors that unfortunately are not uncommon. A number of years ago, in this author's first position as a research director (at an institution that I shall decline to name), I was asked to implement a research project, previously designed by a principal investigator (PI) who was senior to me at the time. The purpose of the project was to evaluate the impact of an in-hospital patient education program after a first myocardial infarction. Four hospitals were involved in the study: two intervention sites and two controls ("business as usual"). In the first phase, patients at Hospital A received the new educational program and patients in Hospital B did not. In the replication phase, patients at Hospital C received the new intervention and patients at Hospital D did not. The instrument chosen to evaluate depression was the Beck Depression Scale and the instrument chosen to evaluate anxiety was the State-Trait Anxiety Scale. The study design compared responses before and after the educational program by site. Being schooled in psychometrics, I was concerned about the reliability and validity of these instruments for this population but was told that these had been extensively used and previously validated in other patient populations. I also had concerns about the quality of the experiences that patients were receiving at the control hospitals but was told that "for political reasons," we could not ask too many questions. Additionally, I had concerns about the implementation of the educational intervention but was told that this was firmly under the control of the nurse coordinator. I next argued for a pilot before launching this very costly and lengthy research project but was told that there was no time and that the PI did not wish to "waste patients."

And so the intervention proceeded according to protocol for well over 2 years. No interim analysis ever was performed because the PI thought that would be too expensive and waste time. When the primary data finally were analyzed, there were no detectable differences whatsoever between the outcomes obtained in the experimental versus control hospitals. The PI was horrified and did not understand how this could have happened. When the process data were analyzed post hoc, we learned that, due to staffing problems at the experimental sites, many nurses who were entrusted to implement the educational intervention had attended few, if any, in-service sessions about the intervention. Moreover, even though the new intervention had a beautifully designed curriculum that had been packaged in a glossy binder, it became known only after the fact that quality patient education also had taken place at Control Hospital B, and we never knew what was done at Control Hospital D, again, "for political reasons."

A final problem concerned the instrumentation. Though, in fact, both the Beck Depression and State-Trait Anxiety Scales had been validated, the validation had not been performed on patients shortly after an acute myocardial infarction. An analysis of baseline scores revealed that most patients were neither depressed nor anxious, apparently due to the unanticipated effects of sedation or denial. Thus, low scores on these primary measures (which clearly were administered too soon after the index event) could not possibly improve due to what are called "floor effects." Needless to say, the private foundation that funded this study was less than thrilled, and none of you have ever seen it in published form. Examples like these abound in research but usually are not reflected in the literature because aborted or incomplete research investigations are never published, and those failing to demonstrate statistically significant differences (or associations) are published far less often than those that do—a phenomenon known as publication bias [31], further discussed in Chap. 9.

A number of years ago, a pediatric emergency fellow at another area hospital approached me for assistance with a dataset that she had compiled over a 4-month period. The data profiled the presenting complaints, diagnoses, and disposition of a series of children who had presented to an emergency room after having complained of largely nonserious illnesses during school. I asked her for a copy of her protocol, but she told me that she did not have one because her study was a chart review, based on de-identified anonymous data and, therefore, was "IRB Exempt." I next asked her for a written copy of her research plan to which she responded, "I never developed one because my clinical mentor told me that it wasn't necessary, and I didn't know that I needed one." I asked her what schools the children had come from and who had made the decision to bring them to the emergency room, but she couldn't answer these questions because that information was not routinely included in the medical chart, which was the source of all of her data. I asked her why she had selected a retrospective chart review as her study design, and she answered that the charts were readily available and that she hadn't thought about any other approach. I asked her why she thought the research study was worth doing, to which she responded, "I'm not sure, but maybe the data will encourage emergency physicians to better counsel parents and school officials who refer relatively healthy children to the emergency room and, thus, cut down on inappropriate visits."

Feeling sorry for her, I helped her to sort out whatever data that she had, and to write an abstract and manuscript that appeared to be respectable, at least superficially. The abstract was accepted at an international meeting (which had somewhat less stringent standards than domestic meetings in her specialty), but when she submitted her manuscript for publication in an academic journal, it was rejected. The reviewers correctly argued that without knowing who made the decision to bring the child to the emergency room, the study had failed its primary objective, which was to furnish information that potentially could alter decision-making patterns for this patient population. Had the fellow developed a proper research plan in the first place, she would have better conceptualized her study and saved months of her time on what was essentially a fruitless undertaking.

The moral posed by these stories is that adequate planning is vital for achieving research objectives and for minimizing the risk of wasting time and resources. As Marks correctly argues, "The success of a research project depends on how well thought out a project is and how potential problems have been identified and resolved before data collection begins" [30].

In subsequent chapters, we will consider many of the fundamental concepts, principles, and issues involved in planning and implementing a well-designed study. It is hoped that awareness of these factors will help you to achieve your research objectives, minimize your risk of wasting time and resources, and result in a more rewarding research experience.

Take-Home Points

- Research is a rigorous problem-solving process whose ultimate goal is the discovery of *new* knowledge.
- Research may include the description of a *new* phenomenon, definition of a *new* relationship, development of a *new* model, or application of an existing principle or procedure to a *new* context.
- Research is systematic, logical, empirical, reductive, replicable and transmittable, and generalizable.
- Research can be classified according to a variety of dimensions: basic, applied, or translational; hypothesis generating or hypothesis testing; retrospective or prospective; longitudinal or cross-sectional; observational or experimental; quantitative or qualitative.
- The ultimate success of a research project is heavily dependent on adequate planning.

References

1. Calvert J, Martin BR (2001) Changing conceptions of basic research? Brighton, England: Background document for the Workshop on Policy Relevance and Measurement of Basic Research, Oslo, 29–30 Oct 2001. Brighton, England: SPRU.
2. Leedy PD. Practical research. Planning and design. 6th ed. Upper Saddle River: Prentice Hall; 1997.
3. Tuckman BW. Conducting educational research. 3rd ed. New York: Harcourt Brace Jovanovich; 1972.
4. Tanenbaum SJ. Knowing and acting in medical practice. The epistemological policies of outcomes research. J Health Polit Policy Law. 1994;19:27–44.
5. Richardson WS. We should overcome the barriers to evidence-based clinical diagnosis! J Clin Epidemiol. 2007;60:217–27.
6. MacCorquodale K, Meehl PE. On a distinction between hypothetical constructs and intervening variables. Psych Rev. 1948;55:95–107.
7. The National Commission for the Protection of Human Subjects of Biomedical and Behavioral Research: The Belmont Report: Ethical principles and guidelines for the protection of human subjects of research. Washington: DHEW Publication No. (OS) 78–0012, Appendix I, DHEW Publication No. (OS) 78–0013, Appendix II, DHEW Publication (OS) 780014; 1978.
8. Coryn CLS. The fundamental characteristics of research. J Multidisciplinary Eval. 2006;3:124–33.
9. Smith NL, Brandon PR. Fundamental issues in evaluation. New York: Guilford; 2008.
10. Committee on Criteria for Federal Support of Research and Development, National Academy of Sciences, National Academy of Engineering, Institute of Medicine, National Research Council. Allocating federal funds for science and technology. Washington, DC: The National Academies; 1995.
11. Busse R, Fleming I. A critical look at cardiovascular translational research. Am J Physiol Heart Circ Physiol. 1999;277:H1655–60.
12. Schuster DP, Powers WJ. Translational and experimental clinical research. Philadelphia: Lippincott, Williams & Williams; 2005.
13. Woolf SH. The meaning of translational research and why it matters. JAMA. 2008;299:211–21.
14. Robertson D, Williams GH. Clinical and translational science: principles of human research. London: Elsevier; 2009.
15. Goldblatt EM, Lee WH. From bench to bedside: the growing use of translational research in cancer medicine. Am J Transl Res. 2010;2:1–18.
16. Milloy SJ. Science without sense: the risky business of public health research. In: Chapter 5, Mining for statistical associations. Cato Institute. 2009. http://www.junkscience.com/news/sws/sws-chapter5.html. Retrieved 29 Oct 2009.
17. Gawande A. The cancer-cluster myth. The New Yorker, 8 Feb 1999, p. 34–37.
18. Kerlinger F. [Chapter 2: problems and hypotheses]. In: Foundations of behavioral research 3rd edn. Orlando: Harcourt, Brace; 1986.
19. Ioannidis JP. Why most published research findings are false. PLoS Med. 2005;2:e124. Epub 2005 Aug 30.
20. Andersen B. Methodological errors in medical research. Oxford: Blackwell Scientific Publications; 1990.
21. DeAngelis C. An introduction to clinical research. New York: Oxford University Press; 1990.
22. Hennekens CH, Buring JE. Epidemiology in medicine. 1st ed. Boston: Little Brown; 1987.
23. Jekel JF. Epidemiology, biostatistics, and preventive medicine. 3rd ed. Philadelphia: Saunders Elsevier; 2007.
24. Hess DR. Retrospective studies and chart reviews. Respir Care. 2004;49:1171–4.
25. Wissow L, Pascoe J. Types of research models and methods (chapter four). In: An introduction to clinical research. New York: Oxford University Press; 1990.
26. Bacchieri A, Della Cioppa G. Fundamentals of clinical research: bridging medicine, statistics and operations. Milan: Springer; 2007.
27. Wood MJ, Ross-Kerr JC. Basic steps in planning nursing research. From question to proposal. 6th ed. Boston: Jones and Barlett; 2005.
28. DeVita VT, Lawrence TS, Rosenberg SA, Weinberg RA, DePinho RA. Cancer. Principles and practice of oncology, vol. 1. Philadelphia: Wolters Klewer/Lippincott Williams & Wilkins; 2008.
29. Portney LG, Watkins MP. Foundations of clinical research. Applications to practice. 2nd ed. Upper Saddle River: Prentice Hall Health; 2000.
30. Marks RG. Designing a research project. The basics of biomedical research methodology. Belmont: Lifetime Learning Publications: A division of Wadsworth; 1982.
31. Easterbrook PJ, Berlin JA, Gopalan R, Matthews DR. Publication bias in clinical research. Lancet. 1991; 337:867–72.

Developing a Research Problem

2

Phyllis G. Supino and Helen Ann Brown Epstein

Origins of Research Problems

A well-designed research project, in any discipline, will begin by conceptualizing the problem—in its most general sense, an unresolved issue of concern (e.g., a contradiction, an unproven relationship, an unclear mechanism, a puzzling or enigmatic state) that warrants investigation. This intellectual activity arguably is the most critical part of the study, and many researchers consider it to be the most difficult. This is particularly true in the early stages of a developing science when theoretical frameworks are poorly articulated and when there is little in the literature about the topic. Although formal rules and procedures exist to guide the development of the research design, data collection protocol, and statistical approach, there are few, if any, guidelines for conceptualizing or identifying research problems, which may take years of thought and exploration to define.

P.G. Supino, EdD (✉)
Department of Medicine, College of Medicine, SUNY Downstate Medical Center, 450 Clarkson Avenue, Box 1199, Brooklyn, NY 11203, USA
e-mail: phyllissupino@aol.com

H.A.B. Epstein, MLS, MS, AHIP
Clinical Librarian, Samuel J. Wood Library and C.V. Starr Biomedical Information Center, Weill Cornell Medical College, New York, NY, USA

In his discussion of how problems are generated in science, Kerlinger described the personal and, often, unsettling nature of the birth of the research problem:

> The scientist will usually experience an obstacle to understanding, a vague unrest about observed and unobserved phenomena, a curiosity as to why something is as it is. His first and most important step is to get the idea out in the open, to express the problem in some reasonably manageable form. Rarely or never will the problem spring full-blown at this stage. He must struggle with it, try it out, live with it.... Sooner or later, explicitly or implicitly, he states the problem, even if his expression of it is inchoate or tentative. In some respects, this is the most difficult and most important part of the whole process. Without some sort of statement of the problem, the scientist can rarely go further and expect his work to be fruitful [1].

Kerlinger's comments point up an important but, nonetheless, poorly recognized fact. Namely, one of the most challenging aspects of the research process is to develop the idea for the research in the first place.

So, from where do research problems come? In general, most spring from the intellectual curiosity of the investigator and, of necessity, are shaped by his or her critical reasoning skills, experience, and environment. Probably the most common source of clinical research problems is the plethora of practical issues that clinicians confront in managing patients which mandate data-driven decisions. For example, among cardiologists, there has been long-standing interest in optimizing management of patients with known or suspected coronary disease. What are the best

P.G. Supino and J.S. Borer (eds.), *Principles of Research Methodology: A Guide for Clinical Investigators*, DOI 10.1007/978-1-4614-3360-6_2, © Phyllis G. Supino and Jeffrey S. Borer 2012

algorithms and diagnostic modalities for differentiating symptoms of myocardial ischemia from symptoms that mimic ischemia? When should such patients be medically managed and when should they undergo invasive therapeutic procedures? What is the risk-benefit ratio of percutaneous coronary angioplasty vs. coronary artery bypass grafting? How often and how should patients undergoing these procedures be evaluated after intervention? What patient-level, societal, and economic factors influence these decisions? Issues such as these have enormous public health implications and have spawned hundreds of research studies.

Research problems also can be generated from observations collected in conjunction with medical procedures [2]. A radiologist might have a set of interesting data collected in conjunction with a new imaging modality (e.g., full-field digital mammography) and might wish to know how much more sensitive and specific this new modality is vs. older technology for breast cancer screening. Alternatively, he might be interested in a new application of an existing modality. A thoracic surgeon may have outcomes data available from two competing surgical techniques. The process of critically thinking about these data, sharing them with colleagues, and obtaining their feedback can lead to interesting questions for analysis and stimulate additional research.

Another source of research problems is the published scientific literature, where an observed exception to the findings of past research or accepted theory, unresolved discrepancies between studies, or a general paucity of quality data on a clinically significant topic can motivate thinking and point to an opportunity for future study. In addition, most well-crafted manuscripts typically document limitations in the investigation (e.g., potential selection bias, inadequate sample size, low number of endpoint events, loss to follow-up) and may suggest areas for future research. Thus, thoughtful review of published research can point to gaps in knowledge that potentially could be filled by new investigations designed to refine or extend previous research.

Research problems also can be suggested by governmental and private funding agencies which publish requests for proposals (RFPs) or applications (RFAs) to address understudied areas affecting the public health. These publications will explicitly identify a problem that the agency would like an investigator to address, provide a background and context for the problem, stipulate a study population (as well as on occasion, specify the approach to be taken), and indicate the level of support offered to the potential investigator.

Finally, research problems can be fostered by environments that stimulate an open interchange of ideas. These environments include scientific sessions conducted by professional societies and organizations, grand rounds given at hospitals and medical schools, and other conferences and seminars. In recent years, methodological approaches such as brainstorming, Delphi methods, and nominal group techniques [3–5] have been developed and sometimes are utilized to facilitate the rapid generation (and prioritization) of research problems by individuals and groups.

Characteristics of Well-Conceived Research Problems

Although the genesis of a research problem is a complex, variable, and an inherently unpredictable process, fortunately, there are generally agreed-upon criteria, described below, for evaluating the merits of the problem once it has been generated [6–8]. Attention to these at the outset will ensure a solid footing for the remainder of the investigation.

The Problem Should Be Important

The most significant characteristic of a good research problem is importance. A clinical research problem is considered important if its resolution has the potential to clarify a significant issue affecting the public health and, ultimately, cause the clinician (or health-care policy maker) to make a decision or undertake an action that he or she would not have made or undertaken had the problem not been addressed. The greater the need for clarification and the larger the number of individuals potentially impacted (i.e., the greater the disease burden), the more important the problem. For this reason, when research proposals are submitted to a funding agency or when research manuscripts are submitted to a journal for publication, perceived importance of the problem is heavily weighted during the peer-review process. Indeed, importance of the problem typically overshadows other criticisms such as incomplete consideration of the literature, suboptimal methodology, and poor writing style, as these flaws often can be remedied. Studies that merely replicate other studies, with no significant alteration in methods, content, or population (or that reflect only a minor incremental advance over previous information) are considered unimportant and tend to fare poorly in the peer-review process. This is true even if the study is well designed. This point is illustrated below by the divergent comments actually made by a reviewer in response to two different manuscripts submitted for publication to a cardiology journal:

- *Manuscript #1*: "This is a superb contribution which *adds importantly* to our knowledge about the pathophysiology of heart failure. The results of this well-focused study are of *great clinical importance.*" (Recommendation: *Accept*)
- *Manuscript #2*: Comment: "Despite a great deal of very precise and laborious effort and the generation of an extraordinary mass of numbers … little forethought was given to the focus or *importance* of the questions to be asked …. The finding is not unexpected, having been suggested by several earlier studies which have evaluated the issue of regional performance in different ways … (Thus,) the authors' observations *add little that is important or useful* to the currently available literature." (Recommendation: *Reject*)

Evaluating the importance of a research problem requires considerable knowledge of and experience in the discipline. For this reason, the new investigator should seek the assistance of mentors and other experts early on to maximize the likelihood that the proposed research will be fruitful.

The Problem Should Be Interesting

As Hully and Cummings have noted, a good research problem, especially if suggested by someone else, must be interesting to the investigator to provide "the intensity of effort needed for overcoming the many hurdles and frustrations of the research process" [7]. It also should be interesting to:

- The investigator's peers and associates to attract collaborators
- Senior scientists at the investigator's institution who can provide necessary mentorial support to guide the study (if the investigator is relatively junior)
- Potential sponsors to motivate them to fund the study (if outside funding is sought)
- Fellow researchers within the larger scientific community who, ultimately, will read and judge its findings
- Individuals outside the scientific community (e.g., clinicians in private practice, policy makers, the popular media, and consumers) who, optimally, will consider, disseminate, and/or utilize the eventual products of the research (if the problem is applied or translational in nature)

Gauging the potential interest of a research problem is difficult because, as Shugan has noted, "no research findings are innately interesting." Instead, they are interesting only relative to a particular audience within some context that they define [9]. While research can be interesting simply because it is new, in general, a research problem will tend to be viewed as noteworthy if it impacts a wide audience, has the potential to cause significant change in what members of that audience will do [9] (i.e., has "importance"), and is clearly framed within the context of a current "hot-button" issue (or an older but nonetheless viable issue). Before investing substantial time pursuing a research problem, it is advisable that new researchers check with their mentors and/or other experienced investigators with broad insights into the general area of inquiry to confirm that the problem satisfies these criteria and, thus, is likely to be interesting to others [10].

The Problem Should Lead to Clear, Researchable Questions

Many workers in the field use the terms "research problem" and "research question" interchangeably. Others view the research problem as an assertion about an issue of perceived importance that implies a gap in knowledge from which questions may be developed (the position taken in this chapter). Whichever view is held, there is general consensus that a research problem should be clearly defined (see section "Crafting the Problem and Purpose Statements" at the end of this chapter) and serve as a springboard for questions whose answers can be found by conducting a study [7, 10–12]. Ellis and Levy [13] argue that research questions are important because they serve to operationalize the goals of the study by narrowing them into specific areas of inquiry. Leedy and Ormand [14] assert that attaining answers to research questions both satisfies the goals of the study and generally contributes to problem solving within the area of interest. Kerlinger and Lee [15] further contend that an investigation has meaning only when there is a clear nexus between the answers obtained to the research questions and the primary research problem. Like the problem itself, the questions should be clear, concise, optimally lead to testable hypotheses, and collectively capture the overall goal or purpose of the research project. In so doing, they serve to guide the methodology used in the study. The reader should note that a distinction is drawn between a "research question" and practical or methodological questions that arise during the design or implementation phases of the research (e.g., How many subjects are needed to provide sufficient power for testing the hypothesis or to achieve a given level of precision for estimating a population parameter? Which approaches are best for enhancing patient recruitment, improving follow-up, and reducing the likelihood of missing data? Given the investigator's constraints, what study design(s) should be used to control for threats to valid inference? Which statistical approach or approaches are most appropriate given the nature of the data?) These and related methodological issues are discussed, in depth, in other chapters of this book.

The Problem Should Be Feasible

A research problem (or a research question) should be feasible in two respects. As Sim and Wright [16] have noted, it should be feasible on a "conceptual-empirical" level, meaning that the concepts and propositions embodied in the research should be susceptible to empirical evaluation. As indicated in Chap. 1, it is the empirical quality of research that differentiates it from other problem-solving processes. Accordingly, it is important that the research question(s) central to the problem be answerable and that answers to the question(s) be generated by the acts of data collection and analysis (i.e., be produced empirically). These criteria are sometimes difficult to satisfy. In order for a question to be answerable, it must be clear, precise, and have a manageable set of possible answers (the latter criterion also relates to the issues of feasibility and scope, described below). The answer or answers also must be inherently knowable and measurable. The question, "how many angels can dance on the head of a pin" is philosophically interesting, but it is neither knowable nor measurable since there is no way to count angels, assuming that they existed in the first place. The question also must be framed in such a way that it will be obvious what type of data are needed to answer it, and it must be possible to collect empirical evidence that, when analyzed, will make a convincing argument when interpreted in relation to that question. In order for empirical evidence to be gathered, suitable subjects (for a clinical study) or material (for a preclinical study) must be available, and valid and reliable instruments must exist or be developed for measurement of the elements that comprise the question. If these elements cannot be measured, the question cannot be answered empirically. Examples of problems that would be difficult to evaluate are:

- How well do patients adjust to life following an initial myocardial infarction?
- Following death of the cancer patient, how well do spouses handle their grief?

Both "adjustment" and "handling grief" clearly are difficult to evaluate by empirical means, unless operational definitions and objective measures are developed for both terms. In a similar vein, questions soliciting opinions (e.g., what should be done to improve the health of a specific population?) and value-laden questions such as "should terminally ill comatose patients be disconnected from life support?" certainly are important and make excellent subjects for argument. However, they (like any question including the word "should") are not always assessable empirically and may require special methods for data gathering (e.g., qualitative techniques).

The problem also should be feasible on a practical level [16]. An investigator must decide, early on, if he or she has the resources to address it within a realistic time frame and at a reasonable cost. A primary determinant of feasibility is the scope of the proposed problem. In planning a research study, it is important to avoid selecting a problem that is too broad because a single investigation cannot possibly provide all relevant information about a problem. The process of identifying the problem can raise ancillary questions that may be of interest to the investigator, but it is important to prioritize these and reserve some for future research so that the time and resources of the investigator are not strained. An axiom in research planning is that it is better to provide quality answers to a small number of questions than to provide inferior information in volume. For example, should an investigator wish to study the effect of drug therapy on patients with heart disease, the question "What is the effect of drug therapy on patients with poor heart function?," while conceptually interesting and clinically important, is much too broad for one study and, in fact, would require hundreds of investigations to answer adequately. The investigator would do well to narrow the problem to include a given class of drugs (e.g., adrenal steroids), a specific index of heart function (e.g., left ventricular performance), and a specific population (e.g., patients with chronic severe aortic regurgitation). On the other hand, the problem should not be too narrowly defined. A question such as "what are the effects of Inderal on the change in ejection fraction from rest to exercise in 75-year-old Queens residents?" probably would result in a criticism of the study as trivial.

The scope of a study can be gauged by the number of subproblems (discrete areas of inquiry within the investigation) needed to express the main problem. If the number of subproblems exceeds six, there is high likelihood that the problem is too broad. In contrast, if an investigator is unable to define a minimum of two subproblems, it may be too narrow [17].

The issue of scope of the problem has direct practical implications for the researcher. Even if the problem is important and empirically testable, the investigator must balance these factors against the cost of doing the research. Long before data are collected, the researcher must decide whether he or she has the time or resources to collect and analyze the data.

Factors affecting time include:

- The interval needed for subject accrual
- The time involved in administering the intervention (if the research is experimental)
- The time involved in collecting data on inputs such as risk factors (if the research is observational)
- The time involved in assessing outcome

Factors potentially affecting resources include:

- Costs of accruing and managing subjects (purchasing and housing of animals for a preclinical study, reimbursing human subjects for participation in a clinical research study)
- Cost of the intervention (if any)
- Costs of measurement procedures
- Cost of data collection, processing, and analysis
- Costs of equipment, supplies, and travel
- Technical expertise (the investigator's own research skills or access to skilled collaborators or consultants)

One way an investigator can determine feasibility is by conducting a pilot study. A pilot study (sometimes called a "feasibility study") typically attempts to determine whether it is possible to address the research problem (or subproblems) under conditions approximating those of the larger, proposed study but with a smaller number of subjects over an abbreviated period of time. The pilot can provide information about the complexities of patient recruitment and the appropriateness of data collection procedures (including acceptability of the research instruments to the study subjects and approaches to detecting endpoints and resolving issues associated with follow-up), and obtain preliminary estimates of morbidity and event rates (among other variables) that can be useful in informing sample size calculations for future investigations. Occasionally, the pilot will produce preliminary answers to the proposed research questions. If the investigator concludes that examining the problem is unaffordable or is unfeasible time-wise, he or she should consider modifications that may include:

- Delimiting the scope of the problem
- Broadening the inclusion criteria
- Relaxing the exclusion criteria
- Adding additional study sites
- Altering the study design used to address the problem (e.g., from a prospective to a retrospective design or from parallel group comparison to a repeated measures design to permit assessment of outcomes with fewer subjects [the pros and cons of these approaches are discussed in further detail in Chap. 5])

If successful, the results of a pilot study can be helpful in convincing a potential funding agency that the proposed research is feasible and, depending on the nature of the preliminary data, that the hypotheses are likely to be confirmed by a larger study conducted by the same investigators.

Another way to "try out" a research question is to present an idea or preliminary data in a poster or "emerging ideas" section of a professional meeting. Thoughts exchanged during a "curbside chat" may crystallize an idea and may lead to valuable networking connections. Social media, like wikis (collaborative, directly editable websites) and blogs (online personal journals), are rich platforms to float ideas and exchange comments. An example of a wiki is *Medpedia*: an open platform connecting people and information to advance medicine (see www.medpedia.com). Useful blogs include *Medical Discoveries* (www.medicalhealthdiscoveries.com), Public Library of Science (PLoS Blog, accessible at http://blogs.plos.org), *Discovery Buzz* (http://discoverybuzz.com/blog), and *Trust the Evidence* (http://blogs.trusttheevidence.net).

Examination of the Problem Should Not Violate the Ethical Standards of the Scientific Community

The investigator may be interested in a problem that has significant scientific or medical importance, but addressing it might expose patients to significant risk. For example, a psychiatrist might be interested in the effects of a particular psychotropic drug on patients with obsessive compulsive disorder. She believes that examination of this problem is both clinically relevant and scientifically important because review of the existing literature suggests that the agent not only has the potential for reducing symptoms but also might provide insights into the underlying processes related to this illness. Pilot data, however, suggest that this drug is highly addictive and, in addition, may adversely affect certain organ systems. Thus, despite scientific merit, the conclusions generated might be at the expense of the overall well-being of the subject. According to accepted standards of scientific conduct, the study should not be done. These rules apply in industrial, as well as in academic, settings. Thus, in the USA, when a pharmaceutical company launches a new drug, it is required by the Food and Drug Administration to perform highly regulated trials of feasibility (phase I) and safety (phase II), before proceeding to a large, randomized phase III efficacy trial. Generally, if the drug produced significant toxicity in patients prior to or during the phase III trial, the investigation would be aborted at that time, despite otherwise beneficial effects. Similar guidelines are followed in most Western European countries. Likewise, prior to conducting research in most academic medical centers, an investigator is required to obtain approval of his or her research protocol from that center's institutional review board (IRB), particularly when that protocol poses more than minimal risk to the subject. During this approval process, the ethical considerations entailed in studying the problem are heavily weighed. In clinical studies, these typically include:

- *Proportionate risk*: Is the risk to the subject outweighed by the potential benefit to that subject? If your IRB concludes that it is not, the study would not be permitted to go forward, despite its possible benefit to the same patient in the future or to society in general.
- *Informed consent*: Is the subject truly aware of the aims of the study? If so, is the subject also aware of the potential for any adverse consequences that might arise due to his or her participation? Several years ago, it came to light that a research investigation, undertaken at a medical center in New York, had been conducted on 28 adult schizophrenics who were not advised that they were participating in a study in which psychosis was temporarily induced [18]. The ethics of performing research on such vulnerable subjects, without their full knowledge, triggered a firestorm of controversy that caused their IRB to mandate an entirely new approach to studies of this nature.
- *Role reversal*: Would the investigator be willing to trade places with the subject? Would he or she be willing to suffer the same pain, discomfort, or, at the very least, inconvenience as the subject, as a result of participating in his or her own research study?
- *Integrity of the design (validity)*: Is the study designed well enough to warrant the expenditure of time and effort, or the potential risk to the patient (i.e., is it likely to yield valid answers to the questions being asked?) If not, not only may the investigators be wasting their own time and that of their subjects, they also may be producing results that have the potential to mislead the medical community and, ultimately, their patients.

These and other ethical problems will be explored more fully in Chap. 12.

Types of Research Questions

Research questions in any discipline may be categorized in multiple ways. Trochim [19] has argued that all research questions may be classified as "descriptive" (What is occurring? What exists?), relational (What is the association between two or more variables? Is the predictive value of one variable greater than or independent of another variable?), or causal (Does a treatment, program, policy, etc., affect one or more outcomes?). Blaikie [20] contends that all research questions can be classified as inquiries about "what," "why," or "how." According to this trichotomy, "what" questions describe presence, magnitude, and variations of characteristics in individuals, patterns in the relationships among these characteristics, and associated outcomes; "why" questions ask about causes of, or reasons for, the existence of phenomena, explanations about relationships between events, and mechanisms underlying various processes, whereas "how" questions deal with methods for bringing about desired changes in outcomes via intervention. Research questions also can be classified according to the type of inferences to be drawn. In medicine, for example, questions characteristically target issues about magnitude of disease burden, prevention, or patient management. Thus, questions may be asked about prevalence and incidence of a disease (or diseases) in a population:

- What influenza virus was most dominant in 2010?
- How many types of respiratory illness have been identified among the World Trade Center Disaster first responders?
- How many cases of breast cancer that were identified in Long Island, New York, occurred in Suffolk County?
- Is resistant tuberculosis on the rise in New York City?
- Is AIDS in Africa still considered to be an epidemic?

Questions also can focus on issues of primary prevention:

- Does use of margarine instead of butter protect against hypercholesterolemia and hypertriglyceridemia?
- Does use of hormone replacement after menopause protect against the development of cardiovascular diseases among women?
- Is physical fitness protective against osteoporosis?

- Does application of dental sealants actually prevent the development of tooth decay?
- Have current local and global interventions and services reduced the transmission and acquisition of HIV infection?

Questions of most interest to clinicians, however, typically center on issues related to the clinical management of patients with known or suspected diseases. Borrowing from an evidence-based practice framework, these can be subcategorized as questions about screening/diagnosis, treatment, prognosis, etiology, or harm (from treatment) [21]. Examples are given below:

- What is the most cost-effective way to differentiate children who are at risk for developmental delays from those who are not? (screening)
- What are the sensitivity, specificity, and positive and negative predictive values of positron emission tomography [PET] among women with suspected coronary artery disease? What is the diagnostic accuracy of PET vs. other available tests such as thallium scintigraphy? (diagnosis)
- What is the best (most effective, tolerable, cost-effective) currently available chemotherapy regimen for acute myeloid leukemia? (treatment)
- Is combination therapy better than single agent therapy for benign prostatic hypertrophy? (treatment)
- What is the probable clinical course of patients with aortic stenosis? (prognosis)
- Which patients with chronic, severe aortic regurgitation progress most rapidly to surgical indications? (prognosis)
- Is autoimmunity causally related to the development of Crohn's disease? Is it also implicated in the development of lupus and rheumatic arthritis? (etiology)
- Do enzymes involved in the synthesis of the extracellular matrix play a role in the development of fibrotic diseases and cancer? (etiology)
- What is the magnitude of risk for adverse outcome of carotid endarterectomy among the elderly? (harm)
- What is the in-hospital mortality associated with valvular replacement? Is it greater with concomitant coronary artery bypass grafting? (harm)

Role of the Literature Search

Even if the research problem was sparked by previously published research, once its basic elements have been defined, it is necessary to conduct a comprehensive search of the literature to acquire a thorough knowledge of relevant earlier findings, ongoing research, or new theories. Although there is no set rule governing the optimal time frame for a literature search or the number of publications to be included, there is general consensus that the search should be of sufficient length and breadth to include existing pertinent seminal and landmark studies [22] as well as current studies in the field (i.e., those conducted within the past 10 years). A proper literature search will help the investigator to determine answers to the following questions:

- Has the problem been previously addressed? If so, was it adequately studied?
- Are the proposed hypotheses, if any, supported by current theory or knowledge?
- Does the methodology cited in the literature provide guidance on available instrumentation for measuring variables?
- Are the results of prior studies informative for calculation of sample size and power?
- Did previous investigators describe the limitations of their research or suggest areas for future study?

Seeking answers to these questions early in the planning process will enable the investigator to determine whether performance of the present study is feasible, whether it is likely to significantly contribute to the existing knowledge base (thus supporting the need for the study), and also whether it may provide guidance on the construction of hypotheses and choice of study design. In addition, creating an automatic search profile early in the planning process will keep the investigator informed about the latest research related to his or her problem. The search profile will generate updated lists of new literature and provide alerts to these updates via e-mail or RSS feed on a daily, weekly, or monthly basis, as desired. The updates also can be used to alert the investigator to research performed by other investigators and provide an opportunity for collaboration.

Like other aspects of a research project, the performance of a proper literature search requires a significant investment of time and effort. This is true in part because the results of most scientific investigations (particularly those reflecting recent work or primary literature) are dispersed over a myriad of e-mail communications, meeting abstracts, web documents, and periodicals, rather than organized collectively in books or other single sources of research. Traditionally, if an investigator needed to learn more about earlier related work, he or she would begin by examining key references cited in known relevant published studies. Today, continuing this principle of "it only takes one good article to get you going," online systems like PubMed from the National Library of Medicine, ISI Web of Knowledge™ from Thomson Reuters the EBSCOhost family of databases from EBSCO Publishing, and the databases of Ovid Technologies, Wolters Kluwer Health, and Google Scholar, generate a list of possible important citations and invite you to click on the "related articles link," or "times cited link" to find similarly indexed papers or cited references from these papers to locate additional relevant citations. A summary of selected core online resources are provided in Table 2.1.

Most investigators will choose to search MEDLINE, the premier bibliographic databases from the National Library of Medicine. It is available by searching PubMed, ISI Web of Knowledge, EBSCOhost, and Ovid plus many other free or fee-based searching systems. The database covers the life sciences with a concentration in biomedicine. Bibliographic citations with author abstracts and linking to full text of many articles come from more than 5,400 biomedical journals published in the USA and around the world. Most citations are written in English with English abstracts. MEDLINE contains over 21 million citations dating back to the mid 1940s. For more information about PubMed, see www.pubmed.gov. Many of the MEDLINE citations in PubMed link to the Gene, Nucleotide, and Protein databases from the National Center for Biotechnology Information (NCBI) for coverage of molecular biology. Google Scholar® pulls in freely available scholarly literature from PubMed and other sources, with some linking to the full text of the articles.

MEDLINE may not provide adequate information about a research problem. Thus, many investigators consider searching EMBASE in lieu of or in addition to MEDLINE (which now is included within EMBASE). EMBASE is created by Excerpta Medica and produced by Elsevier. One can subscribe to it individually from Elsevier or through Ovid from Wolters Kluwer Health in three separate databases: EMBASE, EMBASE Drugs and Pharmacology, and EMBASE Psychiatry. There are over 24 million indexed records from more than 7,500 current, mostly peer-reviewed journals covering biomedical and pharmacological literature. In addition, there is extensive coverage of meeting abstracts. Like MeSH from MEDLINE, EMBASE uses a hierarchical classification of subject headings called "EMTREE" that can be expanded. EMBASE can be searched with significant words, significant phrases, and EMTREE terms. Links to full text of the journal articles are available from many medical libraries.

An investigator may also consider searching BIOSIS Previews®, Biological Abstracts, and Zoological Record together as a package from ISI Web of Knowledge, a product of Thomson Scientific. This resource represents a comprehensive index to the life sciences and biomedical research, including meeting abstracts, journals, books and patents, and contains more than 18 million records taken from more than 5,000 international resources from 90 countries (1926 to present). BIOSIS Previews is available by searching the Ovid suite of databases and ISI Web of Knowledge.

Web of Science's Science Citation Index Expanded, part of ISI Web of Knowledge from Thomson Reuters covers scientific literature from 1900 to present. An investigator can search

Table 2.1 Selected core online resources

Name of resource	Description	Link to full text	Producer	Fee
BIOSIS	Bibliographic database: suite includes Biological abstracts (1926–present) BIOSIS previews (1926–present) Zoological record (1864–present)	Yes	Thomson Reuters Ovid Technologies—Wolters Kluwer	Yes
CINAHL	Bibliographic database for nursing and allied health disciplines	Yes	EBSCOhost	Yes
Cochrane Library	Family of systematic reviews, RCTs, health technology assessments, economic assessments	Yes	Wiley Ovid Technologies—Wolters Kluwer	Yes
EMBASE	Bibliographic database with international coverage Emphasis on biomedicine and drugs	Yes	EMBASE—available from various vendors	Yes
MEDLINE	Bibliographic database of clinical medicine	Yes	National Library of Medicine—available from various vendors	No
PsycInfo	Bibliographic database of scholarly journal articles, book chapters, and dissertations in behavioral science and mental health	Yes	American Psychological Association—available from various vendors	Yes
PubMed	Premier database of biomedical literature primarily MEDLINE (1947–present)	Yes	National Library of Medicine	No
Social Science Citation Index	Bibliographic database with links to citations in bibliography and items cited	Yes	Thomson Reuters	Yes
Web of Science	Bibliographic database indicating number of References, number of times cited (1900–present)	Yes	Thomson Reuters	Yes

this resource by subject topics and keywords. The citation display features a summary abstract, a bibliography, and publications that have cited that paper. As with many systems today, full text of the paper as well as related article citations also may be linked. A citation map can be generated to visually display for two generations the references in the bibliography and cited papers.

If the investigator is interested in behavioral science research, the American Psychological Association offers a suite of databases, PsycINFO®, PsycARTICLES®, PsycBOOKS®, PsycCritiques®, and PsycEXTRA®. Information can be found on psychology and related disciplines (e.g., psychiatry, nursing, neuroscience, law, education, sociology, social work). Available in a variety of formats (e.g., journal articles, books or book chapters, dissertations, technical and annual reports, government reports, conference presentations, consumer brochures, magazines, among others), PsycINFO can be searched with words, phrases, and terms from the Psyc thesaurus. Like MeSH, the terms are arranged in alphabetical and hierarchical order.

Web of Science's Social Science Citation Index can be explored for those interested in social sciences research. Almost 2,500 journals are indexed, representing 50 social science and related disciplines, including anthropology, urban studies, industrial relations, law, linguistics, substance abuse, public health, and information and library sciences, among others. Like Science Citation Index, the citation display features a summary abstract, bibliography, and publications that have cited the paper; full text of the paper and related article citations also may be linked. This database also can be searched with words and phrases.

The EBSCOhost family of databases covers the humanities and social sciences. It also includes CINAHL-Cumulated Index to Nursing and Allied Health Literature. This database provides indexing for nearly 3,000 journals from the fields of nursing and allied health, including librarianship, and contains more than 2.2 million records dating back to 1981. Like MEDLINE, EMBASE, and PsycINFO®, one searches CINAHL with significant words and phrases as well as CINAHL descriptors that can be expanded. Searchers can add citations to a folder, permitting them to be printed, e-mailed, or saved. Also, like other databases, CINAHL links to cited references.

Finally, for those seeking the latest information on evidence-based health care, the Cochrane Library is an excellent source of systematic reviews (discussed in depth in Chap. 9), RCTs, and health technology and economic assessments. It is produced by the Cochrane Collaboration, a worldwide effort dedicated to systematically reviewing the effectiveness of health-care interventions, and is available from Wiley and Wolters Kluwer Health via Ovid. Though the Cochrane Library can be searched with words, phrases, and MeSH descriptors, its central database of randomized trials is extensive (mandating a more precise searching strategy), whereas its database of systematic reviews contains fewer than 5,000 elements (requiring a broader search strategy). If the searcher is able to identify a systematic review that contains a reasonable number of trials from which valid and consistent inferences have been drawn, it may provide most of the literature needed to support a research project.

Although web-based bibliographic programs have become increasingly "user-friendly" by encouraging the searcher to place significant words, phrases, and database subject terms in a search box, the search process itself remains a combination of science and art which requires practice and patience. In view of this, some investigators may opt to complete an online tutorial, sign on to a web-based training session, attend an in-person course at their local library, or consult with a librarian for training and search planning. Some investigators will team up with a searching professional to run the search together or, after a rigorous interview (in which the goals of the study are carefully discussed), will have the searching professional perform the search. For those without access to such instructional resources, we offer the following recommendations:

- Frame your search topic in the form of a specific question or statement.
- Depending on your choice of search system(s), plan your search strategy accordingly with significant words, phrases, and database subject headings or descriptors.

- Decide whether empirical and/or theoretical literature is to be included:
  - Empirical literature comprises primary research reports (e.g., observational studies, controlled trials) and systematic reviews of research.
  - Theoretical literature includes descriptions of concepts, models, and theoretical frameworks.
- Identify preferred literature sources, for example, articles, book chapters, and dissertations.
- Determine the amount of information needed and the temporal period of interest.
- Evaluate the likelihood of finding specific information about your topic. If you think the topic is voluminous, use a more narrow approach to search the literature. If you think the topic will yield a small amount of literature, use a broader approach.
- Display and review all citations with as much text, searching terms, and related links as possible. Many articles will be available in full text directly from the searching system.
- If you determine that your retrieval is inadequate for your needs, consider modifying your search strategy and running your search again.
- Obtain and organize all source documents.

Once the key references have been compiled, these should be carefully reviewed to identify the methodologies employed, conclusions drawn, and limitations of the selected studies. It is of paramount importance that the investigator carefully read the entire published study and any accompanying editorials, comments, and letters, rather than rely on information given in an abstract or in published reviews of the literature written by others. This is because abstracts and review articles provide only incomplete information; in addition, the perspective of the reviewing author may bias the interpretation of primary findings contained in the review articles.

The information contained within each reference should be related to the problem statement to form a nexus between the earlier studies and the current research project. If the investigator determines that the literature supports the need to study the proposed problem, he or she can proceed with confidence, knowing that pursuit of the research project (if properly designed and implemented) is likely to modify or extend the existing body of knowledge. Moreover, information gained from the literature review (including successes or failures of previous published work) can, as indicated earlier, prove invaluable for refining the problem (if necessary), buttressing or revising hypotheses, and validating or modifying the approach taken.

Crafting the Problem and Purpose Statements

Once the problem has been conceptualized and the literature search completed, the investigator is in a position to communicate to interested parties (e.g., mentors, colleagues, potential sponsors) the nature, context, and significance of the problem, including, typically, the type and size of the affected population, what is known and not yet known, and the consequences of the lack of knowledge (i.e., the implied or directly stated), thus elucidating the active challenge to be addressed and justifying the logical argument underlying the study. These elements are incorporated collectively into a "problem statement," a declarative set of assertions, interwoven with literature support, which customarily appears in the *Introduction* of the research report or in the *Background and Significance* section of a research proposal (though, as Polit et al. [12] have observed, the problem statement rarely is labeled as such and must be "ferreted out"). As a general rule, a well-constructed problem statement should be written as concisely as possible for optimal clarity yet contain sufficient information to make a viable argument in support of the study and elicit interest [13]. Abbreviated problem statements, condensed into a sentence or two with minimal supporting argumentation, commonly are provided in the beginning of the abstract accompanying the main body of the research report or research proposal. (Ellis and Levy [13] refer to these reductions as "statements of the problem" to differentiate them from fully developed problem statements with appropriate argumentation.)

If the study is broad, it is recommended that the investigator divide the main problem into subproblems, each of which addresses a single issue. It is important that the sum of the content

Table 2.2 Examples of well-defined problem statements from two research reports

PROBLEM STATEMENT #1: Fleming et al., Circulation, 2008 [23]	PROBLEM STATEMENT #2: Walker et al., CMAJ 2000 [24]
"Atrial fibrillation (AF), the most common complication after cardiac surgery, is associated with significant morbidity, increased mortality, longer hospital stay, and higher hospital costs .... Because ventricular dysfunction is common following cardiac surgery, inotropic drugs are often necessary to improve hemodynamic status; however, the effect of inotropic drugs on postoperative AF has not been extensively studied .... Milrinone has been reported to be associated with a lower risk of postoperative AF compared to dobutamine use, but milrinone increases the risk of atrial arrhythmias in patients with acute exacerbation of chronic heart failure"	"Asymptomatic bacteriuria ... is common in institutionalized elderly people. The prevalence increases with age, occurring in up to 50% of elderly women and 35% of elderly men who reside in long-term facilities .... Despite lack of benefit, institutionalized older adults with asymptomatic bacteriuria are frequently treated with antibiotics. This practice is of particular concern given the deleterious effects of antibiotics, including the potential for the development of antibiotic resistance and adverse reactions seen in this population. Why antibiotics continue to be prescribed for asymptomatic bacteriuria is unclear"

Table 2.3 Examples of well-defined statements of purpose from two published research studies

PURPOSE STATEMENT #1: Fleming et al., Circulation, 2008 [23]	PURPOSE STATEMENT #2: Walker et al., CMA 2000 [24]
"The aim of this analysis was to *test* the hypothesis that the use of inotropic drugs is associated with an increased risk of postoperative AF in cardiac surgery patients participating in an ongoing randomized, double blinded, placebo controlled trial"	"The aim of our study was to *explore* the perceptions, attitudes, and opinions of physicians and nurses involved in the process of prescribing antibiotics for asymptomatic bacteriuria in institutionalized elderly people"

reflected in the subproblems equates to no more or no less than the content reflected in the main problem. Like the main problem, the subproblems should be stated clearly and be related to each other in a meaningful way so that the research will maintain coherence.

Two examples of well-defined problem statements are given in Table 2.2. The first (shown in the left column) is drawn from a quantitative study by Fleming et al. [23] about the impact of milrinone on risk for atrial fibrillation after cardiac surgery. The second (shown in the right column) is a qualitative study by Walter et al. [24] addressing reasons for prescription of antibiotic therapy among the asymptomatic institutionalized elderly with bacteriuria. Note, in each case, the problem statement makes the argument that there is an important unresolved issue that should be addressed, and sets the stage for what the investigator intends to do to facilitate a solution.

The problem statement typically is followed by a "statement of purpose" (usually the last sentence or two in the *Introduction* of the research report or given as a list in the *Specific Aims* of the research proposal), which succinctly identifies what the investigator intends to do (the type of inquiry) to resolve the unknowns explicated in the problem statement. Although, like the problem statement, the statement of purpose typically is not labeled as such, it is easily identifiable as it includes the words "purpose" ("the purpose of the study was/is ...."), "goal" (the goal of the study was/is ...."), or, alternatively, "intent," "aim," or "objective" [12]. In a quantitative study, the statement of purpose also identifies the key variables to be examined and/or interrelated (parameters to be estimated, hypotheses to be tested), the nature of the study population (who is included), and, occasionally, the nature of the study design; in a qualitative investigation, the purpose statement commonly will include the phenomenon or phenomena under study (rather than hypotheses), as well as the study group, community, or setting [12]. Shown in Table 2.3 are the purpose statements from the Fleming and Walker studies. In both cases, the reader will note that the statements of purpose flow directly from the problem statements.

As Polit et al. have noted (and as illustrated above), the use of verbs in a purpose statement is key to determining the thrust of the inquiry and also helps to differentiate quantitative from qualitative studies [12]. The former typically include terms such as "compare," "contrast," "correlate," "estimate," and "test," whereas the

Table 2.4 Examples of research questions restated from two statements of purpose

PURPOSE STATEMENT #1: RESTATED AS A RESEARCH QUESTION Fleming et al., Circulation, 2008 [23]	PURPOSE STATEMENT #2: RESTATED AS A RESEARCH QUESTION Walker et al., CMA 2000 [24]
"Does the use of inotropic drugs increase risk of postoperative AF in cardiac surgery patients?"	"What are the perceptions, attitudes, and opinions of physicians and nurses involved in the process of prescribing antibiotics for asymptomatic bacteriuria in institutionalized elderly people?"

latter include terms such as "describe," "explore," "understand," "discover," and "develop." Verbs such as "prove" or "show" should be avoided in purpose statements of research studies as these can be construed as indicative of investigator bias [12].

As noted above, a statement of purpose can be expressed in declarative form. However, some investigators instead will frame the purpose of their study interrogatively as one or more research questions (each addressing a single concept) that are directed at the "unknowns" in the problem statement. Alternatively, these questions can be added to a global statement of purpose to improve clarity and specificity. As Polit et al. contend, research questions "invite an answer and help focus attention on the kinds of data that would have to be collected to provide that answer" [12]. Listed in Table 2.4 are research questions that could have been framed by Fleming et al. and Walker et al. to address the targets of inquiry in their studies.

However written, both the problem and purpose of the study (or the research questions) should be apparent to the reader in the *Introduction* of the research report (or in the *Background, Significance,* and *Specific Aims* of the research proposal) and should possess sufficient clarity for the reader to understand them without the presence of the author. Unfortunately, this is not always the case. Consider the statements articulated by Houck and Hampson in the introduction to their study about carbon monoxide poisoning following a winter storm during the 1980s, when charcoal briquettes commonly were used for heating in certain areas of the USA:

> A major epidemic of carbon monoxide poisoning occurred after a severe winter storm struck western Washington State during the morning of 20 January 1993. Charcoal briquettes and gasoline-powered generators were principal sources of CO. Although previous reports have described CO poisoning following winter storms in the Eastern United States, the large number and wide distribution of cases following this storm are unique. Unintentional carbon monoxide (CO) poisoning is a substantial health problem in the US, causing an estimated 11,547 deaths from 1979 through 1988. The US Consumer Product Safety Commission estimates that there was an average of about 28 charcoal-related deaths per year from 1986 through 1992. Charcoal briquettes are not an uncommon source of CO poisoning in Washington State: 16% of the 509 unintentional poisoning cases that required hyperbaric oxygen treatment between October 1982 and October 1993 involved charcoal. Our investigation suggests that CO poisoning following severe winter storms should be anticipated. It also suggests that preventive messages are important public health messages, but that they should be understandable to those in the community who neither read nor speak English. [25]

Does the *Introduction* contain a clear statement of the problem so that it is evident why the investigation was important? Is there a statement of purpose (or a set of questions) that explains what the investigators did to address the problem? Do the authors' introductory statements prepare the reader to follow the rest of the paper? After all, that is the principal role of the *Introduction* in a research manuscript. (For further details about the role and proper construction of the Introduction of the scientific paper, the reader is referred to Chap. 13.) Note, the authors have provided the reader with a general background statement and also have presented their conclusions in their *Introduction*, repeating information already given in their *Abstract*. However, other than suggesting that their data were unique, the rationale and aims of their study have not been articulated, and their research questions remain undefined even after reading their comments. The moral illustrated by this example is that for the published paper to engage and edify the reader, the research problem, purpose, and/or research questions must be unambiguously stated early in the research report.

When there is poor definition of problem and purpose, not only may the reader become confused, but these deficiencies may adversely impact the study methodology because all subsequent steps in the research process (e.g., construction of the research questions or hypotheses, development of the research design, collection and analysis of data) are guided by the statements of problem and purpose statements. Houck and Hampson were fortunate. When their article was written, there were relatively few experienced peer reviewers in their discipline (emergency medicine). This may well have helped the authors' efforts to gain publication.

More commonly, deficiencies in the wording of these statements and their connection to the remainder of the paper can be a primary cause of a manuscript being rejected for publication, or being sent back to the author for revision, following the peer-review process. The following criticisms, made by a reviewer in response to two different submissions to a cardiology journal, are illustrative of this point:

- *Submission #1: Comment*: "The *focus* of the study is not clearly apparent, even from the last paragraph which specifically describes the goals. The first page does not point directly to the study hypothesis." (Recommendation: Consider after revision)
- "In its current form, the manuscript resembles a mystery story with a good outcome more than a scientific study. Thus, while indicating the general aim of the authors, the *Introduction* misstates the specific goals required by the apparent design of the reported work, thus *misfocusing* the reader." (Recommendation: Consider after revision)

In sum, all research (whether basic or applied, quantitative or qualitative, hypothesis generating or hypothesis testing, retrospective or prospective, observational or experimental) may be considered as a response to a problem (an ambiguity, gap in knowledge, or other perplexing state) that requires resolution. In thinking through the problem and communicating it to others, the investigator must provide a clear and convincing argument that indicates why the problem must be addressed (the problem statement), articulate a solution to the problem to clarify the ambiguity or fill the gap in knowledge (the purpose statement or research questions), and tie these statements to the methods used. The challenge to the investigator is to define and interrelate these elements well enough to justify the research study and maximize the likelihood that the findings will be understood, appreciated, and utilized.

Take-Home Points

- A well-designed research project, in any discipline, begins with conceptualizing the problem.
- Research problems in clinical medicine may be stimulated by practical issues in the clinical care of patients, new or unexpected observations, discrepancies and knowledge gaps in the published literature, solicitations from government or other funding sources, and public forums such as scientific sessions, grand rounds, and seminars.
- Well-conceived research problems are important, interesting, feasible, and ethical and serve as a springboard for clearly focused questions.
- Research questions most relevant to clinicians include those pertaining to disease prevalence/incidence, prevention, detection (diagnosis or screening), etiology, prognosis, and outcomes of treatment (benefit or harm).
- A comprehensive literature search, conducted early in the planning process, can help to determine whether the proposed study is feasible, whether it is likely to substantively contribute to the existing knowledge base, and whether it can provide guidance in the construction of hypotheses, determination of sample size, and choice of study design.
- Proper framing of the problem and purpose statements is essential for communicating and justifying the research.

References

1. Kerlinger F. Foundations of behavioral research: educational and psychological inquiry. New York: Holt, Reinhart and Winston; 1964.
2. Eng J. Getting started in radiology research: asking the right question and identifying an appropriate population: critical thinking skills symposium. Acad Radiol. 2004;11:149–54.
3. Albrecht MN, Perry KM. Home health care: delineation of research priorities and formation of a national network group. Clin Nurs Res. 1992;1:305–11.
4. Davidson P, Merritt-Gray M, Buchanan J, Noel J. Voices from practice: mental health nurses identify research priorities. Arch Psychiatr Nurs. 1997;11: 340–5.
5. Gallagher M, Hares T, Spencer J, Bradshaw C, Webb I. The nominal group technique: a research tool for general practice? Fam Pract. 1993;10:76–81.
6. Beitz JM. Writing the researchable question. J Wound Ostomy Continence Nurs. 2006;33:122–4.
7. Hulley SB, Cummings SR. Designing clinical research. 1st ed. Baltimore: Williams and Wilkins; 1988.
8. Gliner JA, Morgan GA. Research methods in applied setting. An integrated approach to design and analysis. Mahwah: Lawrence Erlbaum Associates; 2000.
9. Shugan SM. Defining interesting research problems. Market Sci. 2003;22:1–15.
10. Hulley SB, Cummings SR, Browner WS, Grady DG, Newman TB. Designing clinical research. 3rd ed. Philadelphia: Lippincott Williams and Wilkins; 2007.
11. Tuckman BW. Conducting educational research. New York: Harcourt Brace Jovanovich; 1972.
12. Polit DF, Beck CT, Hungler BP. Essentials of nursing research. Methods, appraisal, and utilization. Philadelphia: Lippincott, Williams & Wilkins; 2001.
13. Ellis TJ, Levy Y. Framework of problem-based research: a guide for novice researchers on the development of a research-worthy problem. Inform Sci: Int J Emerg Transdiscipl. 2008;11:17–33.
14. Leedy PD, Ormond JE. Practical research: planning and design. 8th ed. Upper Saddle River: Prentice Hall; 2005.
15. Kerlinger FN, Lee HB. Foundations of behavioral research. 4th ed. Holt: Harcourt College; 2000.
16. Sim J, Wright C. Research in health care. Concepts, designs and methods. Cheltenham: Nelson Thornes; 2000.
17. Leedy PD. Practical research planning and design. 2nd ed. New York: MacMillan; 1980.
18. Sharav VH. The ethics of conducting psychosis-inducing experiments. Account Res. 1999;7:137–67.
19. Trochim, WM.: The research methods knowledge base. 2nd ed. Internet WWW page at URL: www.socialresearchmethods.net/kb/. Version current as of 20 Oct 2006.
20. Blaikie NWH. Designing social research: the logic of anticipation. Malden: Blackwell; 2000.
21. Sackett DL, Straus SE, Richardson WS, Haynes RB. Evidence-based medicine: how to practice and Teach EBM. 2nd ed. Edinburgh/New York: Churchill-Livingstone; 2000.
22. Burns N, Grove SK. The practice of nursing research. Conduct, critique and utilization. 5th ed. St. Louis: Elsevier Saunders; 2005.
23. Fleming GA, Murray KT, Yu C, Byrne JG, Greelish JP, Petracek MR, Hoff SJ, Ball SK, Brown NJ, Pretorius M. Milrinone use is associated with postoperative atrial fibrillation following cardiac surgery. Circulation. 2008;118:1619–25.
24. Walker S, McGeer A, Simor AE, Armstrong-Evans M, Loeb M. Why are antibiotics prescribed for asymptomatic bacteriuria in institutionalized elderly people? CMAJ. 2000;163:273–7.
25. Houck PM, Hampson NB. Epidemic carbon monoxide poisoning following a winter storm. J Emerg Med. 1997;15:469–73.

The Research Hypothesis: Role and Construction

3

Phyllis G. Supino

Wrong hypotheses, rightly worked from, have produced more results than unguided observation

—Augustus De Morgan, 1872[1]—

Overview

Once a problem has been defined, the investigator can formulate a hypothesis (or set of hypotheses, if there are multiple subproblems) about the outcome of the study designed to resolve the problem. A hypothesis (from the Greek, *foundation*) is a logical construct, interposed between a problem and its solution, which represents a proposed answer to a research question. It gives direction to the investigator's thinking about the problem and, therefore, facilitates a solution. Unlike facts and assumptions (presumed true and, therefore, not tested in the study) or theory (a relatively well-supported unifying system explicating a broad spectrum of observations and inferences, including previously tested hypotheses), the research hypothesis is a reasoned but tentative proposition typically expressing a relation between variables. For it to be useful and, more importantly, assessable, it must generate predictions that can be tested by subsequent acquisition, analysis, and interpretation of data (i.e., through formal observation or experimentation). When the results of the study are as predicted, the hypothesis is supported. As noted below, such support does not necessarily indicate verification of the hypothesis. Consistent replication of predictions in subsequent studies may be needed if the hypothesis is to be accepted as a theory or a component of a theory. If results are not as predicted, the hypothesis is rejected (or, at minimum, revised or removed from active consideration until future developments in science and/or technology provide new tools for retesting). As Leedy has stated, a "hypothesis is to a researcher what a point of triangulation is to a surveyor: it provides a position from which he may orient his exploration into the unknown and a checkpoint against which to test his findings" [2]. The paramount role of the hypothesis for guiding biomedical investigations was first highlighted by the eminent physiologist Claude Bernard (1813–1878) [3]. In the current era, hypotheses are considered fundamental to rigorous research, and biomedical studies without hypotheses have been largely abandoned in favor of those designed to generate or test them [4].

P.G. Supino, EdD (✉)
Department of Medicine, College of Medicine,
SUNY Downstate Medical Center, 450 Clarkson Avenue,
Box 1199, Brooklyn, NY 11203, USA
e-mail: phyllissupino@aol.com

Hypotheses Versus Assumptions

It is important to recognize the difference between a hypothesis and an assumption. These terms share the same etymological root and are often confused. An assumption is accepted as fact in designing or justifying a study (though it is likely to have been the subject of previous research).

P.G. Supino and J.S. Borer (eds.), *Principles of Research Methodology: A Guide for Clinical Investigators*,
DOI 10.1007/978-1-4614-3360-6_3,

Thus, the investigator does not set out to test it. Examples of assumptions include:

- Radionuclide cineangiography measures ventricular performance.
- Chest x-rays measure the extent of lung infiltrates.
- The SF-36 measures general health-related quality of life.
- Medical education improves knowledge of clinical medicine.
- An apple a day keeps the doctor away (the most famous [albeit untested] assumption of them all).

In contrast, the hypothesis is an expectation that an investigator will attempt to confirm through observation or experiment. Examples in clinical medicine include:

- Among patients with chronic nonischemic mitral regurgitation (insufficiency), survival will be better among those whose valves have been repaired or replaced than among those who have been maintained on medical therapy.
- Among patients hospitalized with community-acquired pneumonia, posthospital course will be better among those with a low-risk profile than among those with a high-risk profile before hospitalization.
- Life expectancy will be greater among individuals consuming low-calorie diets than among those consuming high-calorie diets.
- Health-related quality of life is better among those whose mitral valves have been repaired than among those whose mitral valves have been replaced.

Hypothesis Generation: Modes of Inference

There is a paucity of empirical data regarding the way (or ways) in which hypotheses are formulated by scientists and even less information about whether these methods vary across disciplines. Nonetheless, philosophers and research methodologists have suggested three fundamentally different modes of inference: deduction, induction, and abduction [5]. These differ primarily according to (1) whether the origin of the hypothesis is a body of knowledge or theory (the "rationalist" perspective), an empirical event (the "inductivist" perspective), or some combination of the two (the "abductivist" perspective); (2) the logical structure of the argument; and (3) the probability of a correct conclusion.

Hypothesis by Deduction

Deduction (from the Latin *de* ["out of"] and *dūcerė* ["to draw or lead"]) is one of the oldest forms of logical argument. It was introduced by the ancient Greeks who believed that acquisition of scientific knowledge (insight into the principles and character of "natural substances" and their causes) could be achieved largely by the same logical processes used to prove the validity of mathematical propositions [6]. Today, deduction remains the predominant mode of formal inference in research in mathematics and in the "fundamental" sciences, but it also plays an important role in the empirical sciences. A deductively derived hypothesis arises directly from logical analysis of a theoretical framework, previously developed to provide an explanation of events or phenomena. It is considered to be non-ampliative because, while it helps to provide proof of principle, it adds nothing new beyond the theory. The validity of a theory can never be directly examined. Therefore, scientists wishing to evaluate it, or to test its utility within a given (perhaps new) context, will formulate a conjecture (hypothesis) that can be subjected to empirical appraisal. In forming a hypothesis by deduction, the investigator typically moves from a general proposition to a more specific case that is thought to be subsumed by the generalization (i.e., from theory to a "conceptual" hypothesis or from a "conceptual" hypothesis to a precise prediction based on the hypothesis). Deductive arguments can be conditional or syllogistic (e.g., categorical [*all*, *some*, or *none*], disjunctive [*or*], or linear [*including a quantitative or qualitative comparison*]) and contain at least two premises (statements of "evidence") and a conclusion. A well-known categorical syllogism and example are given below:

All As are B (e.g., All men are mortal)
C is an A (e.g., Socrates is a man)
∴ C is a B (e.g., Socrates is mortal)

If the premises of a deductive argument are *true* and the reasoning used to reach the conclusion is *valid* (i.e., the *form* of the argument is correct), it will necessarily follow that the conclusion is *sound* (i.e., the premises, if true, guarantee the conclusion). If the form of the deductive argument is invalid (i.e., the premises are such that they do not lead to the conclusion: e.g., Socrates is mortal, all cats are mortal, ∴ Socrates is a cat) and/or the premises are untrue (e.g., all mortals are men [or cats]), the conclusion will be unsound. It should be noted that deductive reasoning is the only form of logical argument to which the term "validity" is appropriate.

The theory from which the hypothesis is derived can be specific to the discipline or it can be "borrowed" from another discipline. Polit and Beck [7] provide two examples of deductively formulated hypotheses, germane to nursing, derived from general reinforcement theory which posits that behaviors that are rewarded tend to be learned or repeated:

1. Nursing home residents who are praised (reinforced) by nursing personnel for self-feeding require less assistance in feeding than those who are not praised.
2. Pediatric patients who are given a reward (e.g., a balloon or permission to watch television when they cooperate during nursing procedures) tend to be more cooperative during those procedures than unrewarded peers.

Deduction also is used to translate broad hypotheses such as these to more specific operational hypotheses (i.e., working hypotheses or predictions) that can be directly tested by observation or experiment. When empirical support is obtained for a hypothesis, this, in turn, strengthens the theory or body of knowledge from which the hypothesis was deduced.

Hypothesis by Induction

Not all hypotheses are derived from theory. Frequently, in the empirical sciences, patterns, trends, and associations are observed serendipitously in clinical settings or in preclinical laboratories or, purposively, through exploratory data analysis or other hypothesis-generating research. Sometimes, they may result from specific findings gleaned from the research literature. These observations may be generalized to produce inductively derived hypotheses that may serve as the basis for predicting future events, phenomena, or patterns. Induction (from the Latin in [meaning "into"] and *dūcerė* ["to draw or to lead"]) is defined by Jenicek and Hitchcock as "any method of logical analysis that proceeds from the particular to the general" [8] and represents the logical opposite of deduction which, as noted above, typically proceeds from the general to the specific. Induction can be used not only to formulate hypotheses but to confirm or refute them, which may be its most appropriate use, as noted below (see Abduction). Inductive reasoning, which is based heavily on the senses rather than on intellectual reflection, was popularized by the English philosopher and scientist, Sir Francis Bacon (1561–1626) [9], who proposed it as the logic of scientific discovery, a position that, subsequently, has been vigorously disputed by the Austrian logician, Sir Karl Popper (1902–1994) [10] and other philosophers of science. There are various forms of inductive inference. One of the most common is enumerative induction (or inductive generalization). Jenicek and Hitchcock [8] describe it as a mode by which "one concludes that all cases of a specified kind have a specified property on the basis of observation that all examined cases of that kind have the property" [8]. It is called "enumerative" because it itemizes cases in which some pattern is found and, *solely for this reason* (i.e., without the benefit of a theoretical framework), forecasts its recurrence. Other forms of induction include argument from analogy (forming inferences based on a shared property or properties of individual cases) or prediction (drawing conclusions about the future cases from a current sample), causal inference (concluding that association implies causality), and Bayesian inference (given new evidence [data], using probability theory [Bayes' theorem] to alter belief in a hypothesis).

All inductive arguments contain multiple premises that provide grounds for a conclusion but do not necessitate it (in contrast to a deductive argument where the premises, if true, entail the conclusion). In other words, a conclusion drawn from an inductive argument is probable (at best), even if its premises are correct. For this reason, all inductive arguments, while ampliative, are considered to be logically *invalid* and are judged, instead, according to their "strength" (i.e., whether they are "inductively strong" or "inductively weak"). The strength of an inductive generalization is determined by the number of observations supporting it and the extent to which the observations reflect all observations that could be made. The more (consistent) observations that exist, the more likely the conclusion is correct (inconsistent observations, of course, reduce the argument's inductive strength). The typical form of an inductive generalization is given below:

A_1 is a B
A_2 is a B
(All As I have observed are Bs)
∴ All As are Bs

Like deductive arguments, inductive generalizations can be categorical, that is, represent conclusions about "all" (as above), "no," or "some" members of a class, or they may involve quantitative arguments, for example, "50% of all coins I have sampled are quarters; therefore, 50% of all coins coming from the same lot that I have sampled *probably* are quarters" (or, as a clinical example, "30% of the patients I have examined are obese; therefore, 30% of patients sampled from the same population as those who I have examined *probably* are obese").

Not all inductive hypotheses used by scientists have been formulated by scientists; some, in fact, owe their origin to folklore. For example, by the late eighteenth century, it was common knowledge among English farm workers that when humans were exposed to cows infected with cowpox (vaccinia), they became immune to its more severe human analogue, smallpox. The English surgeon, Edward Jenner (1749–1823), used this "hypothesis" as the basis of a series of scientific experiments, using exudates from an infected milkmaid, to develop and formally test a vaccine against this disease [11]. He became famous for using vaccination as a method for preventing infection, though there is growing recognition that the first successful inoculations against smallpox actually were performed by a farmer, Benjamin Jesty, some 20 years earlier, who vaccinated his family using cowpox taken directly from a local cow [12]. It also has been claimed that Charles Darwin used inductive reasoning when generalizing about the shapes of the beaks from finches from the various Galapagos Islands [13] and when forming conjectures from observations based on the breeding of dogs, pigeons, and farm animals at home (inferences that formed underpinnings of his theory of evolution) and that Gregor Mendel used the same form of reasoning to conceptualize his "law of hybridization" [14]. Even if these claims are true (and there is far from universal agreement on this matter), inductive generalizations typically are regarded as inferior to hypothesis-generating methods that involve more theoretical reasoning, that consider variations in circumstances (i.e., possible confounding factors) that may account for spurious patterns, and that provide possible causal explanation for observed phenomena. Moreover, recent research in cognition and the relatively new field of neural modeling suggest that simple induction "across a limited set of observations" may have a far smaller role in scientific reasoning than previously realized [15].

Hypothesis by Abduction

Of the three primary methods of reasoning, the one that has been most implicated in the creation of novel ideas, including scientific discoveries, is the logical process of *abduction* (from the Latin *ab* [meaning "away from"] and *dūcerė* ["to draw or to lead"]). It also is the most common mode of reasoning employed by clinicians when making diagnostic inferences. Abduction was introduced into modern logic by American philosopher and mathematician, Charles Sanders Peirce (1839–1914) [16], and remains an important, albeit controversial, topic of research among philosophers of science and students of artificial intelligence. It refers to the process of formulation and acceptance *on probation* of a hypothesis to explain a surprising observation. Thus, hypotheses formed by abduction (unlike those formed by induction) are always explanatory. (The reader should note that other synonyms for, and definitions of, abduction exist, e.g., "retroduction," "reduction," "inference to the *best* explanation," etc., the latter reflecting the evaluative and selective functions that also have been associated with this term.) Abductive reasoning entails moving from a *consequent* (the observation or current "fact") to its *antecedent* (presumed cause or precondition) through a general rule. It is considered "backward" because the inference about the *antecedent* is drawn from the *consequent*.

Peirce devoted his earliest work (before 1900), as did Aristotle long before him, to furthering the development of syllogistic theory to express logical relations. During this early period, abduction (then termed by him as *hypothesis*) was taken to mean the use of a *known* "rule" to explain an observation ("result"); accordingly, his initial efforts were devoted to demonstrating how the hypothesis relates to the premises of the argument and how it differs from the logical structure of other forms of reasoning (i.e., deduction or induction). In his essay, *Deduction, Induction, Hypothesis*, Peirce presents an abductive syllogism:

Rule: "All the beans from this bag are white."
Result: "These beans are white."
Case: "These beans are from this bag." [16]

In this argument, the "rule" and "result" represent the premises (background knowledge and observation, respectively [the order is arbitrary]) and the "case" represents the conclusion (here, the hypothesis). Had this argument been expressed deductively, the "case" would have been the second premise, and the "result," the conclusion (i.e., "all the beans from this bag are white, these beans are from this bag; therefore, these beans are white"). It should be obvious to the reader that the abductive argument is logically less secure than a deductive argument (or even an inductive argument). It represents a *possible* conclusion only (after all, the beans might come from some other bag—or from no bag at all). Therefore, like an inductive argument, it is ampliative though logically invalid. Its strength is based on how well the argument accounts for all available evidence, including that which is seemingly contradictory.

As Peirce's work evolved, he shifted his efforts to developing a theory of inferential reasoning in which abduction was taken to mean the generation of *new* rules to explain *new* observations. In so doing, he focused on, what some have termed, the "creative character of abduction" [17]. Peirce argued that abduction had a major role in the process of scientific inquiry and, indeed, was the only inferential process by which new knowledge was created—a view that was, and continues to be, hotly debated by the philosophical community. In his later work, Peirce described the logical structure of abduction as follows:

The surprising fact, C, is observed.
But if A were true, C would be a matter of course.
Hence, there is reason to suspect that A is true. [18]

The "surprise" (the stimulus to the abductive inference) arises because the observation is viewed, at that moment in time, as an anomaly, given the observer's preexisting corpus of knowledge (theory base) which cannot account for it. The lack of compatibility between the observation and expectation introduces a type of cognitive dissonance that seeks resolution through the adoption of a coherent explanation. In Peirce's opinion, the explanation might be nothing more than a guess (Peirce believed that humans were "hardwired" with the ability for guessing correctly) that, unlike an inductive generalization, enters the mind "like a flash" [18] or, what is commonly termed, as a "eureka moment" or an "ah ha!" experience. Because a guess (insightful or not), by its very nature, is speculative (and, as noted above, is a relatively insecure form of reasoning), Peirce recognized that an abductive hypothesis must be rigorously tested before it could be admitted into scientific theory. This, he

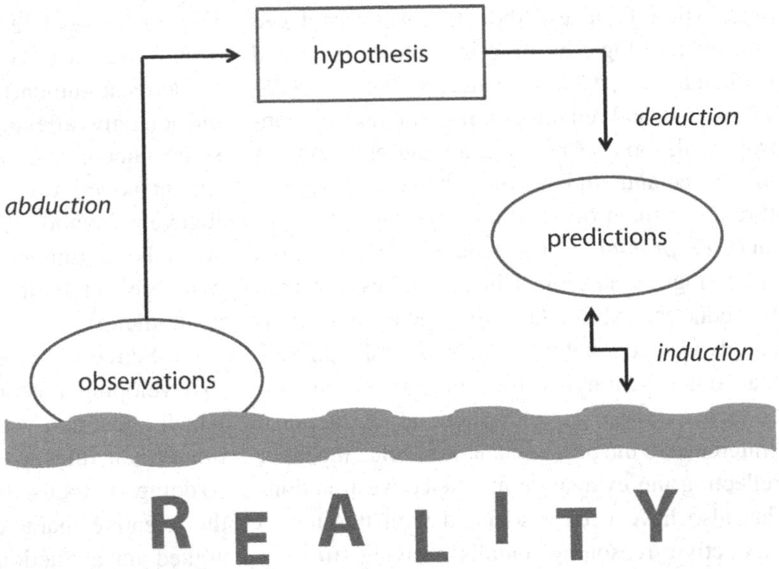

Fig. 3.1 The three stages of scientific inquiry (*From* Abduction and Induction. Essays on their Relation and Integration, Flach PA and Kakas AC. Abductive and Inductive Reasoning: Background and Issues, Chap. 1, pp. 1–27, Copyright 2000, *with permission from Klewer Academic Publishers*)

reasoned, is accomplished by using deduction to explicate the consequences of the hypothesis (i.e., the predictions) and induction to form a conclusion about the likelihood of their truthfulness, based on experimental verification. According to Peirce, these are the primary roles of deduction and induction in the scientific process. Figure 3.1 illustrates the Peircian view of the relation between abduction, deduction, and induction as interpreted by Flach and Kakas [19].

Countless abductively derived hypotheses, principles, theories, and laws have been put forward in science. Many, if not most, owe to the serendipitous consequences of an unexpected observation made while looking for something else [20]. Well-known examples of such "happy accidents" include:

- Archimedes' principles of density and buoyancy
- Hans Christian Oersted's theory of electromagnetism
- Luigi Galvani's principle of bioelectricity
- Claude Bernard's neuroregulatory principle of circulation
- Paul Gross' protease-antiprotease hypothesis of pulmonary emphysema

Although, as Peirce points out, all three modes of inference (abduction, deduction, and induction) are used in the process of scientific inquiry, each requires different skills. As scholars have noted, deduction requires the capacity to reason logically and inductive reasoning requires understanding of the statistical implications of drawing conclusions from samples to populations. In contrast, as Danmark et al. have noted, abduction requires the "discernment of new relations and connections not immediately obvious" [21]—in other words, to "think outside the box." For this reason, the best abductive hypotheses in science have been made by those who not only are observant, wise, and well grounded in their disciplines but who also are imaginative and receptive to new ideas. This view was, perhaps, best expressed by Louis Pasteur (1822–1895) when he argued, "In the fields of observation, chance favors only prepared minds" [22]. Accordingly, developing the "prepared mind," in general, and enhancing the capacity to reason abductively, deductively, and inductively, in particular, should be among the most important goals of those seeking to effectively engage in the process of scientific discovery.

Characteristics of the Research Hypothesis

Irrespective of how it is formulated (or the problem or discipline for which it is formulated), a research hypothesis should fulfill the following five requirements:

1. *It should reflect an inference about variables.*
The purpose of any hypothesis is to make an inference about one or more variables. The inference can be as simple as predicting a single characteristic in a population (e.g., mean height, prevalence of lung cancer, incidence of acute myocardial infarction, or other population parameter) or, more commonly, it represents a supposition about an association between two or more variables (e.g., smoking and lung cancer, diet and hypertension, age and exercise tolerance, etc.). It is, therefore, important for the investigator to understand what is meant by a variable and how it functions in the setting of a hypothesis.

    In its broadest sense, a variable is any feature, attribute, or characteristic that can assume different values (levels) within the same individual at different points in time or can differ from one member of the study population to another. Typical variables of interest to biomedical researchers include subject profile characteristics (e.g., age, weight, gender, etiology, stage of disease), nature, place, duration of naturally occurring exposures (e.g., risk factors, environmental influences) or purposively applied interventions, and subject outcomes or responses (e.g., morbidity, mortality, symptom relief, physiological, behavioral, or attitudinal changes) among others.

    It is important to recognize that a characteristic that functions as a variable in one study does not necessarily serve as a variable in another. For example, if an investigator wished to determine the relation of gender to prevalence of diabetes, it would be necessary to study this problem in a group comprising males and females, some with and some without this disease. Because intersubject differences exist for both characteristics, gender and diabetes would be considered study variables, and a hypothesis could be constructed about their association. However, if all patients in a study group were women with diabetes, no hypothesis could be developed about the relation between gender and diabetes since these attributes would be invariable. (Fuller discussion of nature and role of variables, and their relation to the hypothesis, is presented later in this chapter.)

2. *It should be stated as a grammatically complete, declarative sentence.*
A hypothesis should contain, at minimum, a subject and predicate (the verb or verb phrase and other parts of the predicate modifying the verb). The statements "relaxation (subject) decreases (verb) blood pressure (object, or predicate noun)," "depression (subject) increases (verb) the rate of suicide (predicate)," and "consumption of diet cola (subject) is related to (verb phrase) body weight (object, or predicate noun)" are illustrative of hypotheses that meet this requirement. In these examples, the subject and predicate modifiers reflect the variables to be related, and the verb (or verb phrase) defines the nature of the expected association.

3. *It should be expressed simply and unambiguously.*
For a hypothesis to be of value in a study, it must be clear in meaning, contain only one answer to any one question, and reflect only the essential elements of solution. The reason is that the hypothesis guides all subsequent research activities, including selection of the population and measurement instruments, collection and analysis of data, and interpretation of results. For example, the hypothesis "right ventricular performance is the best predictor of survival among patients with valvular heart disease, but is less important in others" would be difficult to validate. First, what is meant by right ventricular performance? Does this refer to ejection fraction at rest, at exercise, or the change from rest to exercise, or to some other parameter? Second, what is the meaning of "best"? Does it signify ease of measurement or does is it relate to the strength of statistical

association? Third, to what is right ventricular performance compared? Is the contrast between right ventricular performance and clinical descriptors, anatomic descriptors, other functional descriptors, or between all of these? Fourth, what type of "valvular heart disease" is being studied? Is it regurgitant, stenotic, or both? Does it involve the mitral, aortic, or some other heart valve? Finally, what is meant by "less important"? Who (or what) are the "others"? As is true for the research problem, the clearer and less complex the statement of the hypothesis, the more straightforward the study and the more useful the findings.

4. *It should provide an adequate answer to the research problem.*

   For a hypothesis to be adequate, it must address, in a satisfactory manner, both the content and scope of the central question; that is, whether the problem is narrow or broad, simple or complex, evaluation of the hypothesis(es) should result in the full resolution of the research problem. For this reason, it is recommended that the investigator formulate at least one hypothesis for every subproblem articulated in the study. Equally important, a hypothesis must be plausible; for this condition to be satisfied, the hypothesis should be based on prior relevant observation and experience, buttressed by consideration of existing theory, and should reflect sound reasoning and knowledge of the problem at hand. In contrast, speculations which have either no empirical support or legitimate theoretical basis, even if interesting, constitute poor hypotheses and typically yield weak or uninterpretable study outcomes. Finally, if the hypothesis is explanatory in nature (rather than an inductive generalization), all else being equal, it should represent the simplest of all possible competing explanations for the phenomenon or data at hand [23], a principle known as Occam's razor or *entia non sunt multiplicanda praeter necessitatem* (Latin for "entities must not be multiplied beyond necessity").

5. *It should be testable.*

   A hypothesis must be stated in such a way as to allow for its examination which, in the biomedical and other empirical sciences, is achieved through the acts of observation or experimentation, analysis, and judicious interpretation. If one or more of the elements comprising the hypothesis is not present in the population or sample, or if a phenomenon or characteristic contained within the hypothesis is highly subjective or otherwise difficult to measure, the hypothesis cannot be properly evaluated. For example, the statement "female patients cope better with stress than male patients" would be a poor hypothesis if the investigator did not have access to both male and female patients or was unable to generate acceptable definitions and measures to evaluate "coping" and "stress." An even more egregious example is the hypothesis "prognosis following diagnosis of ovarian cancer is related to the patient's survival instinct," as it would be extremely difficult to develop empirical data in support of a "survival instinct"—assuming it did exist.

For many years, philosophers of science have argued about what constitutes evidence in science or support for a scientific hypothesis. By the mid-twentieth century, the tenets of logical positivism (or logical empiricism) dominated the philosophy of science in the United States as well as throughout the English-speaking world [24], replacing the Cartesian emphasis on rationalism as a primary epistemological tool. Strongly eschewing metaphysical and theological explanations of reality, the logical positivists argued that a proposition held meaning only if it could be "verified" (i.e., if its truth could be determined conclusively by observable facts). Early critics of logical positivism, most notable among them Karl Popper, believed that "verifiability" was too stringent a criterion for scientific discovery. This, he argued, was due to the logical limitations inherent in inductive reasoning, namely, the deductive invalidity of forming a generalization based on the observation of particulars, and the attendant uncertainty of such an inference. Thus, while both positive *existential* claims (e.g., "there is at least one white swan") and negative universal claims

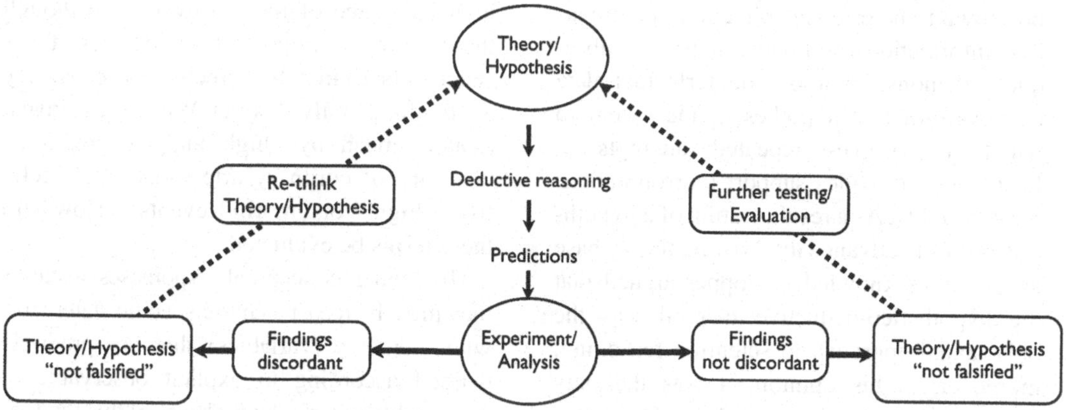

Fig. 3.2 The hypothetico-deductive model: Popper's view of the role of falsification in scientific reasoning

(e.g., "not all swans are white") could be confirmed by finding, respectively, at last one white swan or one black swan, it would be impossible to verify a positive universal claim (e.g., *all* swans are white). To accomplish that, one would have to observe every swan in existence, at all times and in all places, or risk being wrong.

According to Popper, the hallmark of a testable claim is its capacity to be *falsified* [25]. In his view, falsification (*not* verification) is the criterion for demarcation between those hypotheses, theories, and other propositions that are scientific versus those that are not scientific. This, of course, did not mean that a scientific hypothesis or theory must be false; rather, if it were false, it could be shown to be so. Returning to our earlier example, all that would be required to disprove the claim "all swans were white" is to find a swan that is not white. Indeed, this inductive inference, based on the observation of millions of white swans in Europe, was shown to be false when black swans were discovered in Western Australia in the eighteenth century [26]—an event that was not unnoticed by Popper. It provided clear support for his assertion that no matter how many observations are made that appear to confirm a proposition, there is always the possibility that an event not yet seen could refute it. Similarly, any scientific hypothesis, theory, or law could be falsified by finding a single counterexample.

Popper's greatest contribution to science was his characterization of scientific inquiry, based on a cyclical system of conjectures and refutations (a form of critical rationalism) widely known as the "hypothetico-deductive method" [27]. A schematic of Popper's view of this method is shown in Fig. 3.2. Consistent with Popper's writing on the subject, the terms *hypothesis* and *theory* are used interchangeably as both are viewed as tentative, though most workers in the field currently reserve the latter term for hypotheses (or related systems of hypotheses) that have received consistent and long-standing empirical support.

The reader will note that the hypothetico-deductive method begins with an early postulation of a hypothesis. The investigator then uses deductive logic to form predictions from the hypothesis that should be true if the hypothesis is, in fact, correct. The nature of the predictions can vary from study to study, but they share the common attribute of being unknown before data collection. The predictions are then evaluated by formal experimentation or observation. Assuming a properly designed study, those predictions that are discordant with data falsify the hypothesis, which is then discarded or revised, leading to additional study. Although a hypothesis can never be shown to be true via collection of compatible information (as Popper noted, a subsequent demonstration of counterfactual data can overturn any hypothesis), the extent to which it survives repeated attempts at falsification provides support (corroboration) for its validity. As a result, testing of a hypothesis serves to advance the existing theory base and body of knowledge. Popper argued that the hypothetico-deductive method was the only sound approach to scientific reasoning; moreover, in his opinion, it was the only method by which science made any progress.

Although Popper did not originate the hypothetico-deductive method, he was the first to explicate the central role of falsification versus confirmation of a hypothesis in the developing science. While his arguments have been criticized by other philosophers of science who assert that scientists do not necessarily reason that way [28], his views remain prominent in modern philosophy and continue to appeal to many modern scientists [29]. Today, the Popperian view of the hypothetico-deductive method, with its emphasis on testing to falsify a proposed hypothesis, generally is taken to represent an ideal (if not universal) approach to curbing excessive inductive speculation and ensuring scientific objectivity, and is considered to be the primary methodology by which biological knowledge is acquired and disseminated [30].

Types of Hypotheses

Hypotheses can be classified in several ways, as shown below.

1. *Conceptual Versus Operational Hypotheses*
   Hypotheses can vary according to their degree of specificity or precision and theoretical relatedness. Hypotheses can be written as broad or general statements, in which case they are termed *conceptual hypotheses*. For example, an investigator may hypothesize that "a high-fat diet is related to severity of coronary artery disease" or another may conjecture that "depression is associated with a relatively high incidence of morbid events." Although these may be important hypotheses, these statements cannot be directly tested as they are fundamentally abstract. What do the investigators mean by "high fat," "depression," "severity of coronary artery disease," "relatively high," or "morbid events"? How will these terms be evaluated?

   To render conceptual hypotheses testable, they must be recast as more specific statements with elements (variables) that are precisely defined according to explicit observable or measurable criteria. Hypotheses of this type are referred to as *operational hypotheses* or, alternatively, specific hypotheses or predictions and represent the specific (observable) manifestation of the conceptual hypothesis that the study is designed to test. Once the study is designed, data will be collected and analyzed to determine whether they are concordant or discordant with the operational hypothesis which, ultimately, will be reinterpreted in terms of its broader meaning as a conceptual hypothesis. Figure 3.3 below illustrates a simplified version of the *hypothetico-deductive method*, as conceptualized by Kleinbaum, Kupper, and Morgenstern [31] depicting the relation of conceptual and operational hypotheses to the design and interpretation of the study.

   Construction of operational hypotheses represents an important preliminary step in the development of the research design, data collection strategy, and statistical analysis plan and is described in greater detail in subsequent sections of this chapter.
2. *Single Variable Versus Multiple Variable Hypotheses*
   Some investigations are undertaken to determine whether a mean, proportion, or other parameter from a sample varies from a specified value. For example, a group of obstetricians may have read a report that concludes that, throughout the nation, the average length of stay following uncomplicated caesarian section is 5 days. They may have reason to believe that the length of stay for similar patients at their institution differs from the national average and would like to know if

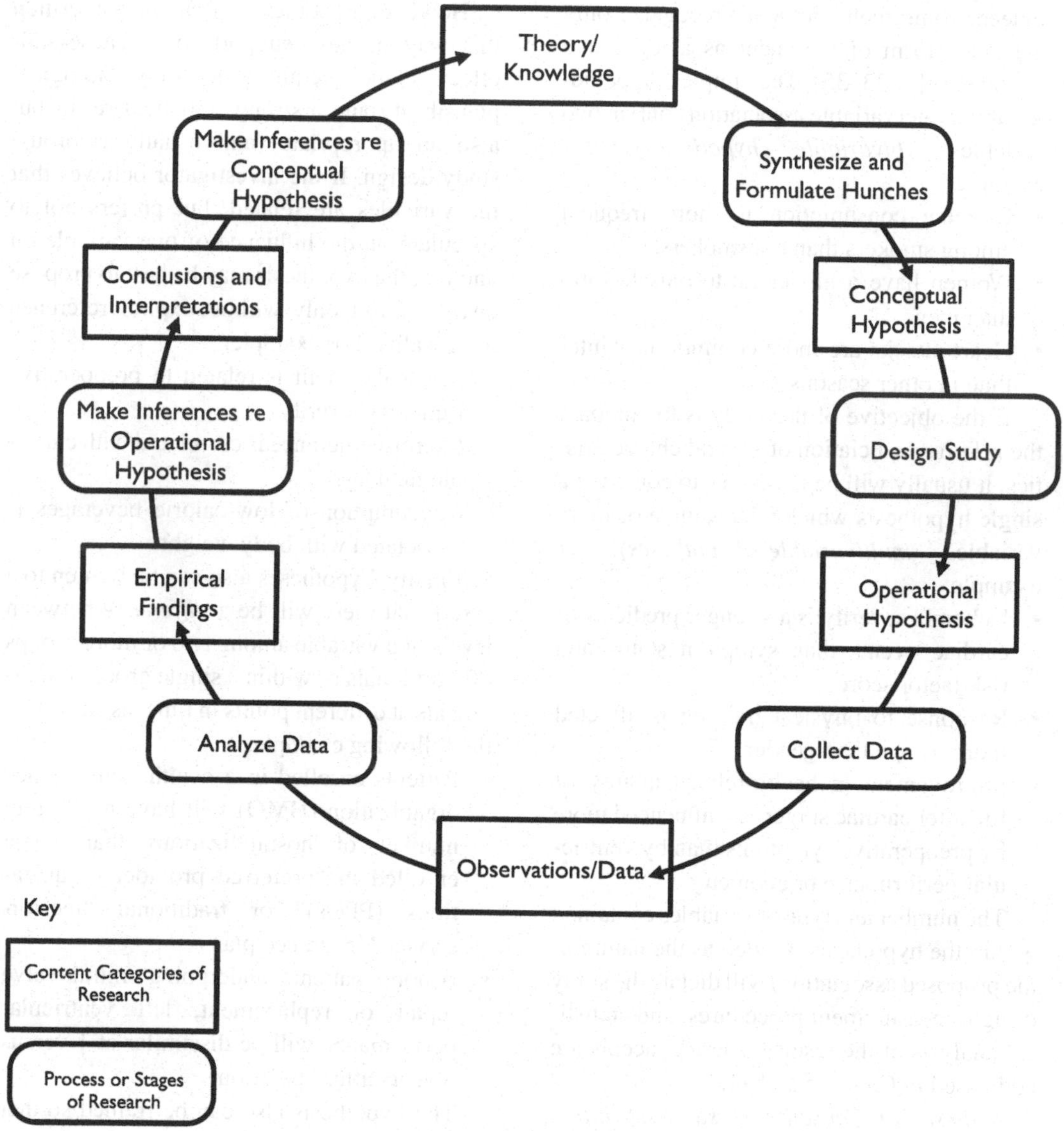

Fig. 3.3 Interrelation of conceptual hypotheses, operational hypotheses, and the hypothetico-deductive method (Reprinted with permission Kleinbaum DG, Kupper LL, Morgenstern H. *Epidemiologic Research: Principles and Quantitative Methods, Fig. 2.2: An Idealized Conceptualization of the Scientific Method* (New York: Van Nostrand Reinhold 1982), p. 35)

their belief is correct. To study the question, they must first recast their question as a hypothesis including the stipulated variable, select a representative sample of patients from their institution, and compare data from their sample with the national average (stipulated value) using an appropriate one-sample statistical test. (The reader should note that the only variable being tested within this hypothesis is length of stay. In this case, caesarian section is only a descriptor of the target population because all data to be examined are from patients undergoing this procedure.)

However, the objective of most hypotheses is not to draw inferences about population parameters but to facilitate evaluation of a proposition that two or more variables are systematically related in some manner [32].

Indeed, some methodologists recognize only the latter form of argument as a legitimate hypothesis [7, 33–35]. The simplest hypotheses about intervariable association contain two variables (*bivariable hypotheses*), for example:

- Caffeine consumption is more frequent among smokers than nonsmokers.
- Women have a higher fat-to-muscle ratio than men.
- Heart attacks are more common in winter than in other seasons.

If the objective of the study is to compare the *relative* association of several characteristics, it usually will be necessary to construct a single hypothesis which relates three or more variables (*multivariable hypotheses*), for example:

- Ischemia severity is a stronger predictor of cardiac events than symptom status and risk factor score.
- Response to physical training is affected more by age than gender.
- Improvement in health-related quality of life after cardiac surgery is influenced more by preoperative symptoms than by ventricular performance or geometry.

The number and type of variables contained within the hypothesis (as well as the nature of the proposed association) will dictate the study design, measurement procedures, and statistical analysis of the results. These concepts are addressed in Chaps. 5 and 11.

3. *Hypotheses of Causality Versus Association or Difference*

The relation posited between variables may be cast as one of *cause-and-effect*, in which case the researcher hypothesizes that one variable affects or influences the other(s) in some manner. For example:

- Estrogen produces an increase in coronary flow.
- Smoking promotes lung cancer.
- Patient education improves compliance.
- Coronary artery bypass grafting causes a reduction in the number of subsequent cardiac events.

However, hypotheses often are not written this way because support for a cause-and-effect relation requires not only biological plausibility and a strong statistical result but also an appropriate (and usually rigorous) study design. If the investigator believes that the variables are related, but prefers not to speculate on the influence of one variable on another, the hypothesis may be cast to propose an *association* only, without explicit reference to causality. For example:

- Surgical benefit is related to preoperative ischemia severity.
- Exercise tolerance is correlated with chronological age.
- Consumption of low-calorie beverages is associated with body weight.

Finally, hypotheses also can be written to a assert that there will be a *difference* between levels of a variable among two or more groups of individuals or within a single group of individuals at different points in time, as shown by the following examples:

- Patients enrolled in a health maintenance organization (HMO) will have a different number of hospitalizations than those enrolled in "preferred provider organizations (PPOs)" or traditional "fee-for-service" insurance plans.
- Among patients undergoing mitral valve repair or replacement, left ventricular performance will be dissimilar at 1 versus 3 years after operation.

The hypothesis also can be framed so that the nature of the association (e.g., linear, curvilinear, positive, inverse, etc.) or difference ("larger" or "smaller," "better" or "poorer," etc.) will be specified (see below, Alternative hypotheses [directional]).

4. *Mechanistic Versus Nonmechanistic Hypotheses*

Hypotheses can be written so as to provide a mechanism (i.e., an explanation) for an asserted relationship or prediction, or they can be written without defining an underlying mechanism. *Mechanistic hypotheses* are common in preclinical research which typically attempts to define biochemical and physiological causes of disease or dysfunction and pathways amenable to therapeutic intervention.

Shown below are two examples of mechanistic hypotheses that were evaluated in two different preclinical investigations: (Note the use of the phrase "as a result of" in the first hypothesis evaluating the impact of endothelial nitric oxide synthase [eNOS] and "due to" in the second hypothesis evaluating antagonism of endothelin [ET]-induced inotropy. Italics have been added for emphasis.)

- "Gender-specific protection against myocardial infarction occurs in adult female as compared to male rabbits *as a result of* eNOS upregulation" [36].
- "ET-induced direct positive inotropy is antagonized in vivo by an indirect cardiodepressant effect *due to* a mainly ETA-mediated and ET-induced coronary constriction with consequent myocardial ischemia" [37].

In clinical research, hypotheses more commonly are *nonmechanistic* (i.e., framed without including an explicit explanation). Shown below are two published literature examples:

- "Patients with medically unexplained symptoms attending the clinic of a general adult neurologist will have delayed earliest and continuous memories compared with patients whose symptoms were explained by neurological disease" [38].
- "Patients with acute mental changes will be scanned more frequently than other elder patients" [39].

The reader will note that these hypotheses do not include the mechanism for memory variations in these patient populations (first example) or the reasons why elderly patients with acute mental changes should be scanned more frequently than comparable patients without such changes (second example). In situations like this, it is critical that the justification be clear from the introductory section of the research paper or protocol.

5. *Alternative Versus Null Hypotheses*

The requirement that a hypothesis should be capable of corroboration or unsupportability ("falsification") reflects the fact that two outcomes always can arise out of a study of any single research problem. Thus, prior to collecting and evaluating empirical evidence to resolve a problem, the investigator will posit two opposing assertions. The first assertion will indicate the supposition for which support actually is sought (e.g., that there *is* a difference between a population parameter and an expected value or, more commonly, that there is some form of relation between variables within a particular population); the other will indicate that there *is no* support for this supposition. This first type of assertion is termed the *alternative hypothesis* and is generally denoted H_A or H_1. The alternative hypothesis can be differentiated further according to its quantitative attributes. As an example, in a study evaluating the impact of beta-adrenergic antagonist treatment (β-blockade) on the incidence of recurrent myocardial infarctions (MIs), an investigator could frame three contrasting alternative hypotheses:

1. The proportion of recurrent MIs among comparable patients treated with versus without β-blockade is *different*.
2. The proportion of recurrent MIs among patients treated with β-blockade is *less than* that among comparable patients treated without β-blockade.
3. The proportion of recurrent MIs among patients treated with β-blockade is *greater than* that among comparable patients treated without β-blockade.

The first of these statements is termed a *nondirectional hypothesis* because the nature of the expected relation (i.e., the direction of the intergroup difference in the proportion of recurrent infarctions) is not specified. The second and third statements are termed *directional* hypotheses since, in addition to positing a difference between groups, the nature of the expected difference (positive or negative) is predefined. Generally, the decision to state an alternative hypothesis in a directional versus nondirectional manner is based on theoretical considerations and/or the availability of prior empirical information. (In statistics, a nondirectional hypothesis is usually referred to as a two-tailed or two-sided hypothesis; a directional hypothesis is referred to as a one-tailed or one-sided hypothesis.)

As noted, the hypothesis reflects a tentative conjecture which, to gain validity, ultimately must be substantiated by experience (empirical evidence). However, even objectively measured experience varies from time to time, place to place, observer to observer, and subject to subject. Thus, it is difficult to know whether an observed difference or association was produced by random variation or actually reflects a true underlying difference or association in the population of interest. To deal with the problem of uncertainty, the investigator must implicitly formulate and test what, in essence, is the logical opposite of his or her alternative hypothesis (i.e., that the population parameter is the same as the expected value or that the variables of interest are not related as posited). Thus, the investigator must attempt to set up a straw man to be knocked down. This construct (which need not be not stated in the research report), is termed a *null* (or no difference) hypothesis and is designated H_0. A null hypothesis asserts that any observable differences or associations found within a population are due to chance and is assumed true until contradicted by empirical evidence. In the single variable (one-sample) hypothesis, the assertion is that the parameter of interest is not different from some expected population value, whereas in a bivariable or multivariable hypothesis, the assertion is that the variables of interest are <u>un</u>related to some factor or to each other.

A null hypothesis is framed by inserting a negative modifier into the statement of the alternative hypothesis. In the examples given above, the following null statements could be developed:

1. The proportion of recurrent MIs among comparable patients treated with versus without β-blockade is *not* different.
2. The proportion of recurrent MIs among patients treated with β-blockade is *not* less than that among comparable patients treated without β-blockade.
3. The proportion of recurrent MIs among patients treated with β-blockade is *not* greater than that among comparable patients treated without β-blockade.

Only after both the null and alternative hypotheses have been specified, and the data collected, can an appropriate test of statistical significance be performed. If the results of statistical analysis reveal that chance is an unlikely explanation of the findings, the null hypothesis is rejected and the alternative hypothesis is accepted. Under these circumstances, the investigator can conclude that there is a statistically significant relation between the variables under study (or a statistically significant difference between a parameter and an expected value). On the other hand, if chance cannot be excluded as a probable explanation for the findings, the null, rather than the alternative, hypothesis must be accepted. It is important to note that acceptance of the null hypothesis does not mean that the investigator has demonstrated a true lack of association between variables (or equation between a population parameter and an expected value) any more than a verdict of "not guilty" constitutes proof of a defendant's innocence in a legal proceeding. Indeed, in criminal law, such a verdict means only that the prosecution, upon whom the burden of proof rests, has failed to provide sufficient evidence that a crime was committed. Similarly, in research, failure to overturn a null hypothesis (particularly when the alternative hypothesis has been argued) generally is taken to mean that the investigator, upon whom the burden of "proof" (or, more appropriately, corroboration) also rests, has failed to demonstrate the expected difference or association. Null results may reflect reality, but they may also be due to measurement error and inadequate sample size. For this reason, *negative studies*, a term for research that yields null findings, are far less likely to gain publication than studies that demonstrate a statistically significant association [40, 41]. (See Chap. 9 for a more detailed discussion of "publication bias.")

Constructing the Hypothesis: Differentiating Among Variables

As indicated earlier, hypotheses most commonly entail statements about variables. Variables, in turn, can be differentiated according to their level of measurement (or scaling characteristics) or the role that they play in the hypothesis.

Level of Measurement

Variables can be classified according to *how well* they can be measured (i.e., the amount of information that can be obtained in a given measurement of an attribute). One factor that determines the informational characteristics of a variable is the nature of its associated measurement scale, that is, whether it is nominal, ordinal, interval, or ratio—a classification system framed in 1946 by Stevens [42]. Understanding these distinctions is important because scaling characteristics influence the nature of the statistical methods that can be used for analyzing data associated with a variable.

1. *The Nominal Variable*
   Nominal variables represent names or categories. Examples include blood type, gender, marital status, hair color, etiology, and presence versus absence of a risk factor or disease, and vital status. Nominal variables represent the weakest level of measurement as they have no intrinsic order or other mathematical properties and allow only for qualitative classification or grouping. Their lack of mathematical properties precludes calculation of measures of central tendency (such as means, medians, or modes) or dispersion. When all variables in a hypothesis are nominal, this limits the types of statistical operations that can be performed to tests involving cross-classification (e.g., tests of differences between proportions). Sometimes, variables that are on an ordinal, interval, or ratio scale are transformed into nominal categories using cutoff points (e.g., age in years can be recoded into old versus young; height in meters to tall versus short; left ventricular ejection fraction in percent to normal versus subnormal).
2. *The Ordinal Variable*
   Ordinal variables are considered to be semi-quantitative. They are similar to nominal variables in that they are comprised of categories, but their categories are arranged in a meaningful sequence (rank order), such that successive values indicate more or less of some quantity (i.e., relative magnitude). Typical examples of ordinal variables include socioeconomic status, tumor classification scores, New York Heart Association (NYHA) functional class for angina or heart failure, disease severity, birth order, perceived level of pain, and all opinion survey scores. However, distances between scale points are arbitrary. For example, a patient categorized as NYHA functional class IV may have more symptomatic debility than one categorized as functional class II, but he or she does not necessarily have twice as much debility; indeed, he or she may have considerably more than twice as much debility. Appropriate measures of central tendency for ordinal variables are the mode and median (rather than the mean or arithmetic average) or percentile. Similarly, hypothesis tests of subgroup differences based on ordinal outcome variables are limited to nonparametric approaches employing analysis of ranks or sums of ranks.
3. *The Interval Variable*
   Interval variables, like ratio variables (below), are considered quantitative or metric variables because they answer the question "how much?" or "how many?" Both may take on positive or negative values. A common example of an interval variable is temperature on a Celsius or Fahrenheit scale. Both interval and ratio variables provide more precise information than ordinal variables because the distances between successive data values represent true, equal, and meaningful intervals. For example, the difference between 70°F and 80°F is equivalent to the difference between 80°F and 90°F. However, the zero point on an interval scale is arbitrary (note, freezing on a Celsius scale is 0° but is 32° on a Fahrenheit scale) and does not necessarily

connote absence of a property (in this case, absence of kinetic energy). When analyzing interval data, one can add or subtract but not multiply or divide. Most statistical and operations are permissible, including calculation of measures of central tendency (e.g., mean, median, or mode), measures of dispersion (e.g., standard deviation, standard error of the mean, range), and performance of many statistical tests of hypotheses including correlation, regression, t-tests, and analysis of variance. However, due to the absence of a true zero point, ratios between values on an interval scale are not meaningful (though ratios of differences can be computed).

4. *The Ratio Variable*
   Like interval variables, the distances between successive values on a ratio scale are equal. However, ratio variables reflect the highest level of measurement because they contain a true, nonarbitrary zero point that reflects complete absence of a property. Examples of ratio variables include temperature on a Kelvin scale (where zero reflects absence of kinetic energy), mass, length, volume, weight, and income. When ratio data are analyzed, all arithmetic operations are available (i.e., addition, subtraction, multiplication, and division). The same statistical operations that can be performed with interval variables can be performed with ratio variables. However, ratio variables also permit meaningful calculation of absolute and relative (or ratio) changes in a variable and computation of geometric and harmonic means, coefficients of variation, and logarithms.

Quantitative variables (interval or ratio) can be either continuous or discrete. Continuous variables (e.g., weight, height, temperature) differ from discrete variables in that the former may take on any conceivable value within a given range, including fractional values or decimal values. For example, within the range 150–151 lbs, an individual theoretically can weigh 150 lbs, 150.5 lbs or 150.95 lbs, though the capacity to distinguish between these values clearly is limited by the precision of the measurement device. In contrast, discrete variables (e.g., number of dental caries, number of white cells per cubic centimeter of blood, number of readers of medical journals, or other count-based data) can take on only whole numbers. Nominal and ordinal variables are intrinsically discrete, though in some disciplines (e.g., behavioral sciences), ordinally scaled data often are treated as continuous variables. This practice is considered reasonable when ordinal data intuitively represent equivalent intervals (e.g., visual analogue scales), when they contain numerous (e.g., 10 or more) possible scale values or "orderings" [43], or when shorter individual measurement scales are combined to yield summary scores. The reader should note, however, that in other disciplines and settings, treating all data as continuous data is controversial and generally is not recommended [44].

Role in the Research Hypothesis

Another method of classifying variables is based on the specific role (function) that the variable plays in the hypothesis. Accordingly, a variable can represent (1) the putative cause (or be associated with a causal factor) that initiates a subsequent response or event, (2) the response or event itself, (3) a mediator between the causal factor and its effect, (4) a potential confounder whose influence must be neutralized, or (5) an explanation for the underlying association between the hypothesized cause and effect. Viewed this way, variables may be independent, dependent, or may serve as moderator, control, or intervening variables. Understanding these distinctions is crucial for constructing a research design, executing a statistical program, or communicating effectively with a statistician.

1. *The Independent Variable*
   The independent variable is that attribute within an individual, object, or event which affects some outcome. The independent variable is conceptualized as an input in the study that may be manipulated by the investigator (such as a treatment in an experimental study) or reflect a naturally occurring risk factor. In either case, the independent variable is viewed as *antecedent* to some outcome and is presumed

to be the cause, or a predictor of that outcome, or a marker of a causal agent or risk factor. We call this type of variable "*independent*" because the researcher is interested only on its impact on other variables in the study rather than the impact of other variables on it. Independent variables are sometimes termed *factors* and their variations are called *levels*.

If, for example, if an investigator were to conduct an observational study of the effects of diabetes mellitus on subsequent cardiac events, the independent variable (or factor) would be history of diabetes, and its variants (positive or negative history) would be levels of the factor. As a second example, in an intervention study examining the relative impact of inpatient versus outpatient counseling on patient morbidity after a first MI, the independent variable (factor) would be the counseling, and its variants (inpatient counseling vs. outpatient counseling) would correspond to the alternative levels of the factor. The reader should note that in both of these hypothetical examples, there was only one independent variable (or factor) and that each factor had two levels. It is possible and, in fact, common for studies to have several independent variables and for each to have multiple factor levels (indeed, the number of factor levels in dose–response studies is potentially infinite). Care needs to be exercised as researchers often confuse a factor with two levels for two factors. Levels are always components of the factor. Understanding this distinction is essential for conducting statistical tests such as analysis of variance (ANOVA).

2. *The Dependent Variable*
In contrast to the independent variable, the dependent variable is that attribute within an individual or its environment that represents an *outcome* of the study. The dependent variable is sometimes called a response variable because one can observe its presence, absence, or degree of change as a function of variation in the independent variable. Therefore, the dependent variable is always a measure of *effect*.

As an example, suppose that an investigator wished to study the effects of adrenal corticosteroid therapy on systolic performance among patients with heart failure. In this study, systolic performance would be the dependent variable; the investigator would measure its degree of improvement or deterioration in response to introducing versus not introducing steroid treatment. Because it is a measure of effect, the dependent variable can be observed and measured but, unlike the independent variable, it can never be manipulated.

Independent and dependent variables are relatively simple to identify within the context of a specific investigation, for example, a prospective cohort or an experimental study or a well-designed retrospective study in which one variable clearly is an input, the second is a response or effect, and an adequately defined temporal interval exists between their appearance. However, when research is cross-sectional, and variables merely are being correlated, it is sometimes difficult or impossible to infer which is independent and which is dependent. Under these circumstances, variables are often termed "covariates."

3. *The Moderator Variable*
Often, an independent variable does not affect all individuals in the same way, and an investigator may have reason to believe that some other variable may be involved. If he or she wishes to systematically study the effect of this other variable, rather than merely neutralize it, it may be introduced into the study design as a moderator variable (also known as an "effect modifier"). The term moderator variable refers to a secondary variable that is measured or manipulated by the investigator to determine whether it *alters* the relationship between the independent variable of central interest and the dependent (response) variable. The moderator variable may be incorporated into a multivariate statistical model to examine its interactive effects with the independent variable or it may be used to provide a basis for stratifying the sample into two or more subgroups within which the effects of the independent variable may be examined separately.

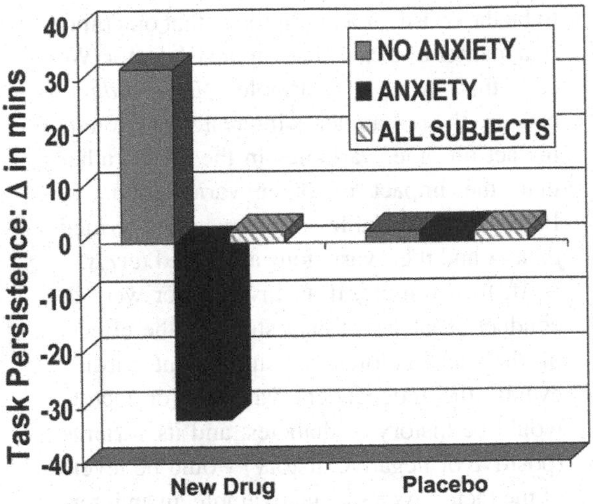

Fig. 3.4 A hypothetical example of the effects of a moderator variable: influence of chronic anxiety on the impact of a new drug for patients with attention deficit hyperactivity disorder

For example, suppose a psychiatrist wishes to study the effects of a new amphetamine-type drug on task persistence in patients with attention deficit hyperactivity disorder (ADHD) who have not responded well to current medical therapy. She believes that the drug may have efficacy but suspects that its effect may be diminished by the comorbidity of chronic anxiety. Rather than give the new drug to patients with ADHD who do not also have anxiety and placebo to patients with ADHD plus anxiety, to avoid confounding, she enrolls both types of patients, randomly administers drug or placebo to members of each subgroup, and measures task persistence among all subjects at a fixed interval after onset of therapy. In this hypothetical study, the independent variable would be type of therapy (factor levels: new drug, placebo), the dependent variable would be task persistence, and chronic anxiety (presence, absence) would be the moderator. Figure 3.4 illustrates the importance of a moderator variable. If none had been used in the study, the data would have led the investigator to conclude that the new drug was ineffective as no overall treatment effect would have been observed for the ADHD group (left panel, diagonal patterned bar), with change in task persistence for the entire treated group similar to subjects on placebo (right panel). However, as noted, the new drug was not ineffective but instead was *differentially* effective, promoting greater task persistence among patients without associated anxiety but decreasing task persistence among those with anxiety, as hypothesized.

A cautionary note is in order. Although moderator variables can increase the yield or accuracy of information from a study, an investigator needs to be very selective in using them as each additional factor introduced into the study design increases the sample size needed to enable the impact of these secondary factors to be satisfactorily evaluated. During the study planning process, the investigator must determine the likelihood of a potential interaction, the theoretical or practical knowledge to be gained by discovery of an interaction, and decide whether sufficient resources exist for such evaluation.

4. *The Control Variable*

In this last example, the investigator chose to evaluate the interactive effects of a secondary variable on the relation of the independent and dependent variables. Others in similar situations might choose not to study a secondary independent variable, particularly if it is viewed as extraneous to the primary hypothesis or focus of the study. Additionally, it is impractical to examine the effects of every ancillary variable. However, extraneous variables cannot be ignored because they can confound study results and render the data uninterpretable. Variables such as these usually are treated as control variables.

A control variable is defined as any potentially confounding aspect of the study that is manipulated by the investigator to neutralize its effects on the dependent variable. Common control variables are age, gender, clinical history, comorbidity, test order, etc. In the hypothetical example given above, if the psychiatrist had wanted to control for associated anxiety and not evaluate its interactive effects, she could have chosen patients with similar anxiety levels or, had his or her study employed a parallel design (which it did not), she could have made certain that different treatment groups were counterbalanced for that variable.

5. *The Intervening Variable*
   Just as the moderator variable defines *when* (under what conditions) the independent variable exerts its action on the dependent variable, the "intervening variable" may help explain *how* and *why* the independent and dependent variables are related. This can be especially important when the association between independent and dependent variables appears ambiguous. There is general consensus that the intervening variable underlies, and accounts for, the relation between the independent and dependent variable. However, historically, workers in the field have defined them in different (and often contradictory) ways [45]. For example, Tuckman describes the intervening variable as a hypothetical internal state (construct) within an individual (motivation, drive, goal orientation, intention, awareness, etc.) that "theoretically affects the observed phenomenon but cannot be seen, measured, or manipulated; its effect must be inferred from the effects of the independent and moderator variables on the observed phenomenon" [35]. In the previous hypothetical example which examined the interactive effects of drug treatment and anxiety on task persistence, the intervening variable was *attention*. In educational research, the intervening variable between an innovative pedagogical approach and the acquisition of new concepts or skills is *the learning process* impacted by the former. In clinical or epidemiological research, the intervening variable can represent a disease process or physiological parameter that links an exposure or purposively applied intervention to an outcome (e.g., secondhand smoking causes lung cancer by inducing *lung damage*; valvular surgery increases LV ejection fraction by improving *contractility*.). Others such as Baron and Kenny [46] view an intervening variable as a factor that can be measured (directly or by operational definitions, described later in this chapter), fully derived ("abstractable") from empirical findings (data), and statistically analyzed to demonstrate its capacity to *mediate* the relation between the independent and dependent variables. As an example, Williamson and Schulz [47] measured and evaluated the relation between pain, functional disability, and depression among patients with cancer. They determined that the observed relation of pain to depression was due to diminution of function, operationally defined as activities of daily living (the intervening or mediating variable), which, in turn, caused depression. Similarly, Song and Lee [48] found that depression mediated the relation of sensory deficits (the independent variable in their study) to functional capacity (their dependent variable) in the elderly. (For a comprehensive discussion of mediation and statistical approaches to test for mediation, the reader is referred to MacKinnon 2008 [49].) Whether viewed as a hypothetical construct or as a measurable mediator, an intervening variable is always intermediate in the causal pathway by which the independent variable affects the dependent variable and is useful in explaining the mechanism linking these variables and, potentially, for suggesting additional interventions.

Below are two hypotheses from cardiovascular medicine in which constituent variables have been analyzed and labeled according to their role in each hypothesis.

Hypothesis 1: "Among patients with heart failure who have similar clinical histories, those receiving adrenal corticosteroid treatment will demonstrate a greater improvement in systolic performance than those not receiving steroid treatment."

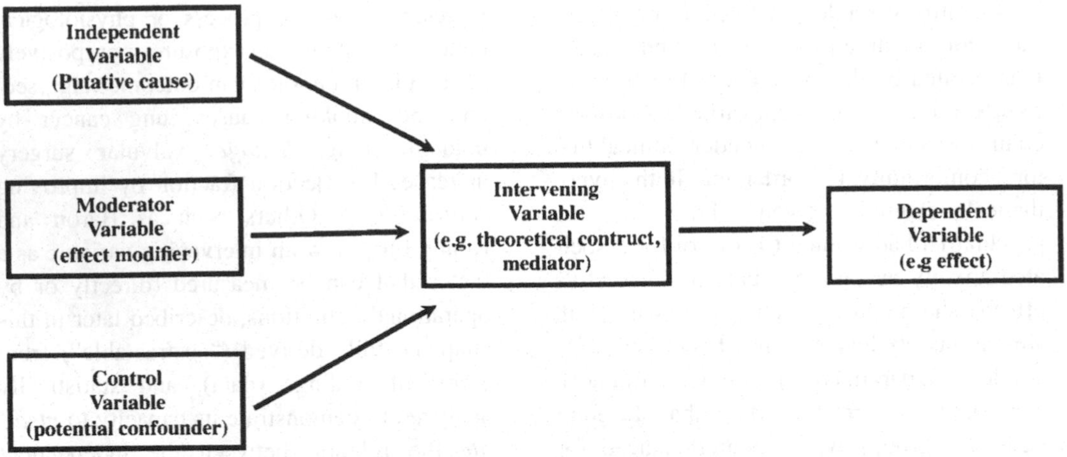

Fig. 3.5 Interrelation among variables in a study design

- *Independent variable*: adrenal corticosteroid treatment
- *Factor levels:* 2 (treatment, no treatment)
- *Dependent variable*: systolic performance
- *Control variable*: clinical history
- *Moderator variable*: none
- *Intervening variable*: change in magnitude of the inflammatory process

Hypothesis 2: "Patients with angina who are treated with β-blockade will have a greater improvement in their capacity for physical activity than those of the same sex and age who are not treated with β-blockade; this improvement will vary as a function of severity of initial symptoms."

- *Independent variable*: β-blockade treatment
- *Factor levels*: 2 (treatment, no treatment)
- *Dependent variable*: capacity for physical activity
- *Moderator* variable: severity of initial symptoms
- *Control variables*: sex and age
- *Intervening variable*: alteration in myocardial work

In sum, many research designs, particularly those intended to test hypotheses about cause or prediction and effect, contain independent, dependent, control, and intervening variables. Some also contain moderator variables. Figure 3.5 illustrates their interrelationship.

Role of Operational Definitions

As indicated earlier, one of the characteristics of a hypothesis that sets it apart from other types of statements is that it is *testable*. The hypotheses discussed thus far are conceptual. A conceptual hypothesis cannot be directly tested unless it is transformed into an operational hypothesis. To accomplish this, operational definitions must be developed for each element specified in the hypothesis.

An operational definition identifies the *observable* characteristics of that which is being studied. Its use imparts specificity and precision to the research, enabling others to understand exactly how the hypothesis was tested. As a corollary, it enables the scientific community to evaluate the appropriateness of the methodology selected for studying the problem. Operational definitions are required because a concept, object, or situation can have multiple interpretations. While double entendre is one basis of Western humor, inconsistent (or vague) definitions within a study are not comical as they typically lead to confused findings (and readers). Imagine, for example, what might occur if one member of an investigative team, studying the relative impact of two procedures for treating hemodynamically important coronary artery disease, defined "important" as >50% luminal diameter narrowing of one or more coronary vessels and another, working in the same study, defined it as ≥70% luminal diameter narrowing; or if one investigator studying new onset angina used 1 week as the criterion for "new" and another used 1 month. Operational definitions can describe the manipulations that the investigator performs (e.g., the intervention), or they can describe behaviors or responses. Still others describe the observable characteristics of objects or individuals. Once the investigator has selected appropriate operational definitions (this choice is entirely study dependent), all hypotheses in the study can be "operationalized."

A hypothesis is rendered operational when its broadly (conceptually) stated variables are replaced by operational definitions of those variables. Hypotheses stated in this manner are called *operational hypotheses*, *specific hypotheses*, or *predictions*.

Let us consider two hypotheses previously given in this chapter:

"Patients with heart failure who are treated with adrenal corticosteroids will have better systolic performance than those who are not" is sufficiently general to be considered a conceptual hypothesis and, as such, is not directly testable. To render this hypothesis testable, the investigator could operationally define its constituent elements as follows:

- Heart failure = "secondary hypodynamic cardiomyopathy"
- Adrenal corticosteroids = "cortisol"
- Better systolic performance = "higher left ventricular ejection fractions at rest"

The hypothesis, in its operational form, would state: "Patients with secondary hypodynamic cardiomyopathy who have received cortisol will have higher ventricular ejection fractions at rest than those who have not received cortisol treatment."

Similarly, the hypothesis that "patients with angina who are treated with β-blockers will have a greater improvement in their capacity for physical activity than those not treated with β-blockers, and that this improvement will vary as a function of initial symptoms," while complex, is still general enough to be considered conceptual. To render this hypothesis testable, its constituent elements could be defined as follows:

- β-blockers = "propranolol" (assuming that the investigator was specifically interested in this drug)
- Capacity for physical activity = "New York Heart Association functional class"
- Severity of symptoms = angina class 1–2 versus angina class 3–4

This hypothesis, in its operational form, would be stated: "Patients with angina who are treated with propranolol will have greater improvement in New York Heart Association functional class than those not treated with propranolol, and this improvement will vary as a function of initial angina class (1–2 vs. 3–4)." In this form, the hypothesis could be directly tested, although the investigator would still need to specify measurement criteria and develop an appropriate design.

Any element of a hypothesis can have more than one operational definition and, as noted, it is the investigator's responsibility to select the one that is most suitable for his or her study. This is an important judgment because the remaining research procedures (i.e., specification of subject inclusion/exclusion criteria, the nature of the intervention and outcome measures, and data analysis methodology) are derived from operational hypotheses. Investigators must be careful to use a sufficient number of operational definitions so that reviewers will have a basis upon which to judge the appropriateness of the methodology outlined in submitted grant proposals and manuscripts, so that other investigators will be able to replicate their work, and so that the general readership can understand precisely what was done and have sufficient information to properly interpret findings.

Once operational definitions have been developed and the hypothesis has been restated in operational form, the investigator can conduct the study. The next step will be to select a research design that can yield data to support optimal statistical hypothesis testing. The strengths, weaknesses, and requirements of various study designs will be discussed in Chaps. 4 and 5.

Take-Home Points

- A hypothesis is a logical construct, interposed between a problem and its solution, which represents a proposed answer to a research question. It gives direction to the investigator's thinking about the problem and, therefore, facilitates a solution.
- There are three primary modes of inference by which hypotheses are developed: deduction (reasoning from a general propositions to specific instances), induction (reasoning from specific instances to a general proposition), and abduction (formulation/acceptance *on probation* of a hypothesis to explain a surprising observation).
- A research hypothesis should reflect an inference about variables; be stated as a grammatically complete, declarative sentence; be expressed simply and unambiguously; provide an adequate answer to the research problem; and be testable.
- Hypotheses can be classified as conceptual versus operational, single versus bi- or multivariable, causal or not causal, mechanistic versus nonmechanistic, and null or alternative.
- Hypotheses most commonly entail statements about "variables" which, in turn, can be classified according to their level of measurement (scaling characteristics) or according to their role in the hypothesis (independent, dependent, moderator, control, or intervening).
- A hypothesis is rendered operational when its broadly (conceptually) stated variables are replaced by operational definitions of those variables. Hypotheses stated in this manner are called operational hypotheses, specific hypotheses, or predictions and facilitate testing.

References

1. De Morgan A, De Morgan S. A budget of paradoxes. London: Longmans Green; 1872.
2. Leedy Paul D. Practical research. Planning and design. 2nd ed. New York: Macmillan; 1960.
3. Bernard C. Introduction to the study of experimental medicine. New York: Dover; 1957.
4. Erren TC. The quest for questions—on the logical force of science. Med Hypotheses. 2004;62:635–40.
5. Peirce CS. Collected papers of Charles Sanders Peirce, vol. 7. In: Hartshorne C, Weiss P, editors. Boston: The Belknap Press of Harvard University Press; 1966.
6. Aristotle. The complete works of Aristotle: the revised Oxford Translation. In: Barnes J, editor. vol. 2. Princeton/New Jersey: Princeton University Press; 1984.
7. Polit D, Beck CT. Conceptualizing a study to generate evidence for nursing. In: Polit D, Beck CT, editors. Nursing research: generating and assessing evidence for nursing practice. 8th ed. Philadelphia: Wolters Kluwer/Lippincott Williams and Wilkins; 2008. Chapter 4.
8. Jenicek M, Hitchcock DL. Evidence-based practice. Logic and critical thinking in medicine. Chicago: AMA Press; 2005.
9. Bacon F. The novum organon or a true guide to the interpretation of nature. A new translation by the Rev G.W. Kitchin. Oxford: The University Press; 1855.
10. Popper KR. Objective knowledge: an evolutionary approach (revised edition). New York: Oxford University Press; 1979.
11. Morgan AJ, Parker S. Translational mini-review series on vaccines: the Edward Jenner Museum and the history of vaccination. Clin Exp Immunol. 2007;147: 389–94.
12. Pead PJ. Benjamin Jesty: new light in the dawn of vaccination. Lancet. 2003;362:2104–9.
13. Lee JA. The scientific endeavor: a primer on scientific principles and practice. San Francisco: Addison-Wesley Longman; 2000.
14. Allchin D. Lawson's shoehorn, or should the philosophy of science be rated, 'X'? Science and Education. 2003;12:315–29.
15. Lawson AE. What is the role of induction and deduction in reasoning and scientific inquiry? J Res Sci Teach. 2005;42:716–40.
16. Peirce CS. Collected papers of Charles Sanders Peirce, vol. 2. In: Hartshorne C, Weiss P, editors. Boston: The Belknap Press of Harvard University Press; 1965.
17. Bonfantini MA, Proni G. To guess or not to guess? In: Eco U, Sebeok T, editors. The sign of three: Dupin, Holmes, Peirce. Bloomington: Indiana University Press; 1983. Chapter 5.
18. Peirce CS. Collected papers of Charles Sanders Peirce, vol. 5. In: Hartshorne C, Weiss P, editors. Boston: The Belknap Press of Harvard University Press; 1965.

19. Flach PA, Kakas AC. Abductive and inductive reasoning: background issues. In: Flach PA, Kakas AC, editors. Abduction and induction. Essays on their relation and integration. The Netherlands: Klewer; 2000. Chapter 1.
20. Murray JF. Voltaire, Walpole and Pasteur: variations on the theme of discovery. Am J Respir Crit Care Med. 2005;172:423–6.
21. Danemark B, Ekstrom M, Jakobsen L, Karlsson JC. Methodological implications, generalization, scientific inference, models (Part II) In: explaining society. Critical realism in the social sciences. New York: Routledge; 2002.
22. Pasteur L. Inaugural lecture as professor and dean of the faculty of sciences. In: Peterson H, editor. A treasury of the world's greatest speeches. Douai, France: University of Lille 7 Dec 1954.
23. Swineburne R. Simplicity as evidence for truth. Milwaukee: Marquette University Press; 1997.
24. Sakar S, editor. Logical empiricism at its peak: Schlick, Carnap and Neurath. New York: Garland; 1996.
25. Popper K. The logic of scientific discovery. New York: Basic Books; 1959. 1934, trans. 1959.
26. Caws P. The philosophy of science. Princeton: D. Van Nostrand Company; 1965.
27. Popper K. Conjectures and refutations. The growth of scientific knowledge. 4th ed. London: Routledge and Keegan Paul; 1972.
28. Feyerabend PK. Against method, outline of an anarchistic theory of knowledge. London, UK: Verso; 1978.
29. Smith PG. Popper: conjectures and refutations (Chapter IV). In: Theory and reality: an introduction to the philosophy of science. Chicago: University of Chicago Press; 2003.
30. Blystone RV, Blodgett K. WWW: the scientific method. CBE Life Sci Educ. 2006;5:7–11.
31. Kleinbaum DG, Kupper LL, Morgenstern H. Epidemiological research. Principles and quantitative methods. New York: Van Nostrand Reinhold; 1982.
32. Fortune AE, Reid WJ. Research in social work. 3rd ed. New York: Columbia University Press; 1999.
33. Kerlinger FN. Foundations of behavioral research. 1st ed. New York: Hold, Reinhart and Winston; 1970.
34. Hoskins CN, Mariano C. Research in nursing and health. Understanding and using quantitative and qualitative methods. New York: Springer; 2004.
35. Tuckman BW. Conducting educational research. New York: Harcourt, Brace, Jovanovich; 1972.
36. Wang C, Chiari PC, Weihrauch D, Krolikowski JG, Warltier DC, Kersten JR, Pratt Jr PF, Pagel PS. Gender-specificity of delayed preconditioning by isoflurane in rabbits: potential role of endothelial nitric oxide synthase. Anesth Analg. 2006;103:274–80.
37. Beyer ME, Slesak G, Nerz S, Kazmaier S, Hoffmeister HM. Effects of endothelin-1 and IRL 1620 on myocardial contractility and myocardial energy metabolism. J Cardiovasc Pharmacol. 1995;26(Suppl 3): S150–2.
38. Stone J, Sharpe M. Amnesia for childhood in patients with unexplained neurological symptoms. J Neurol Neurosurg Psychiatry. 2002;72:416–7.
39. Naughton BJ, Moran M, Ghaly Y, Michalakes C. Computer tomography scanning and delirium in elder patients. Acad Emerg Med. 1997;4:1107–10.
40. Easterbrook PJ, Berlin JA, Gopalan R, Matthews DR. Publication bias in clinical research. Lancet. 1991;337:867–72.
41. Stern JM, Simes RJ. Publication bias: evidence of delayed publication in a cohort study of clinical research projects. BMJ. 1997;315:640–5.
42. Stevens SS. On the theory of scales and measurement. Science. 1946;103:677–80.
43. Knapp TR. Treating ordinal scales as interval scales: an attempt to resolve the controversy. Nurs Res. 1990;39:121–3.
44. The Cochrane Collaboration. Open Learning Material. www.cochrane-net.org/openlearning/html/mod14-3.htm. Accessed 12 Oct 2009.
45. MacCorquodale K, Meehl PE. On a distinction between hypothetical constructs and intervening variables. Psychol Rev. 1948;55:95–107.
46. Baron RM, Kenny DA. The moderator-mediator variable distinction in social psychological research: conceptual, strategic and statistical considerations. J Pers Soc Psychol. 1986;51:1173–82.
47. Williamson GM, Schultz R. Activity restriction mediates the association between pain and depressed affect: a study of younger and older adult cancer patients. Psychol Aging. 1995;10:369–78.
48. Song M, Lee EO. Development of a functional capacity model for the elderly. Res Nurs Health. 1998; 21:189–98.
49. MacKinnon DP. Introduction to statistical mediation analysis. New York: Routledge; 2008.

Design and Interpretation of Observational Studies: Cohort, Case–Control, and Cross-Sectional Designs

4

Martin L. Lesser

Introduction

Perhaps, one of the most common undertakings in biomedical research is to determine whether there is an association between a particular factor (usually referred to as a "risk factor") and an event. That event might be a disease (e.g., lung cancer) or an outcome in subjects who already have a disease (e.g., sudden death among subjects with valvular heart disease). For example, an investigator might want to know whether smoking is a risk factor for lung cancer or whether oral contraceptive use is a risk factor for a myocardial infarction in women. These kinds of research questions are often answered using specific types of research designs, the two most common being the "case–control" and "cohort" study designs. (In this chapter, we will use the term "disease" interchangeably with "disease outcome" as both represent endpoints of interest.)

While both types of study designs aim to answer the same kind of research question, the method of conducting these designs is quite different. For example, in a cohort study (more specifically a "prospective" cohort study, to be further elucidated below), we might start out by gathering together hundreds of college students who are smokers and follow them over their lifetimes to see what fraction develop lung cancer (i.e., estimate the incidence rate). Likewise, we might follow a similar "cohort" of college nonsmokers to determine their lung cancer incidence rate. In the end, we would compare the incidence rates of lung cancer and, using appropriate statistical methodology, determine whether the incidence rates were significantly different from one another, thereby supporting or not supporting the hypothesis that smoking is associated with lung cancer.

On the other hand, in the "case–control" design, we would begin by selecting individuals who have a diagnosis of lung cancer ("cases") and a group of appropriate individuals without lung cancer ("controls") and "look back" in time to see how many smokers there were in each of the two groups. We would then, once again, using appropriate statistical methods, compare the prevalence rates of a smoking history to determine whether such an association between smoking and lung cancer is supported by the data.

Thus, the essential difference between these two study designs is that, in the cohort design, we first identify subjects with and without a given risk factor and then follow them forward in time to determine the respective disease incidence rates, whereas in the case–control design, we first identify subjects with and without the disease and then determine the fraction with the risk factor in each group.

M.L. Lesser, PhD (✉)
Biostatistics Unit, Departments of Molecular Medicine and Population Health, Feinstein Institute for Medical Research, Hofstra North Shore-LIJ School of Medicine, 350 Community Drive, 1st floor, Manhasset, NY 11030, USA
e-mail: mlesser@nshs.edu

P.G. Supino and J.S. Borer (eds.), *Principles of Research Methodology: A Guide for Clinical Investigators*,
DOI 10.1007/978-1-4614-3360-6_4, © Phyllis G. Supino and Jeffrey S. Borer 2012

In both of these study designs, the timing of the suspected risk factor exposure in relation to the development or diagnosis of the disease is important. Both study designs consider the situation where exposure to the risk factor precedes the disease. While such designs cannot *prove* causality (as will be discussed below), this ordering of exposure and disease is a necessary condition for causality.

A third type of commonly used observational design is the cross-sectional study. As will be discussed below, this design does not specifically examine the timing of exposure and disease.

It should be pointed out that case–control and cohort study designs are not necessarily restricted to the study of risk factors for a *disease*, per se. For example, if we wanted to conduct a study to determine risk factors for a patient dropping out of a clinical trial, we could select cases to be those who dropped out of a clinical trial and controls would be those who did not drop out of the clinical trial. Of course, dropping out of a clinical trial is not a disease (we might refer to it as an "outcome"), yet it can be studied in the context of a case–control study design.

The case–control, cohort, and cross-sectional studies are considered "observational" study designs, which means that no particular therapeutic or other interventions are being purposively applied to the subjects of the study. The subjects of the study simply are being observed in their natural settings to determine, in this example, how many developed lung cancer or how many were smokers. A study design where an intervention is purposively applied to subjects to determine, for example, whether one treatment modality is better than another would be called an "experimental" design or more specific to biomedical research, a "clinical trial" in which the intervention (e.g., drug, device, etc.) is assigned to the subject as per protocol. (For detailed discussions of studies of interventions and how to prepare for them, the reader is referred to Chaps. 5 and 6.)

The important issue of whether to choose a case–control or cohort study design for a particular research study will be discussed later in this chapter. Each has relative advantages and disadvantages that need to be weighed when such a choice is being considered.

Cohort Studies

Basic Notation

In the most general setting, we will hypothesize that exposure (E) to a particular agent, environmental factor, gene, life event, or some other specific factor increases the risk of developing a particular disease (D) or condition. Perhaps, a better way to state the hypothesis would be that "exposure is associated with the disease."

More formally, we might use the following hypothesis testing notation:

H_0: Exposure to the factor is not associated with an increased risk of developing the disease.

H_A: Exposure to the factor increases the risk of developing the disease.

In statistical terms, H_0 and H_A are the null and alternative hypotheses, respectively. (A discussion of hypothesis specification and testing can be found in Chaps. 3 and 11 in this text.) As in most hypothesis testing problems, the objective is to refute the null hypothesis and demonstrate support for the alternative hypothesis.

It is important to note the hypotheses relating E and D do not use the word "cause" because in observational studies, we cannot prove causality; we can only hope to show that an association exists between E and D which may not necessarily be causal. We will have more to say about establishing causality from observational studies later in this chapter.

Selection of Exposed Subjects

In order to conduct a cohort study, one must first select subjects who have been exposed to the hypothesized risk factor. It is not the purpose of this chapter to provide detailed guidance on alternative sampling methodologies, which is discussed in greater detail in Chap. 10. Here, our goal is to provide general guidance as to how to sample subjects and from where they might be sampled, with the specific details left to the reader in consultation, perhaps, with a statistician or epidemiologist.

Definition of the Exposure

To select exposed subjects, there must be a clear definition of what it means to be, or have been, exposed to the risk factor under study. Suppose, for example, a study was conducted to determine the effect of exposure to heavy metals (e.g., gold, silver, etc.) on semen and sperm quality in men during their peak reproductive years. We might enlist the support of a company that works with heavy metals in a factory setting and then obtain seminal fluid samples from men working in that factory. However, we would still need to know what it means to be "exposed." Exposure can be defined in many ways. For example, just working in that factory environment for at least 6 months might be one definition of exposure; another definition might involve the direct measurement of heavy metal particles in the factory or on a detector worn by each factory worker from which a determination of exposure might be made based on some minimum threshold exposure level indicated on the detector. If one were to study the effect of cigarette smoking in pregnant women on the birth weight of newborns, once again, one would need to have a definition of what it means to be a smoker during pregnancy: is having smoked one cigarette during pregnancy enough to define the smoking status or does it need to be a more consistent and higher frequency of cigarettes during the pregnancy? As for measurability, it is desirable but not always possible to define exposure based on some directly measurable quantity.

Sources of Exposed Subjects

Where might exposed subjects be found? Certainly, in the prior example of occupational exposure, one might look to identify potentially exposed subjects from the roster of companies in certain lines of manufacturing or other work, labor unions, or other organizations or groups of individuals that would be associated with a particular occupation and, potentially, with such an exposure. One also might enroll persons living near environmental hazards, persons with certain lifestyles, such as those who regularly attend an exercise gym. In an epidemiologic study of long-term effects of prescription drugs, one might utilize a roster or list of individuals who have been prescribed a certain type of drug. When selecting cohorts of exposed subjects, an attempt should be made to select these cohorts for their ability to facilitate the collection of relevant data, possibly over a long period of time. For example, there are several large-scale prospective cohort studies that involve physicians [1, 2].

Table 4.1 Sources of exposure information

Preexisting records
Interviews, questionnaires
Direct physical examination or tests
Direct measurement of the environment
Daily logs

Sources of Exposure Information

To determine whether or not a subject has been exposed to a particular risk factor, the investigator has several sources of information that might be used for making this determination (Table 4.1). First, preexisting records (medical charts, school records, etc.) might be used for determining whether a particular exposure occurred. While preexisting records may be easy and inexpensive to retrieve, they may be inaccurate with respect to the information that an investigator needs in his or her research investigation because data in the chart was not collected with this research study in mind—rather, the data were collected for clinical reasons only.

A second source of exposure information, that represents an improvement upon preexisting records, is self-reported information (e.g., interviews or questionnaires that may be administered to prospective participants in the cohort study). This approach allows the investigator some flexibility about which questions should be asked and how they should be asked, which might not be available in preexisting records. Of course, conducting interviews or administering questionnaires has associated costs that may be substantially greater than retrieving preexisting records or charts.

Beyond direct interviews and questionnaires, the investigator also can perform physical examinations or tests on individual subjects to determine certain exposures. Direct measurement of environmental variables (e.g., in an occupational exposure type of cohort study) also would be reasonable. Of course, these approaches to determining exposure status generally have higher associated costs and logistical difficulties than do interviews, questionnaires, or use of preexisting records. Finally, the investigator might ask subjects to maintain daily logs of certain activities, environmental exposures, foods, etc., in order to determine levels of exposure over time. Daily logs have the advantage of providing information on a detailed and regular basis but have the shortcoming of being inaccurate due to the self-report nature of a daily log.

In summary, there are many sources of exposure information available to the investigator. The use of a particular source depends on its relative advantages and disadvantages with respect to accuracy, feasibility, and cost.

Selection of Unexposed Subjects (Controls)

The control group for the exposed subject should comprise individuals who have been unexposed to the factor being studied. As will be seen for case–control studies, the proper selection of a control group can be a difficult task.

First, one must have a good definition of exposure in order to operationalize the definition of "unexposed." Obviously, we want the unexposed subjects to be free of the exposure in question but similar to the exposed cohort in all other respects. How an investigator would determine the exposure status of a potential control certainly depends on the type of exposure one is studying. In the example of heavy metal exposure given above, one would probably administer some sort of interview to determine whether the potential control has ever been in an occupation or an environmental situation where there might have been heavy metal exposure. Additionally, there are different degrees of exposure to a risk factor that would need to be considered. For example, in our hypothetical study on heavy metal exposure and male fertility, it might be convenient to select controls from the business offices of the same company which might be located at some distance from the factory. However, if one were to select office workers as potential unexposed controls, the investigator would have to be careful that those potential controls are not regularly exposed to the heavy metal factory. This could happen if, for example, the vice president for quality control, who worked in the business office, made daily tours of the factory and, therefore, was exposed (albeit a small amount of exposure) to the heavy metals.

Table 4.2 Sources of outcome information

Death certificates
Physician and hospital records
Disease registries
Self-report
Direct physical examination or tests

Sources of Outcome Information

Once a cohort study is underway, it is essential for the investigator to determine whether the particular outcome has or has not occurred. Once again, there are various sources of information (Table 4.2), each of which has its advantages and disadvantages from a logistical cost and accuracy perspective. Death certificates often are used to determine cause of death and comorbidities at the time of death for a participating subject. Unfortunately, death certificates can be inaccurate with regard to the specific details of cause of death and, of course, may not capture information about other outcomes that the investigator is seeking.

Physician and hospital records represent good sources of outcome information provided that the subject has maintained contact in that particular health-care or physician system. If the outcome in question was whether a patient suffered a myocardial infarction (MI), there is no guarantee that the patient will be seen for that MI at the investigator's hospital, and therefore, the investigator may not have access to that information based on his or her immediate hospital records.

Disease registries can be useful sources of information, but, once again, they are very similar to physician and hospital records in that disease registries are often specific to a particular hospital or large regional health area. Also, confidentiality issues may preclude the ability to access records in disease registries for subjects.

Self-report (described in detail in Chap. 8) is a relatively inexpensive and logistically simple method for determining outcome but can be inaccurate because patients may not be cognizant of the subtleties of various diseases or outcomes that have been diagnosed. However, written permission from the patient sometimes can be obtained for the investigator to contact the patient's physicians and hospital records in order to make definite ascertainment of whether or not an outcome occurred.

Finally, direct physical examination or tests conducted on the subject might reveal whether an outcome has occurred, of course, depending on the nature of the outcome being studied. Once again, this type of information might be very accurate but could be costly or logistically difficult to obtain in all subjects.

In sum, different sources of outcome information have their advantages and disadvantages relative to accuracy, logistics, and cost and should be weighed carefully by the investigator in designing a cohort study.

Confounding in Cohort Studies

Nature of the Problem

While the identification of a potential unexposed group might seem rather straightforward in many study designs, there is always an underlying problem in the choice of these unexposed "controls," i.e., confounding. Essentially, confounding can be described in two ways. It is the phenomenon that occurs when an exposure and a disease are not associated but a third variable (known as the confounding variable) makes it appear that there *is* an association between exposure and disease. Conversely, confounding can also occur when a third variable makes it appear that there is no association between an exposure and a disease when, in fact, there is.

Table 4.3 Criteria for confounding

1.	The presumed confounder (F) is associated with the exposure (E)
2.	Independent of exposure, F, must be associated with the risk of disease (D)

Before providing concrete examples of confounding, it is important to formally define the concept. Let "E" denote the exposure and "D" denote the disease being studied. A third factor, "F," is called a confounding variable if it meets two criteria: (1) F is associated with exposure, E; and (2) independent of exposure, F, is associated with the risk of developing the disease, D. It should be emphasized that a confounding factor, F, must meet both of these conditions in order to be a confounder. Often, in error, research investigators treat variables as confounders when they only meet one of those criteria (Table 4.3).

As an example of confounding, suppose that an investigator wished to determine whether smoking during pregnancy was a risk factor for an adverse outcome (defined as spontaneous abortion or low birth weight). The investigator would recruit two cohorts of pregnant women, one whose members smoke while pregnant and the other whose members do not. (The finer details of how to identify and recruit these cohorts are not within the scope of this chapter.) The two cohorts are then followed through their pregnancies, and the rates of adverse outcomes are compared (using a measure known as *relative risk*, which will be described later). Further, suppose that the investigator does find an increased risk of adverse outcomes in the smoking group. He submits his results to a peer-reviewed journal but is unsuccessful in gaining publication because one of the reviewers notes that the explanation for the increased risk may not be due to smoking, but, rather, to the effect of a confounding variable, namely, educational status. Why might educational status be a confounder? First, individuals with low educational levels are more likely to be smokers. (This satisfies criterion #1 of the definition of confounding.) Second, irrespective of smoking, women with low educational levels are at greater risk for adverse maternal-fetal outcomes. (This satisfies criterion #2.) Thus, it is unclear whether the increased risk is attributable to smoking, educational level, or both. How does one eliminate the effect of a confounding variable?

Minimizing Confounding by Matching

One solution to the confounding problem in cohort studies is to "match" the exposed and unexposed cohorts on the confounding variables. (This approach will be discussed in greater detail later on in the section on case–control designs.) For example, a smoker who did not achieve a high school education would be paired (or "matched") with a nonsmoker who was also a non-high school graduate. By matching in this way, the representation of education level will wind up being identical in both cohorts; thus, the effect of the confounding variable is eliminated. Of course, matching could be carried out for multiple confounders, but usually, only two or three are considered for practical reasons.

Although matching exposed and unexposed subjects on confounding variables is theoretically desirable, such matching often is not carried out in cohort studies due to sample size, expense, and logistics. Many cohort studies are rather large, and to perform matching can be practically difficult. Matching in small cohort studies also may be limited by the sample size in that it may be difficult to find appropriate matches for the exposed subjects.

Typically, in cohort studies, confounding variables are dealt with in the statistical analysis phase where adjustments can be made for these variables as covariates in a statistical regression model. Also, it should be pointed out that in cohort studies which often are conducted over a long period of time, a subject's confounding variable may change over time, and a more complicated accounting for that change would need to be dealt with in the analysis phase. Matching is more common in case–control studies and will be discussed in greater detail below.

Table 4.4 Bias and related problems in cohort studies

1. Exposure misclassification bias
2. Change in exposure level over time
3. Loss to follow-up
4. Nonparticipation bias
5. Reporting bias

Sources of Bias in Cohort Studies

As in any type of study design, there are potential flaws (or "biases") that may creep into the study design and affect interpretation of the results. As also noted in Chaps. 5 and 8, bias refers to an error in the design or execution of a study that produces results that are distorted in one direction or another due to systematic factors. In other words, bias causes us to draw (incorrect) inferences based on faulty assumptions about the nature of the data.

There are many types of bias that can occur in research designs. Given in Table 4.4 are some of the more common types that would be encountered in cohort studies. (See Hennekens and Buring 1987 [3] for a more complete description.)

1. *Exposure Misclassification Bias*. This type of bias occurs when there is a tendency for exposed subjects to be misclassified as unexposed or vice versa. The example cited above in selection of controls is an example of misclassification bias. In that example, the quality control personnel who work in the "white-collar" business office might be classified as unexposed when, in fact, they are routinely exposed to the heavy metals because they tour the factory twice a day (even though they do not work in the factory). Typically, exposure misclassification bias occurs in the direction of erroneously classifying an individual as unexposed when, in fact, he or she is exposed. This would have the effect of reducing the degree of association between the exposure and the disease. In other words, if, in fact, exposure did increase the risk of disease, it is possible that we would declare little or no association. If the bias went in the other direction (i.e., unexposed subjects are misclassified as exposed), then we run the risk of finding an

association when, in fact, none exists. A solution to the misclassification problem is to have strict, measurable criteria for exposure. Of course, the ability to accurately measure or determine exposure may be limited by available resources.

2. *Change in Exposure Level over Time*. Bias may occur when a subject's exposure status changes with time. For example, a subject in the smoking cohort may quit smoking 10 years after high school. Is that subject in the smoking or nonsmoking cohort? In cases like this, it is common to classify the subject's time periods with respect to smoking or nonsmoking and to use the "person-years" method (see Kleinbaum et al. 1982 [4]) to analyze the data. Using this method, the subject is not classified as exposed or unexposed—only his follow-up time periods. Nevertheless, if "crossover" from one cohort to the other occurs, particularly in one direction only (e.g., smokers become nonsmokers, but nonsmokers do not start to smoke after high school), this may impart a bias that confounds interpretation of the study. For example, if many "quitters" develop lung cancer (presumably because they were exposed for several years), this occurrence might reduce the observed association between smoking and lung cancer.
3. *Loss to Follow-up Bias*. Bias can occur when members of one of the groups are differentially lost to follow-up compared to the other, and the reason for their loss is related, in part, to their level of exposure. Consider the following hypothetical observational study that evaluates newly diagnosed heterosexual AIDS patients. The two cohorts in this example are those patients who were IV drug users (IVDUs) and those who were not. Both cohorts are started on the same antiretroviral therapy at diagnosis. The research question is whether there is a difference between the two groups in viral load at the end of one year.

   As the study progresses, some patients die. To illustrate this bias using an exaggerated scenario, suppose that there are 50 IVDUs (the exposed cohort) and 50 non-IVDUs (the unexposed cohort), and, of the 50 IVDUs, 20 have died before the end of the 1-year follow-up period, leaving only 30 with measured viral load levels at follow-up (as there is no follow-up viral load recorded on the 20 IVDUs who died). The effect of this might be that the 30 IVDUs who completed the 1-year follow-up might have been, in general, "healthier" than the IVDUs who died, leading to a biased comparison.
4. *Nonparticipation Bias*. Nonparticipation bias is somewhat similar to loss to follow-up bias except that the bias occurs at the time of enrollment into the study. Suppose we were conducting a cohort study to determine whether child abuse is a risk factor for psychiatric disorders in teenage years. Although this might be a problematic study to conduct, due to the sensitive nature of the risk factor (i.e., child abuse), one might consider contacting families who were seen at a psychiatric facility once child abuse was discovered and asking them to participate in the study to follow their children through their teenage years to determine their psychiatric status. Controls would be families or subjects without histories of abuse who would be followed in the same way. In a situation such as this, it is likely that many families with histories of child abuse would decline to participate and that those who would participate might be "psychologically healthier," rendering them unrepresentative of the general group of families with child abuse. Furthermore, if this group were, indeed, psychologically healthier, then the incidence of teen psychological disorders might be lower, thus attenuating the true association between child abuse and psychological disorders.
5. *Reporting Accuracy Bias*. Reporting accuracy bias in cohort studies is similar to that in case–control studies. It refers to a situation where either the exposed or unexposed subjects deliberately misreport either their exposure or their outcome status, usually due to the sensitive nature of the variables being studied. (See the section on case–control studies for examples.)

Fig. 4.1 Computing the relative risk

	Disease Yes	Disease No	
Exposure (Yes)	a	b	a+b
Exposure (No)	c	d	c+d
Total	a+c	c+d	a+b+c+d

Incidence of Disease in Exposed Group = a/(a+b)
Incidence of Disease in Unexposed Group = c/(c+d)
Relative risk = RR = [a/(a+b)]/[c/(c+d)]

Computing and Interpreting Relative Risk

The foregoing discussion dealt primarily with issues surrounding the design and interpretation of cohort studies. Between design and interpretation is a phase during which various calculations are carried out to quantify the relationship between the presumed risk factor and the disease under investigation. The most common measure used in cohort studies for quantifying such risk is the "relative risk" (RR). The calculation and interpretation of RR can be illustrated by referring to Fig. 4.1. Here, a and b, respectively, represent the number of exposed subjects who did and did not develop the disease in question. Likewise, c and d represent the unexposed subjects who, respectively, did and did not develop the disease. In a cohort study, one usually selects exposed subjects so that the row total of exposed (a+b) is fixed at some predetermined sample size. Likewise, the sample size for the row of unexposed (c+d) is also fixed. The two row totals do not necessarily have to be equal. This table is often referred to as a 2×2 table– pronounced "two-by-two"– since it contains two rows and two columns corresponding to Exposure and Disease status.

In the exposed group, the fraction of subjects who developed disease (i.e., incidence rate in the exposed) is a/(a+b); the corresponding incidence rate in the unexposed is c/(c+d).

The relative risk is then defined as

$$\begin{aligned} RR &= (\text{incidence rate in exposed})/(\text{incidence rate in unexposed}) \\ &= [a/(a+b)]/[c/(c+d)]. \end{aligned}$$

Typically, one might compare the rates to determine whether they are different, since, if the rates are the same (i.e., RR=1), that effectively tells us that there is no association between the risk factor and the disease. On the other hand, if the rate is greater in the exposed (i.e., RR>1), that would suggest that the risk factor is positively associated with the disease. (RR<1 would suggest that the subjects with the "risk factor" actually have a lower likelihood of disease.) It should be noted that RR is always a positive number unless one or more of the cells in the above 2×2 table contains a zero, in which case it is common to compute the RR by adding ½ to a, b, c, and d and using the formula given above (see Agresti 2002 [5]).

The following example (see Fig. 4.2) computes the RR for a cohort study investigating oral contraceptive use as a risk factor for MI in women. In this example, 1,000 women who used an OC were followed over a period of

Fig. 4.2 Relative risk: an example

Does oral contraceptive use increase the risk of thrombophlebitis?

	Thrombophlebitis Yes	Thrombophlebitis No
OC Use (Yes)	30	970
OC Use (No)	3	997

$$RR = \frac{.03}{0.003} = 10$$

time to see who developed an MI. Likewise, 1,000 OC nonusers were followed in a similar way. The incidence rates of MI were 0.03 and 0.003, respectively, yielding a RR = 10, which means that women who used OC had 10 times a greater risk of MI than nonusers. For determining whether a RR is significantly different from 1, the reader is referred to Kleinbaum et al. 1982 [4].

Prospective Versus Retrospective Cohort Designs

One usually thinks of a cohort study as "prospective" because it looks forward from an exposure to the subsequent development of disease. However, a cohort study can be classified as "retrospective" or "prospective," depending on when it is being conducted with respect to the outcome. If, at the time the investigator initiates the study, the outcome (e.g., disease) has not yet occurred in the study subjects, then the study is "prospective" because the investigator must follow the subjects in real time in order to ascertain outcome status. On the other hand, if the study is conducted after the exposures and outcomes have already occurred, this type of design often is classified as a "retrospective" cohort study.

For example, referring back to the section on confounding, there is general consensus that the study of smoking during pregnancy as a risk factor for adverse maternal-fetal outcomes is of the prospective type because, as described, the investigator must wait from the time of exposure to observe the outcome of the pregnancy. However, suppose that the study were to be conducted by reviewing patient charts from 2 years prior to the initiation of the study and identifying women who smoked and did not smoke during pregnancy at that time. Then, the investigator would determine the pregnancy outcome from the chart data (i.e., the outcomes are already known and documented in the charts). This is an example of what many term a retrospective cohort study. (As noted in Chap. 1, DeAngelis [6] and others would refer to this as a "historical" or "nonconcurrent" cohort study.)

To the reader, the distinction between retrospective and prospective cohort studies may not seem important since the logic of the two approaches is essentially the same. However, in a prospective cohort study, the investigator typically has more quality control of the conduct of the study and how data are to be collected than in a retrospective study because the former is being conducted in real time. In a retrospective cohort study, the investigator is limited by the nature and quality of data already available, which most likely were collected for routine clinical purposes using criteria and standards that are different from those of the current research investigation.

Case–Control Studies

The purpose of a case–control study, like a cohort study, is to determine whether an association exists between exposure (E) to a proposed risk factor and occurrence of a disease (D). The essential difference between the two designs is that in a cohort study, exposed and unexposed subjects are identified and then followed over time to determine the incidence rates of disease in those two groups, whereas in a case–control study, subjects with and without the disease are classified as having or not having been exposed to the proposed risk factor. More simply put, the cohort study follows subjects "forward" in time, whereas the case–control study looks "backward" for an associated factor by first identifying subjects with and without the disease.

Selection of Cases

If we are to conduct a case–control study, then we first need to determine who our "cases" will be and how we will select them for inclusion in the study.

Case Definition

The first step in selecting cases is to define what is meant by a "case." For example, if we were studying lung cancer, we might specify that a case would be any subject with biopsy-proven adenocarcinoma of the lung. If the research question itself necessarily distinguished between small cell and non-small cell lung cancer and only the latter type was to be studied, then we would have to add that to the definition. Other examples of strict definitions might be as follows: if one were studying nutritional factors and their association with MI, we would define a patient to have an MI if the patient exhibits a certain degree of enzyme elevation and has clearly defined prespecified changes on an electrocardiogram.

Homogeneity of Cases

Most diseases vary according to severity or subtype. If we were to include in our study only cases with a very specific subtype and/or severity (e.g., a particular histology of lung cancer), then the study design may benefit from decreased "noise" or variation, but the results may be less generalizable. Furthermore, restriction of the case definition will result in a smaller potential pool of subjects (i.e., smaller sample size). Conversely, if the case definition is expanded to include, say, multiple subtypes of the disease, then the results may be more generalizable, and the subject pool size may increase. However, there will be greater variability, which may reduce the ability to detect an association between E and D (i.e., reduced statistical power). Determining the heterogeneity of case definition is a fine balancing act between addressing the specific research question and sample size considerations.

Sources of Cases

In most research studies, a case of disease will be identified and selected from medical practices or facilities such as hospitals or physician practices. Occasionally, cases of disease can be obtained by using disease registries.

Prevalent Versus Incident Cases

An important consideration in the selection of cases is whether a case is considered a "prevalent" or "incident" case. A subject is said to be a "prevalent case" if the patient has the disease in question regardless of when it was diagnosed. It may have been diagnosed 2 days ago, 2 years ago, or 10 or 20 years ago. But, as long as the subject is available, that subject is considered a prevalent case. An "incident case" refers to a more restrictive criterion. In order to be an incident case, an individual needs to have been diagnosed "recently." "Recently" may have different connotations in different disease entities, but, for example, in a chronic disease like cancer, an incident case might be a case that was diagnosed within the past 2–3 months. On the other hand, for a disease that is rapidly fatal, such as anthrax poisoning, an incident case might be defined as a case that was diagnosed an hour or 2 ago. The essential point to remember in designing case–control studies is, that when selecting cases, we should select incident cases, not prevalent cases. The reasons are as follows.

First, case–control studies often involve the recall of information about past exposures. This type of information often is obtained by interviewing the subject him or herself or by interviewing family members or friends who might have such information. Of course, some exposure information may also be gleaned from patient charts or other documents that exist independent of an interview with a subject. It stands to reason that if the interval of time between diagnosis of the disease and the interview for exposure information is lengthy, then the ability to properly recall exposures will be reduced. Certain exposures such as smoking are not likely to be forgotten, but, for example, if we were studying more complex and/or rare exposures, the ability to accurately recall such exposures and associated details would decrease over time. Thus, the shorter the interval between diagnosis and gathering of exposure information the more likely the recall of information will be accurate.

A second reason for selecting incident cases is illustrated by the following example. Suppose we were studying the association between smoking and lung cancer. We might go to the tumor registry of our hospital and find 1,000 lung cancer cases that were diagnosed over the past 10 years. The next step in our research design would be to contact these subjects and ask them whether or not they were smokers prior to their development of lung cancer. One of the problems associated with this approach is that out of those 1,000 lung cancer cases diagnosed over the past 10 years, many will have expired before we would be able to contact them. Cases that are still alive probably would fall into two broad groups: (a) those who have been recently diagnosed and have not had enough exposure to lung cancer yet to die from the disease and (b) those who were diagnosed in the more distant past but who have survived. The latter group (b) is likely made up of those with lower grade disease or those who have been more successful in combating their disease with therapy. That group may be very different from those who were diagnosed in the more distant past who already have died of their disease. In fact, it is conceivable that smoking may not just be associated with developing lung cancer but may, instead, be associated with its lethality. Thus, it is possible that the smokers are those who died early in the group that was diagnosed in the more distant past whereas nonsmokers are the ones who have survived despite their disease. In this case, when comparing this biased group of cases to non-cancer controls, we would observe an attenuated association between smoking and lung cancer. This bias would provide potentially misleading results.

On the other hand, if one were to simply sample recently diagnosed cases and assuming that the disease is not rapidly fatal (even small cell lung cancer patients would survive to be interviewed), almost all of the available lung cancer cases would be included in the study since, at that point, no one would be lost to follow-up or death. Therefore, the sample would not be biased as it might have been had the sampling methodology been based on prevalent case selection.

Selection of Controls

Perhaps, the most difficult aspect of conducting a case–control study is the selection of controls. In principle, controls should be a group of individuals who are free of the disease or outcome in question (i.e., unexposed) and are as similar in all other respects to the case group.

Definition of Controls

Controls should be free of the disease in question. One of the difficulties in selecting controls is determining how far we should go to ensure that someone is free of the disease or outcome. For example, if we were to select as a control for our lung cancer cases an individual who has never had a diagnosis of lung cancer, do we need to perform a bronchoscopy on that patient for certainty of that fact, or do we simply take his self-report as the truth that he has never had lung cancer? Of course, there are subtleties that arise when subclinical disease exists at the time an individual is being selected as a control. These are fine points that would need to be dealt with in a very careful manner, in consultation with a statistician or an epidemiologist.

At this point, it is instructive to provide an example of where verification of non-disease status might be problematic and require some additional thought about the design of the study. Suppose we were conducting a case–control study to determine whether there is an association between a high fat diet and colon cancer. Specifically, our hypothesis is that colon cancer cases will report a higher frequency of high fat diets than non-cancer controls. To test our hypothesis, we would select our colon cancer cases in some way consistent with the guidelines already stated above and then select controls. One possible source of controls would be adults visiting a large shopping mall. (We might choose to select individuals over 50 years old if our case–control study was designed to answer the question in this population.) Next, we could set up a colon cancer information booth in the mall and invite the passersby to answer a question or two about history of colon cancer and, if they wished, to pick up a fecal occult blood test kit so that they can screen themselves for colon cancer. Those who self-reported that they had never had a diagnosis of colon cancer could be invited to participate as controls for our case–control study. We might use as an exclusion criterion a positive test result on the fecal occult blood test (even though that finding obviously does not equate to a diagnosis of colon cancer).

A member of our investigative team might object to this approach since self-report and fecal occult blood testing, in and of themselves, would not completely verify the disease-free status of someone passing through the shopping mall. Thus, we might be more rigorous in our selection of controls. This might be done by enlisting the collaboration of a gastroenterologist who performs colonoscopies and selecting from his or her colonoscopy practice those subjects who have colonoscopies with a benign or negative outcome. Such outcomes might include diverticulosis, inflammatory bowel disease, a benign polyp, other benign tumors of the colon, etc. If we were to view colonoscopy as a close to foolproof way of determining an individual's colon cancer status, then this would be a better way of selecting controls for such a study than selecting them from visitors to a shopping mall (even though colonoscopy, itself, is not infallible). Of course, subjects who have a diagnosis of colon cancer based on the colonoscopy would be excluded from the control group.

The selection of controls from among those undergoing colonoscopy, nonetheless, could potentiate a different problem, namely, selection bias. Generally speaking, there are two broad groups of individuals who undergo colonoscopy: (a) those who are symptomatic and who are referred by their physician to a gastroenterologist to determine the cause of their rectal bleeding, abdominal pains, cramping, diarrhea, etc., and (b) those who are asymptomatic who undergo colonoscopy for screening purposes only. However, these two groups differ in ways that can influence the results of the investigation. For example, a high fat diet may not be specific to the risk of colon cancer but may be associated with other intestinal problems (e.g., some of the benign conditions cited above). If this association was not appreciated during the study design stage, and individuals from the "symptomatic" group were selected as controls, their rate of high fat diets would be spuriously inflated, thus reducing the observed degree of association between fatty diets and colon cancer. On the other hand, selection of the asymptomatic individuals who undergo cancer screening are more likely to be health-conscious individuals since they are voluntarily attending a screening program. Because these individuals are more health conscious, they may have an "artificially" lower level of fat intake than a standard population of individuals without colon cancer. Accordingly, when we compare the fat intake for this control group against the colon cancer group, we may observe an exaggerated association because of the artificially reduced levels of fat intake in our control group.

There are several ways to address this problem, none of which constitutes a perfect resolution of the issue. In this example, some investigators might employ only one of the control groups with the understanding that the bias would need to be considered when interpreting the results. Thus, for example, if the benign disease group were used as the control and only a small association was observed (i.e., odds ratio [OR] is close to 1), the association would be inconclusive because of the directionality of the bias. However, if a large and statistically significant association (i.e., OR > 1) were found, then, because the bias is working against the hypothesis of positive association, this larger OR would provide evidence in favor of the association. Another approach might be to include both groups as separate controls and, knowing the opposite directions of the bias, compare cases to each control group and draw inferences accordingly.

Sources of Controls

Recall that in a case–control study, cases of disease are most conveniently selected from a medical practice or facility, but controls need not be selected from such sources even though it might also be convenient to do so. Controls also can be selected from the community at-large using sophisticated sampling techniques or by simply placing advertisements in community media to recruit individuals who meet the control criteria. Very often, investigators will collaborate with various work places that will permit access to their employees as potential controls for a particular study. Over the years, departments of motor vehicles often have served as a source of controls for many research studies. Occasionally, close friends, relatives, or neighbors of an individual case will serve as controls. Choosing such individuals can solve a myriad of problems because this type of control sometimes will share the same environmental conditions as the case or have a similar genetic disposition. The approach also facilitates cooperation because, very often, friends, relatives, or neighbors will cooperate with an investigator who is also working with that individual's relative. However, selecting friends and relatives as controls may have adverse consequences because it often "forces" the cases and controls to be similar on the very risk factors being investigated, thus reducing the association between the risk factor and disease. In summary, the selection of controls requires careful thought and knowledge of the underlying subject matter.

Confounding in Case–Control Studies

The Nature of the Problem

The impact of confounding on interpretation of findings from cohort studies has previously been addressed. The reader should note that its adverse effects are not limited to cohort studies but represent a potentially serious problem in case–control designs as well. Schlesselman [7] provides interesting examples of such confounding, which we now describe.

Consider a hypothetical case–control study designed to test the hypothesis of association between alcohol use (E) and lung cancer (D). Cases of lung cancer are selected for study, and a group of controls without lung cancer is identified. Suppose that the rate of alcohol use in the lung cancer cases is found to be significantly greater than that of the controls. The conclusion would be that alcohol use increases the risk of lung cancer. However, one might criticize the study because smoking should have been considered a confounding variable.

Why is smoking a confounding variable? One needs to refer back to the definition. Certainly, smoking is associated with lung cancer (criterion #2), independent of any other factors. However, smoking's association with lung cancer does not, in itself, make it a confounding variable. Smoking must also be associated with alcohol use (criterion #1). How is smoking associated with alcohol use? The answer lies in the fact that individuals who drink alcohol tend to have a higher rate of smoking than individuals who do not drink alcohol. Therefore, smoking is related both to alcohol use (E) and lung cancer (D) and is, therefore, a confounding variable.

As another example of a confounding variable that may obscure an association between a putative risk factor and disease, consider a case–control study to determine whether there is an association between oral contraceptive (OC) use and MI in women. Once again, one would pick cases of women who had suffered a recent MI and determine whether or not they had used OC in, say, the past 5 years. A possible result of this study would be that the level of OC use was not substantially greater in the MI cases than in the non-MI controls, thereby resulting in the conclusion that there is little or no association between OC use and MI. However, once again, smoking could be considered a confounding factor because it meets the two criteria of a confounder: first, smoking is associated with MI. Second, smoking is associated with OC use. Why is this so? The reason is that women who are smokers are less likely to be prescribed an OC than women who are nonsmokers because of the risk of thrombophlebitis and other cardiovascular disorders. In this example, the OC users were underrepresented in the MI case group because there were many smokers in the MI group, many of whom were never prescribed OC. Thus, the confounding effect of smoking potentially masks a relationship (i.e., reduces the association) between OC use and MI.

Although it is important to identify confounders, it is just as important to recognize factors that may appear to be confounders but, in fact, are not. Once again, two examples from Schlesselman [7] are instructive. Consider a case–control study designed to investigate whether a sedentary lifestyle is a risk factor for MI. Cases are those with a recent history of MI and controls are individuals without MI (appropriately chosen). The "exposure" variable is (for simplicity) "sedentary lifestyle" (coded as "no" or "yes"), as derived from some validated measure of physical activity. One might consider levels of fluid intake (F) as a possible confounding variable because physically active, non-sedentary subjects might have higher levels of fluid intake than sedentary subjects; in other words F is associated with E. Accordingly, we would consider matching cases to controls on fluid intake. However, fluid intake is not a true confounder because there is no known or presumed association between fluid intake and MI (D). Thus, matching on fluid intake is not necessary.

Reducing Confounding by Matching

If confounding is an important problem in epidemiologic studies, how do we deal with it? A common solution is matching. Matching is a technique whereby cases and controls are made to appear similar with respect to one or more confounding variables. When cases and controls are properly matched, the representation of the confounding variables is similar in both groups and, therefore, should have no appreciable effect on the results and interpretation of the case–control study.

Most students in the medical sciences are familiar with the idea of matching since they probably have read many studies where matching was employed. However, it is our objective in this chapter to describe the logistics of matching in somewhat more detail. The first step in matching cases to controls is to identify the confounding variables. The next step is to determine the desired method of matching. Typically, one should not match on more than a few variables (i.e., two or three), but this also depends on the sample size in the case–control study and on the distribution of the confounding variables in the samples being studied. Let us consider a simple example where we have determined that age and sex are important confounders. (It is important to emphasize that, while age, sex, race, and socioeconomic status are four of the most commonly encountered confounders, it is not always necessary to match on any of these variables. The reader should be reminded again that in order for a variable to be a confounder, it must meet the *two* criteria given in the definition above.)

1. *Group Versus. Calipers Matching*. When age and sex are potential confounders, one way to match cases and controls is to classify male and female subjects into age groupings (a common method of classification for age is by decades, i.e., age 20–29, 30–39, 40–49, 50–59, or 60 and above). This approach would yield up to 10 different age/sex combinations corresponding to each of the 5 age categories cross-classified with sex (male, female). Therefore, if a case were to be chosen and that particular subject was a 30-year-old male, we would choose a control who was a male in the 30- to 39-year age group; these two individuals (the case and the control) would be naturally matched and paired.

   The reader should note, however, that there is a disadvantage to creating groups on a measured variable such as age. Suppose, in the above example, we required a match for a 30-year-old male, and, based on the pool of potential controls, a 29-year-old male and a 39-year-old male were both available. Using the grouping criteria defined above, the 30-year-old male would have to be matched with the 39-year-old male because they were in the same age category. However, it would make more sense to match a 30-year-old male with a 29-year-old male because the two are closer in age.

A solution to this problem is to use what is known as "calipers" matching whereby, on a measured variable, a control would be matched to a case based on being within a certain number of units away from that case's measurement (hence the use of the term calipers). For example, we might define a rule to match age to within (±) three years. In this case, the 29-year-old male is within three years of the 30-year-old male and would be matched to the 30-year-old male, whereas the 39-year-old male would be outside the defined three-year limit. A compromise between broad grouping and calipers would be to arrange the potentially confounding variable (in this case, age) into narrow categories (e.g., 30–33, 34–37, 38–41, etc.). This would reduce the effect of the disparity that occurred in the example given above involving grouping by decades. When using this method for age matching, the investigator must take care to consider the nature of the study population. For example, if one were matching on age using three-year calipers in a case–control study evaluating utilization of health-care services, a 64-year-old case could be matched to any control ranging from 61 to 67 years old. However, in this example, matching a 64-year-old to, say, a 64-year-old in a health services utilization study might result in matching a non-Medicare subject with a Medicare subject. As these two types of patients might have very different utilization patterns, a bias could be introduced into the study design. Similarly, when conducting research with pediatric patients, it is important to match as closely and precisely to actual age as possible (which is equivalent to making the calipers extremely narrow). For example, one would *not* match children to within three years (e.g., matching a 10-year-old girl to a seven- or 13-year-old girl) since individuals at these ages could have very different outcomes due to variations in socialization, sexual maturity, body size, and other developmental variables. Effective matching, under these circumstances, requires that there be a large pool of available controls to pair with cases.

2. *Individual Versus Frequency Matching.* Another consideration in matching is whether the investigator wishes to use individual versus frequency matching. Typically, with individual matching, one case and one control are matched to one another (1:1 matching). Occasionally, the statistician or epidemiologist will recommend "many-to-one" matching which might involve matching two or three controls to each case. It is uncommon to match more than three controls to a case because it can be shown that the statistical power benefits do not substantially increase after two or three matches to a control. The reader should keep in mind that if he or she conducts a case–control study with 1:1 matching, it is necessary that there be an equal number of cases and controls. A common misstatement that is seen in many research proposals employing case–control studies is, for example, "there will be 50 cases with disease and they will be matched to 20 controls without disease." If the investigator was thinking of performing individual matching, then this statement makes no sense as it would require a constant ratio of controls to cases. Usually, what the investigator intends is that they will select cases and controls so that, for example, the average age (or sex distribution) of both groups is approximately the same. However, this approach is not matching; it is simply determining how comparable the two groups are after they have been selected. Unless one prospectively selects controls in a deliberate way so as to match them directly to a given case, the term "matching" is not appropriate.

When an investigator does not perform individual matching but instead wants to ensure that the confounding variables have the same joint distributions among both cases and controls, the method of choice is "frequency matching." Frequency matching refers to the deliberate and prospective selection of controls so that the joint distribution of the confounding variables is approximately the same in both the case and control groups. As an example, suppose we were performing a case–control study to determine whether maternal smoking during pregnancy was a risk factor for premature birth. Our cases might be 100 premature infants delivered during the past year, and our controls would be drawn from the hundreds of normal term births delivered during the same time period. Further, we have determined that parity (i.e., nulliparous vs. parous) and age (grouped in 3-year intervals) are confounding variables for which matching will be performed. Suppose we have decided that, based on statistical power and resources available to conduct the study, that the number of controls will be 250. Further, suppose that in the case group, 10% of the cases were born to nulliparous 30- to 33-year-old women. We would then identify from our vast pool of term-delivery controls all women who are nulliparous 30- to 33-year-olds. From this pool of candidates, we would randomly select 25 nulliparous 30- to 33-year-old women. By selecting 25 at random, this would assure that 10% of the control group (10% of 250=25) would be nulliparous 30- to 33-year-olds. Likewise, suppose that 16% of the cases are parous 25- to 28-year-old women, then in a similar way we would identify all parous 25- to 28-year-old women who had full-term deliveries and, from that group, randomly select 40 matching controls as 40 would constitute 16% of the control group. If we continued in this fashion, we would obtain a control group that had either precisely or approximately the same joint distribution of parity and age in both cases and controls. It is important to note that to use frequency matching, one would need to know the distribution of the confounding variables in the case group prior to selecting the matched controls. This certainly would be workable in a study such as this where ascertainment of smoking status (the risk factor) could be made by chart review so that one could first constitute the case group and then return to select the control group. Frequency matching may be logistically more difficult to conduct in other types of case–control studies, but the concept is still the same.

3. *Propensity Matching*. A recently developed method for matching cases and controls (which also may also be used for matching exposed and unexposed subjects in a cohort study) is known as "propensity scoring" (Rosenbaum and Rubin [8, 9]). Briefly, this method involves predicting whether a subject is a case or a control based on observed predictor covariates. Thus, one subject may be a case and the other a control, but their "covariate profiles" are similar as reflected by their predicted probability of being in, say, the "case" group. Specifically, the probability of being a "case" (i.e., the propensity score) is computed for each subject in the study (both cases and controls) using a statistical method known as multiple logistic regression (see Chap. 11). Then, cases are matched to controls on the propensity score. So, for example, suppose that in a particular study, the score is being computed as a function of age, sex, smoking status, family history, and socioeconomic status. If a particular case has a score of, for example, 0.75, we would try to match this case to a control that also has a score of 0.75. In this way, cases and controls are matched based on a measure of their similarity. An advantage of the propensity score method is that it allows the investigator to match cases and controls on a single criterion (the score) that is a function of multiple confounding variables, rather than having to match on each of the individual confounders.

Sources of Bias in Case–Control Studies

As in cohort studies, case–control studies are subject to a variety of biases. Given below are some of the more common types that may be encountered.

Recall Bias

Recall bias occurs when one of the groups recalls exposure to the risk factor more accurately than the other group. It is not uncommon for recall bias to manifest itself as cases remembering exposures better than controls. As an example, suppose one were conducting a case–control study to examine risk factors for early childhood leukemia. The cases in such a study might be parents of children with leukemia who were diagnosed before their fourth birthday, and the controls might be parents of children who did not have a diagnosis of leukemia. The investigator interviews both groups of parents with respect to exposure to a variety of potential risk factors. It would not be unlikely that the mother of a young child with leukemia would remember many household exposures better than a mother whose child was healthy since it is human nature to recall antecedent events potentially leading up to a serious disease or traumatic event better than someone who has no reason to remember those events or exposures. Another example of recall bias might be found in a study examining antecedents of lower back pain. Subjects who experience lower back pain probably would have better recall of events related to lifting of heavy objects that may have preceded the diagnosis of the back pain versus those without back pain who may not have any particular reason to remember such events.

Reporting Accuracy Bias

This term refers to lying or deception in the response to questions concerning exposure, as frequently occurs in the setting of case–control studies where sensitive questions are being asked of the subject. A classic example of reporting accuracy bias might be as follows: Suppose one were to conduct a case–control study among women to determine if her number of sex partners during the past year is a risk factor for contracting venereal disease (VD). One might conduct this study at a women's health center and select as cases women with newly diagnosed VD. Controls could be women from the same clinic who do not have a diagnosis of VD. The important question in the epidemiologic interview would be "how many sexual partners have you had in the past year?" The responses in the case group (those with VD) might look as follows: 1, 1, 2, 2, 2, 3, 4, 5, 5, 6, 6, 6, 8, 9, and 10. (The responses have been ordered from smallest to largest in order to better visualize the data.) When the control group is asked to respond to the same question, the results might be 1, 1, 1, 1, 1, 1, 1, 2, 2, and 2. Based on these responses, the average number of sexual partners in the case group would be 4.7 versus 1.3 in the control group, thus suggesting (subject to a formal statistical test) that increased number of sexual partners is a risk factor for venereal disease.

Although, at face value, the interpretation of the results might be as just stated, there is a potential reporting accuracy bias. The bias might occur because women who have VD may be more likely to be truthful about the number of sexual partners they have had, whereas women who are controls may not be, thus causing the average number of sexual partners to be artifactually greater in the case group than in the control group. Why might such a bias exist? One hypothesis is that individuals with a particular disease (in this case, VD) tend to be more candid with their physicians about past medical history and behaviors [10]. In fact, many patients (rightly or wrongly) believe that if they are truthful, then their physicians may be able to better treat their disease than if they are not truthful. Assuming that this women's health center serves women who are married, those with boyfriends, male partners, etc., among the control group might be less likely to be truthful about the number of sexual partners because they would perceive that they have something to lose and nothing to gain by admitting multiple sexual partners. Of course, the ethical conduct of such a study would require an assurance of confidentiality with respect to responses to the epidemiologic questions, but such an assurance does not guarantee that subjects will cooperative when confronted with a highly personal and sensitive question.

Selection Bias

Selection bias in case–control studies occurs when identification and/or inclusion of cases (or controls) depends, in part, on the subject's level of exposure to the risk factor under study.

There are several common forms of selection bias (i.e., detection and referral bias) as discussed below.

1. *Detection Bias*. Detection bias occurs when subjects exposed to the risk factor are more (or less) likely to be screened for the disease. A good example can be found in a hypothetical case–control study to determine whether exogenous estrogen use is a risk factor for endometrial cancer in women. One might choose as cases women with newly diagnosed endometrial cancer and as controls those without a diagnosis of endometrial cancer (suitably matched on various confounding variables). The study would then determine what fraction of cases had been exposed to estrogen (according to some predefined criteria) and similarly for the controls. A problem (potential bias) in this type of study is that when a woman undergoes estrogen therapy, it is likely that she will visit her gynecologist more often than if she does not since she would need to be monitored more frequently for potential side effects, such as vaginal bleeding. Consequently, if the woman were to develop endometrial cancer (irrespective of whether estrogen increased the risk), then it is more likely that the gynecologist will discover it due to the increased surveillance. Thus, when one selects cases for this study, unbeknownst to the investigator, the cases may have a higher likelihood of exposure simply because of the way that they were "selected" to enter the case pool.
2. *Referral Bias*. Referral bias occurs when controls are referred into the "control pool" for reasons that are related to the disease under study. As an example, suppose that a case–control study was being conducted to determine whether caloric intake was a risk factor for coronary artery disease (CAD). Since the investigator works in a hospital, she would like to select her controls, for convenience, from her hospital environment. She reasons that selecting controls from the pulmonary, endocrinology, or renal clinic might create a bias because many of those patients already have heart disease (or are at risk for heart disease), so she decides to select controls from the podiatry clinic around the block. She further reasons that most of the patients visiting the podiatry clinic are presenting for a variety of foot problems unrelated to heart disease or diet. However, she does not realize that some of these patients also have been referred for foot problems related to diabetes, and diabetes, of course, is related both to heart disease and caloric intake. Therefore, in using these subjects as controls (without excluding controls seen for diabetic-related problems) might weaken any true association between diet (caloric intake) and CAD.

   Another type of referral bias relates to the situation where included cases are not truly representative of all cases of the disease. For example, suppose we were investigating a possible increased risk of pediatric inflammatory bowel disease (IBD) among children who were formula-fed during infancy, as opposed to having been breast-fed. If we were to select the IBD cases from a medical practice at a prominent teaching hospital that specializes in pediatric IBD, we might be seeing a disproportionately high number of "severe" cases since it is likely that severe, difficult-to-manage cases would be referred to this center. Furthermore, if, in fact, formula feeding is not a risk factor for *development* of IBD but is a risk factor for *having a more severe case of IBD among those with such a diagnosis*, then it is likely that these cases will have a higher percentage of formula-fed individuals than the non-IBD control group. Accordingly, we would be more likely to conclude that formula feeding is a risk factor for IBD, when it is not.

Computing and Interpreting Measures of Risk

The foregoing discussion dealt primarily with issues surrounding the design and interpretation of case–control studies. Between the design and interpretation of a case–control study is a phase

Fig. 4.3 Computing the odds ratio

	Disease		
	Yes (case)	No (control)	
Exposure (Yes)	a	b	a+b
Exposure (No)	c	d	c+d
Total	a+c	c+d	a+b+c+d

Odds of exposure in the cases = [a/(a+c)] / [c/(a+c)] = a/c
Odds of exposure in the controls = [b/(b+d)] / [d/(b+d)] =b/d
Odds Ratio = OR = (a/c) / (b/d) = (ad)/(bc)

during which various calculations are carried out to quantify the relationship between the presumed risk factor and the disease under investigation. The most common measure used for drawing inferences in a case–control study is the odds ratio (OR). The calculation and interpretation of the OR can be illustrated by reference to Fig. 4.3. Here, a and c, respectively, represent the number of cases who were exposed and not exposed to the risk factor. Likewise, b and d, respectively, represent the number of controls who were exposed and not exposed. In a case–control study, one usually selects cases so that the column total of cases (a+c) is fixed at some predetermined sample size; likewise for the control column (b+d). Frequently, the cases and controls are sampled in equal numbers (so that a+c=b+d), but there are circumstances where equality may not hold, as pointed out in the section on matching.

In the case group, the fraction of subjects who were exposed to the candidate risk factor is a/(a+c); the corresponding proportion exposed in the control group is b/(b+d). Typically, one might compare the two proportions to determine whether they are different since if the proportions are the same, that effectively tells us that the risk factor is not associated with the disease; on the other hand, if the proportion of exposed cases is much larger than that of the controls, that would suggest that the risk factor is associated with the disease.

For various mathematical reasons, it is more convenient to express the risk, not as a difference between proportions but as a ratio of odds. To the unfamiliar reader, the odds of an event occurring is defined as the probability that the event will occur divided by the probability that it will not occur. For example, if the probability of an event is 25%, the odds of the event occurring is 25/75 (or, as some would prefer to express it, 1:3 odds). Thus, the odds of exposure among cases is [a/(a+c)]/[c/(a+c)] whereas the odds of exposure among controls is [b/(b+d)]/[d/(b+d)]. If we denote these quantities by O_1 and O_2, respectively, then $OR = O_1/O_2 = (ad)/(bc)$. Computation of the OR in this fashion always will result in a positive number unless one or more of the cells in the above 2×2 table contains a zero; in the latter instance, it is common to compute the OR by adding ½ to a, b, c, and d and using the same formula [5] employed for computation of the relative risk (RR) in a cohort study. Just as in the interpretation of the RR, if $OR > 1$, this is taken to mean that the exposure to the risk factor increases the risk of disease by that many times or by that "fold" increase. Thus, for example, if $OR = 1.5$, this means that individuals with the risk factor are 1.5 times more likely to get the disease than those without the risk factor. Conversely, if $OR < 1$, exposure to the risk factor is protective. Thus, if $OR = 0.5$, that means that those with the risk factor are half as likely to get the disease as

Fig. 4.4 The odds ratio: an example

Does family history of coronary artery disease increase the risk of myocardial infarction?

	Myocardial Infraction Yes	No
Family History of CAD (Yes)	400	300
Family History of CAD (No)	600	700
Total	1000	1000

OR= (400x700)/(600x300) = 1.56

those without the risk factor. An OR that is "close" to 1.0 means the factor is not associated with risk of disease. Figure 4.4 illustrates computation of the OR for a hypothetical case–control study investigating family history of coronary artery disease (CAD) as a risk factor for myocardial infarction (MI) in men. In this example, OR = 1.56, which means that men with a family history of CAD have a 1.56 times greater risk of MI than those without such a family history.

Case–Control and Cohort Designs: Advantages Versus Disadvantages

As with any scientific study design, there are distinct advantages and disadvantages to their uses. Below, we provide a concise listing of some of the important pros and cons of case–control and cohort designs, as identified by Schlesselman [7].

Cohort Studies

Advantages

- Allow complete information on the subject's exposure, including quality control of data, and experience thereafter
- Provide a clear temporal sequence of exposure and disease.
- Afford an opportunity to study multiple outcomes related to a specific exposure.
- Permit calculation of incidence rates (absolute risk) as well as relative risk.
- Enable the study of relatively rare exposures.
- Methodology and results are easily understood by non-epidemiologists.

Disadvantages

- Not suited for the study of rare diseases because a large number of subjects is required.
- Not suitable when the time between exposure and disease manifestation is very long, although this can be overcome in historical cohort studies.
- Exposure patterns, for example, the composition of oral contraceptives, may change during the course of the study and make the results irrelevant.
- Maintaining high rates of follow-up can be difficult.
- Expensive to carry out because a large number of subjects usually is required.
- Baseline data may be sparse as the large number of subjects often required for these studies does not allow for long interviews.

Case–Control Studies

Advantages

- Permit the study of rare diseases.
- Permit the study of diseases with long latency between exposure and manifestation.

- Can be launched and conducted over relatively short time periods.
- Relatively inexpensive as compared to cohort studies.
- Can study multiple potential causes of disease.

Disadvantages

- Information on exposure and past history primarily is based on interview and may be subject to recall bias.
- Validation of information on exposure is difficult, or incomplete, or even impossible.
- By definition, concerned with one disease only.
- Cannot usually provide information on incidence rates of disease.
- Generally incomplete control of extraneous variables.
- Choice of appropriate control group may be difficult.
- Methodology may be hard to comprehend for non-epidemiologists, and correct interpretation of results may be difficult.

Cross-Sectional Studies

The question addressed by a cross-sectional study is similar to that addressed by case–control or cohort studies: Is there an association between a particular factor and a disease or other event? The essential difference is that in a cross-sectional study, both the disease and exposure are assessed at the same time, with no attention to the timing of the exposure relative to the disease in question. For example, suppose we wanted to know whether artificial sweeteners were a risk factor for diabetes (type II). We could distribute a questionnaire to some large group of subjects, perhaps by direct mail. The questionnaire would ask whether the subject has had a diagnosis of type II diabetes and whether the subject consumes artificial sweeteners. Such a study would provide an estimate of prevalence of both diabetes and of artificial sweetener consumption in the targeted population. However, if the ultimate objective is to know whether artificial sweeteners might have some causal role in diabetes, the data collected via this study design would not shed any light on this question because (given the way the study was conducted) it would not be known whether the sweetener exposure came before or after the diagnosis of diabetes. Obviously, to be implicated in a causal process, the exposure would have had to occur prior to the disease. (This would be a necessary but not sufficient condition for causality [see below].)

Thus, one of the disadvantages of a cross-sectional study is that a causal (or suggested causal) association cannot be determined. Another disadvantage is that rare diseases are difficult to study since a very large number of subjects would be needed to yield a sufficient number of diseased individuals (likewise, if the prevalence of the risk factor was rare). Despite these important drawbacks, cross-sectional designs usually are quicker and less expensive to conduct than case–control or cohort studies since no follow-up is needed. Another advantage of the cross-sectional study is that it can provide some evidence suggesting an association between exposure and disease and, thus, help in designing a more formalized cohort or case–control study.

The Question of Causality

In most studies of risk factors and the occurrence of disease, the ultimate goal is to determine if exposure (E) to the risk factor *causes* the disease (D) in question. In experimental studies (e.g., laboratory experiments with animals or randomized clinical trials in humans), establishing causality is more straightforward than in observational studies, such as case–control or cohort studies. This is because in the experimental situation, many confounding variables can be controlled by the experimenter or by randomization, and, therefore, it becomes a more direct method for establishing causality.

In the observational study, association between E and D can be readily established, but there is no direct method to prove causality. However, epidemiologists [7, 11] have provided a set of guidelines for determining whether there is a causal association between E and D. These guidelines state that, in order to establish causality, all of the five of the following criteria must be satisfied:

1. *Temporal association*. If causation is to hold, then exposure must precede the disease. Sometimes, the time sequence of E and D may be difficult to determine, but this criterion of temporal association is certainly a necessary condition.
2. *Consistency of association*. Loosely translated, this means that different studies of the same risk factor–disease question result in similar, or consistent, results. If results among several "similar" studies were discordant, this would weaken the causality hypothesis.
3. *Strength of association*. The greater the value of the relative risk or odds ratio, the less likely the association is spurious, lending evidence toward the causality hypothesis.
4. *Dose–response relationship*. If it can be shown that the risk of disease increases as the "dose" of the risk factor increases, this makes causality more plausible.
5. *Biological plausibility*. While satisfaction of the above criteria is important, causality ultimately will be more believable if there is some acceptable biological explanation as to *why* such causal association might exist.

In summary, it is not possible to directly prove a causal hypothesis using case–control or cohort study designs. However, the causal hypothesis becomes much more tenable if the above five criteria can be established for the problem at hand.

Take-Home Points

- The use of a proper study design is essential to the investigation of risk factors for disease or other outcomes.
- Observational studies are useful in studying risk factors for disease or clinical outcomes.
- Cohort and case–control study designs are the most common strategies used in observational research, with cross-sectional studies playing a less important role.
- The choice between utilizing a cohort or case–control design depends upon several factors including disease prevalence and/or incidence, data availability and quality, and time required for follow-up.
- Confounding is a potentially serious problem that can affect the interpretation of either a cohort or a case–control study.
- Matching is a method used to reduce the effects of confounding.
- The degree of risk is quantified by the relative risk for cohort studies and the odds ratio for case–control studies.
- There are numerous sources of bias that can affect the interpretation of observational studies.
- In general, causality cannot be directly proven in observational studies, but certain criteria can suggest a causal hypothesis.

References

1. Manson JE, Nathan DM, Krolewsky AS, Stampfer MJ, Willett WC, Hennekens CH. A prospective study of exercise and incidence of diabetes among US male physicians. JAMA. 1992;268:63–7.
2. Colditz GA, Manson JE, Hankinson SE. The nurses' health study: contribution to the understanding of health among women. J Womens Health. 1997; 6:49–62.
3. Hennekens CH, Buring JE. Epidemiology in medicine. Boston: Little, Brown; 1987.
4. Kleinbaum D, Kupper L, Morgenstern H. Epidemiologic research: principles and quantitative methods. Belmont: Lifetime Learning; 1982.
5. Agresti A. Categorical data analysis. 2nd ed. Hoboken: Wiley; 2002.
6. DeAngelis C. An introduction to clinical research. New York: Oxford University Press; 1990.
7. Schlesselman JJ. Case-control studies. New York: Oxford University Press; 1982.
8. Rosenbaum PR, Rubin DB. Constructing a control group using multivariate matched sampling methods that incorporate the propensity score. Am Stat. 1985;39:33–8.
9. Rosenbaum PR, Rubin DB. Reducing bias in observational studies using subclassification on the propensity score. J Am Stat Assoc. 1991;79:516–24.
10. Swan SH, Shaw GM, Schulman J. Reporting and selection bias in case-control studies of congenital malformations. Epidemiology. 1992;3:356–63.
11. MacMahon B, Pugh TF. Epidemiology: principles and methods. Boston: Little, Brown and Company; 1970.

5 Fundamental Issues in Evaluating the Impact of Interventions: Sources and Control of Bias

Phyllis G. Supino

Introduction

The ability to draw valid inferences from data is the cornerstone of research and provides the basis for understanding the new knowledge that research results represent. In clinical research and, most importantly, in trials of therapy, such inferences determine whether the findings have any value in the real world. This chapter will review potential threats to validity of data-based inferences that may result from specific study design elements in assessment of purposively applied interventions and will present critical analyses of several published examples. It draws heavily on the seminal work of Donald T. Campbell and Julian C. Stanley [1] whose analysis, originally developed for the social sciences, provides a cogent theoretical framework for understanding the logical structure, strengths, and weaknesses of alternative study designs.

Potential Threats to Validity

In its broadest sense, validity is defined as the "best available approximation to the truth or falsity of a proposition" [2]. In scientific inquiry, validity refers to whether assertions made in a research study, including those about cause and effect, are likely to be true. Campbell and Stanley argued that two different types of validity, "internal" and "external" (described below), must be considered when evaluating the legitimacy of conclusions drawn from an interventional study. Both forms of validity are protected or jeopardized ("threatened") by the choice of study design and related methodological issues.

Threats to Internal Validity

Internal validity refers to the extent to which evaluators of the research are confident that a manipulated independent variable accounts for changes in a dependent variable. It is the indispensable element for interpreting the experiment. The independent variable is the "treatment" (e.g., drug, surgery) that is applied to study subjects; the dependent variable is the observed outcome (or response). To draw internally valid conclusions from an interventional study, dependence of outcome on treatment must be clearly apparent; other, potentially confounding factors must not be plausibly responsible for outcomes, or their impact must be definitively determinable so that the effect of the intervention can be unambiguously assessed. In other words, demonstration of an association between intervention and outcome, as in an observational study, would be inadequate; cause and effect must be inferable. Thus, the study design must effectively control for competing explanations (i.e., "rival hypotheses") for the findings. For

P.G. Supino, EdD (✉)
Department of Medicine, College of Medicine,
SUNY Downstate Medical Center,
450 Clarkson Avenue, 1199, Brooklyn,
NY 11203, USA
e-mail: phyllissupino@aol.com

P.G. Supino and J.S. Borer (eds.), *Principles of Research Methodology: A Guide for Clinical Investigators*,
DOI 10.1007/978-1-4614-3360-6_5,

the clinician, this would be equivalent to the logic underlying the protocols for ruling out myocardial infarction in the setting of chest pain. Campbell and Stanley identified eight factors that may threaten the internal validity of an interventional study. They referred to these as "internal validity threats" because they can provide competing explanations for observed outcomes and, thus, obscure true causal linkages. It is incumbent on a good investigator to use study designs devoid of these potential internal validity threats insofar as is possible.

1. *Selection Bias*. Selection bias is the improper assignment (allocation) of subjects for comparison. It is one of the most commonly recognized threats to the internal validity of an interventional study. An investigator may inadvertently contribute to this bias by nonrigorous matching (or failed randomization) techniques, or by choosing subjects for the experimental treatment who are believed to be most likely to benefit from it (a form of "referral bias"). For example, in a trial comparing surgery with medical treatment, those with the most favorable clinical profile might be assigned (referred) to the surgical group (based on presumed benefit), while the less robust patients might be assigned to the medically treated group. This approach is almost always optimistically biased in favor of the surgical group, which is why it is so difficult to form confident conclusions from trials conducted in this manner. It is equally incorrect to allow subjects to self-select their treatment assignments because volunteers for experimental treatments have been shown in various studies [3–5] to be different from the total ambient population in terms of personality (e.g., risk tolerance, decisiveness, action orientation), severity of disease or symptoms, and race, among other variables. These characteristics could skew associated outcomes in any direction (though it is generally thought that the direction of the bias induced by self-selection bias, like referral bias, is in favor of the experimental treatment).

   When groups to be compared are not equivalent initially for these or for any other reason, observed differences on outcome measures among the groups may be due to (or at least strongly influenced by) these baseline differences rather than to the intervention. Selection bias sometimes can be neutralized after data collection through statistical processes. However, the best strategy is to preclude the problem by using an appropriate study design to maximize the comparability of the compared groups prior to intervention.

2. *History Effects*. "History effects" are caused by events not related to, or anticipated by, the research protocol that occur during the study and influence outcomes. History effects potentially threaten internal validity when a study is performed in a less than isolated setting, particularly when effects on the dependent variable are assessed before and after the intervention and the temporal interval separating these assessments is relatively long. When history effects occur, measured outcomes may partially or completely reflect the outside event and not the intervention. History effects can be caused by factors such as unintended procedural or environmental changes in the experimental setting, changes in the social climate that can influence attitudes, media campaigns that can increase general knowledge, to newsworthy events relevant to the altered health concerns of subjects in the study, etc. As an example of the latter, if an investigator was evaluating the impact of a breast cancer awareness program to promote increased use of mammography and a well-known pubic figure was diagnosed with breast cancer, it would be difficult to determine whether the ensuring increased use of mammography was due to the program or to the media attention surrounding the public figure's diagnosis. In the clinical setting, history effects can be induced by changes in routine care (e.g., introduction of a new medication or other treatment, alterations in patient management, variations in patient reimbursement rules) that could impact study outcomes. The effects of history are best minimized by closely monitoring

to ensure that ancillary factors not directly integral to the intervention remain equivalent for all compared groups for the duration of the study. History effects also can be minimized by using contemporaneous (parallel) control group designs, where comparators would have equal likelihood of exposure to significant external events extraneous to the experimental setting.

3. *Maturation Effects*. "Maturation effects" are due to dynamic processes within subjects that may change with time and are independent of the intervention (e.g., growing older, progression or regression of illness). Like history, maturation may threaten internal validity when analysis of outcome depends on comparison of pre- and post-intervention measures. It is a particular concern when studies extend over long periods of time (longitudinal studies) during which biological alterations naturally can be expected and, thus, may affect outcomes. The effects of maturation, like selection bias and history effects, are minimized in parallel designs by selecting comparison groups likely to have similar developmental patterns.
4. *Testing Effects*. "Testing effects" are the influences of taking a test, being measured, or otherwise being observed, on the results of subsequent testing, measurement, or observation. Testing effects may occur whenever the testing process is itself a stimulus to change, even in the absence of a treatment. Examples are the act of being weighed during a weight-reduction program, or requiring patients receiving nicotine substitutes to document and periodically report the number of cigarettes they have smoked. In these cases, assuming the subjects are aware of the results of testing, the process of being measured may cause subjects to undertake lifestyle changes that will affect outcome independently of the intervention. Testing effects are potential concerns when measurement assesses knowledge, attitudes, behaviors, and (especially) skills, because the testing itself can provide an opportunity for altering subsequent results through practice or learning. The threat to internal validity can be minimized by using alternate forms of measurement for testing before and after intervention, or by eliminating pre- and post-intervention comparisons from the data analysis plan. Of course, as is true in virtually all interventional research, the latter approach requires demonstration of equivalence of the compared groups before the intervention is applied (i.e., at "baseline," the pre-intervention period, or control condition).
5. *Instrumentation Effects*. "Instrumentation effects" (also known as "instrument decay" or "instrument drift") are caused by changing measurement instruments or observers during the course of a study, or by intra-study changes in the *original* instruments or observers, that may cause systematic error (bias) in measuring the outcome variable. If the error entails consistent overprediction versus baseline, the bias is said to be positive; consistent underprediction is a negative bias [6]. For example, if alternate versions of a test instrument are used before and after an intervention to reduce testing effects, any observed changes may be due to differences in difficulty level (e.g., easier posttests in studies assessing educational impact) or other systematic variations in the alternative instruments, rather than to the intervention. To avoid instrument effects when alternate forms of measurement are employed, they should be previously evaluated to assure equivalence. Parallel problems can occur when observers are changed during the course of study since new observers may use different criteria for scoring and interpreting data than the original observers. Instrumentation effects also can occur when the same instrument (or observer) is used throughout the study since instrument calibration may change with time (or observer attitudes/assessment criteria may change with experience).

Like history and maturation, instrumentation effects are a potential threat to internal validity in any longitudinal study involving serial measurements. They are of particular concern when subjective measures (e.g., interviews or questionnaires) are used; in this situation, care must be taken to assure that instruments have demonstrated high reliability (internal consistency) to ensure stability. However, whether objective or subjective measures are used, observers may alter their interpretation of data as they grow more proficient or fatigued. Thus, instrumentation effects also can be minimized through development of standardized data collection protocols so that any fluctuations in measurement will occur randomly rather than systematically (or when comparing treatments by using the same observers across treatment conditions ["counterbalancing"] to avoid confounding).

6. *Statistical Regression.* "Statistical regression" is the tendency of individuals who scored extremely high or low on initial testing to score closer to the previously established population mean on subsequent retesting, independent of the intervention. This is one of the most often overlooked threats to internal validity, even among investigators who are well trained in statistics. Statistical regression results from measurement error, as extreme or highly deviant scores may arise due to chance. Such deviant scores are less likely to reappear on reevaluation. Regression effects can be minimized by avoiding the selection of a subject pool based on extreme scores, for example, very high blood pressure or low IQ scores. Another useful strategy to avoid regression effects is to obtain multiple measurements on each patient at several different appropriate times prior to intervention, or several measurements at the protocol-mandated baseline and time after intervention, which may then be averaged to optimize reliability of the estimate.
7. *Experimental Mortality.* "Experimental mortality" (or "attrition bias") is caused by the loss of subjects from a study who were originally included at baseline. Because subjects who withdraw may have different attributes than those who remain, their withdrawal may bias pre- to post-intervention comparisons, especially if these attributes are related to the outcome. Experimental mortality can bias outcome even for post-interventional comparisons if dropout is due to some characteristic of an intervention that is not related to the mechanism underlying its presumed efficacy. When comparison groups are used in an experimental design, a mortality bias also is introduced if the subjects lost to follow-up differ diagnostically among these groups. For example, a psychiatrist might wish to follow two groups of psychotic patients, one of which had been given an innovative treatment (the experimental group) while the other had been managed traditionally (the control group) to determine whether the intervention decreased return visits to his/her practice. If more severely ill patients were lost to follow-up in the intervention group than in the control group, the investigator might falsely conclude that reductions in return visits among the intervention group were attributable to the innovative treatment when, in fact, they may have occurred merely as a result of differences in attrition rates due to differences in illness severity. Experimental mortality is best minimized by using large groups of subjects who are geographically stable, accessible to investigators (i.e., have working telephone numbers and valid postal or e-mail addresses), and who are interested in participating in the study, and by developing strategies to facilitate follow-up. When subjects are lost, it is prudent to compare their baseline characteristics with those who remain in study to identify potential bias, and to utilize external vital statistics databases (e.g., the National Death Index) to identify and confirm deaths that may not be known to investigators.
8. *Interaction of Factors.* Sometimes two or more threats to validity can exist concurrently. These may combine to further restrict validity. Two factors that might be expected to combine are selection and maturation. For example, if two groups of patients were not initially equivalent in severity of illness (a selection bias), their illnesses might

progress at different rates (a maturation bias). Thus, one of the two groups might end up sicker, or healthier, than the other, irrespective of any intervention. This threat is best controlled by procedures to minimize individual biases (e.g., randomized allocation to treatment groups).

9. *Experimenter Bias*. In a perfect world, an investigator involved in a quantitative study would be detached and objective, maintaining a highly circumscribed relationship with the subject. In an interventional study, his or her responsibility is to administer or allocate subjects to a treatment and to impartially measure outcomes and other variables of interest. "Experimenter bias," not identified by Campbell and Stanley, occurs when the expectations of the investigator (usually unknowingly and unintentionally) influence the outcome of the study, thereby confounding the results. The profound impact of experimenter bias on internal validity was demonstrated by Rosenthal (1964) in his seminal studies of expectancy on experimenter judgment and learning outcomes conducted during the mid-1960s [7]. The experimenter's expectations typically arise from deeply seated views about his or her study hypothesis and can impact the study in a number of ways. For example, the investigator could subtly communicate expectations (cues) to participants about anticipated outcomes and influence them through the power of suggestion. The investigator could provide extra attention or care to subjects that is outside of the intervention (the latter is also termed "performance bias" when systematically done for members of only one of the comparison groups or "compensatory treatment bias" when specifically applied to controls). The investigator also can bias the study through improper ascertainment or verification of outcomes, for example, by searching more diligently for adverse events in patients with versus without hypothesized risk factors ("detection bias") or by assigning a more favorable rating on a subjective scale to subjects in the experimental versus control arm (a form of instrumentation bias). Experimenter bias is best controlled by techniques that blind both the investigator and the subject to the latter's treatment assignment, by the use of observers from whom the purpose of the study is withheld, and by standardization of the methodology of outcome assessment to ensure that subjects in the control group are evaluated as thoroughly and as frequently as those receiving the intervention.

10. *Subject Expectancy Effects*. The "subject expectancy effect" (also termed "nonspecific effects"), also not identified by Campbell and Stanley, is a cognitive bias that arises when a subject anticipates an outcome (positive or negative) from an intervention, and reports a response to the intervention that is premised on this belief. This is the basis of the "placebo effect," long recognized in clinical medicine. It occurs when a patient responds positively to an inactive intervention (e.g., a pharmacologically inert pill) and appears to improve subjectively and even, occasionally, objectively. This effect on outcome is due to the patient's belief that the intervention is curative. It may be stimulated or reinforced by suggestion of therapeutic benefit by an authority figure (e.g., physician or other investigator, as noted above under Experimenter Bias) and/or by the subject's inherent desire to please him or her. Indeed, the term placebo is derived from the Latin, "I will please." An opposite phenomenon is the "nocebo (Latin for, "I will harm") effect" which occurs when a subject reports negative responses to administration of an inert intervention due to his/her pessimistic expectation that it would produce harmful or unpleasant consequences. Although the magnitude of these subject expectancy effects is variable and somewhat controversial, there is general consensus that they can impact the validity of any study in which the subject is aware of receiving a treatment for which the outcome is subjective (e.g., studies involving pain control or symptom relief). As with experimenter bias, subject expectancy is best

controlled by utilizing study designs that "blind" the subject to his/her treatment assignment. For some type of interventions such as those involving lifestyle changes (e.g., dietary alterations, smoking cessation) or surgical studies, subject blinding may be difficult, if not impossible. (This is also true for those conducting these interventions and other members of the investigational team.) In these instances, blinded assessment of outcomes by external adjudicators could reduce, if not eliminate, expectancy biases. However, in many biomedical studies (e.g., those evaluating the effects of pharmacological agents), subjects (and investigators) can be blinded to treatment assignments through the use of placebos. The incorporation of placebos enables determination of treatment effects above and beyond those arising from subject (or investigator) expectancy. Obviously, placebos work best when they closely approximate the physical characteristics of the active intervention. (This problem is avoided in early phase I clinical trials of therapeutics where both placebo and active drug may be administered intravenously, or when the investigational intervention does not cause characteristic physiological effects that might unmask the treatment assignment.) When the treatment assignment is known to both subject and investigator, it is said to be "unblinded" (or "open"); when only the subject or the investigator (but not both) is unaware of the treatment assignment, the study is said to be "single blinded"; when treatment assignment is unknown both to subject and investigator, the study is said to be "double blinded"; and when it is unknown to the subject, investigator, and others analyzing or monitoring the data, the study is said to be "triple blinded."

Threats to External Validity

"External validity" refers to generalizability, that is, can the study findings be extrapolated to subjects, contexts, and times other than those for which the findings were obtained? Internal validity is a prerequisite for external validity. However, external validity is not assured even when internal validity has been established. In fact, the rigorous controls required to establish internal validity may inadvertently compromise a study's generalizability. The investigator must use a variety of strategies to strike a delicate balance between both concerns, if the study is to be both accurate (internally valid) and have practical utility (be externally valid). The four most common threats to external validity, identified in the seminal works of Campbell and Stanley, are given below.

1. *Reactive Effects of Testing*. The "reactive effects of testing" involve sensitization—or desensitization—of study subjects to interventions caused by the pre-intervention testing that might not be undertaken in the general, nonstudy population. This threat to external validity is most often encountered when pretests are obtrusive and/or outside of the normal experience of the subject. For example, to study the effects of a new nutrition program, an investigator might assess baseline knowledge of food groups and portion control, for the purpose of comparing pre- to post-intervention changes. If the pretest had focused attention on the intervention, any treatment effects that were observed might not be replicable if the pretest was not given. To diminish this bias, the investigator should minimize or, ideally, dispense with the use of pretests. However, as with its internal validity analog (testing effects), this approach is valid only when there is reasonable certainty that the comparison groups are equivalent at baseline. Alternatively, the investigator could opt to use the least obtrusive pre-intervention assessments to minimize reactivity. Special research designs (e.g., the Solomon four-square design), in which pretests are given to some but not all study subjects, can be used to determine the reactive effects of testing on study outcomes.
2. *Interactive Effects of Selection and Treatment*. Sometimes two investigators will run similar studies and obtain different findings. One possible cause of this outcome is the interactive effects of selection and treatment (or "selection-treatment interaction"). The interactive effects of selection and treatment are the

presumed basis of the failure of results found in an intervention study to be generalizable to other subjects to whom that intervention is applied. This failure occurs because the study was conducted on a sample that was not representative of the larger population to which results should be extrapolated. The selection-treatment interaction frequently is seen in clinical research when research subjects are scarce (a common situation) and the investigator is limited to those who present themselves and are willing to participate. In these situations, study subjects typically are selected by convenience, rather than by population-based sampling. A convenience sample includes all, or a portion, of patients who are being seen in a practice, hospital, or clinic, provided they meet the inclusion criteria of the study, and consent to participate. If the subjects selected for the study are, for example, healthier, wealthier, or wiser than the general population, or if they come from a unique geographic area, they may benefit more or less from a treatment, and it may not be possible to replicate the study, or to extrapolate its results to the larger population of interest. In theory, the interactive effects of selection and treatment are best controlled by random selection of subjects from the target population. Because this seldom is possible in clinical research (especially in randomized clinical trials [RCTs] in which strict inclusion/exclusion criteria and possibility of a subject's receiving a placebo sharply narrow the pool of study-eligible patients), the investigator should endeavor to select subjects who have characteristics similar to those to which he or she wishes to extrapolate results. Multicenter studies, drawing from diverse demographic populations, tend to suffer less than single-center studies from this external validity threat. Nonetheless, even small, single-center studies have value provided the investigator identifies and reports potential biases in his or her selection plan and is also careful to limit generalizations to appropriate populations.

3. *Reactive Effects of Experimental Arrangements.* This validity threat is defined as aberrant behavior exhibited by subjects that results solely as a consequence of their participation in an experiment, and that may not occur outside the experimental setting. The reactive effects of experimental arrangements are often confused with "the placebo effect." Although there are cognitive components inherent in both validity threats, the primary difference is that with the reactive effects of experimental arrangements, the subject's bias is based on the idiosyncrasies of the research environment, whereas with the placebo effect, the subject's bias is based on expectations about the treatment (that may or may not be part of a research study). The reactive effects of experimental arrangements were serendipitously discovered in a series of trials evaluating the impact of the work environment on employee productivity, conducted by Harvard University researchers between 1924 and 1932 at the Hawthorne Works, a factory plant of the Western Electric Company in Cicero, Illinois. The initial studies (illumination experiments) varied the level of light intensity to which employees were exposed. When the light intensity increased, worker output (and positive affect) improved but, much to the investigators' surprise, worker performance also improved when lighting intensity was diminished. The same pattern emerged when other environmental factors were manipulated. These unintended outcomes (also known as the "Hawthorne effect") [8] led the researchers to conclude that the mere act of being studied changed the participants' behavior (i.e., brought about a pseudo-treatment effect), confounding inferences about effects of the various interventions imposed upon them. Underlying mechanisms proposed to explain these findings include unintended special attention and benefits that may have been given to subjects by observers, uncontrolled novelty due to the artificiality of the experimental arrangements, and inadvertent responses to subjects from observers leading to learning effects that positively impacted performance. While there is no consensus as to the cause, the reactive effects of experiments

currently are recognized as a potential threat both to external and internal validity in research from various disciplines (e.g., medicine, education, psychology, and management science). Their impact is potentially problematic in any situation in which there is human awareness of participation in a study and in which study outcomes can be motivated by that knowledge. A related threat to validity that is caused by experimental arrangements is known as the "John Henry effect" [9]. This may occur when subjects in the control group, being aware of their treatment assignment, view themselves as competing with subjects in the intervention group and change their behavior (i.e., try harder) in an attempt to outperform them.

Whenever possible, the investigator should take steps to reduce the reactive effects of experimental arrangements to increase the likelihood that the findings from a study will be replicated beyond the experimental context. Methodological options for achieving this objective include (1) minimizing the obtrusiveness of experimental manipulations and measurements, (2) blinding subjects to their treatment assignment (to control for "John Henry effects"), and (3) providing equivalent attention to intervention and control groups, especially in studies involving psychological, behavioral, and educational outcomes. To accomplish this, investigators may include a "Hawthorne control group" that receives an irrelevant intervention to equalize subject contact with project staff.

4. *Multiple Treatment Interference.* A fourth threat to the external validity of an intervention study is "multiple treatment interference," defined as the influence of one treatment on another, which may produce results that would not be found if either were applied alone. Multiple treatment interference is a potential problem in any study in which more than one treatment (or treatment level) is given to, and formally evaluated in, the same subject. The threat applies even when the treatments are given in sequence because treatment effects may carry over and it may not be possible to eliminate the effects of the prior exposure. Under these conditions, it will be difficult to determine how much of the ultimate treatment outcome was attributable to the first treatment and how much was due to the second, thus limiting the applicability of the study findings to the real world in which patterns of treatment availability may not mirror those of study. Multiple treatment interference is very difficult to eradicate. It is best controlled by avoiding the use of within-subject designs. Where this is not possible, the investigator must carefully counterbalance or randomly order treatments across subjects and provide appropriate washout periods.

Elements of the Research Design

In analyzing the anatomy of a study to evaluate the impact of an intervention, it can be very helpful to employ shorthand that displays the major elements of the design, the sequence of events, and certain of the constraints within the design. This shorthand, based largely on the notation developed by Campbell and Stanley, will be used in the remainder of this chapter to examine the strengths and weaknesses of ten alternative study designs.

- The symbol X denotes the intervention (primary treatment or independent variable) that is applied to the subjects in the study. When more than one level of a treatment is included in a design, they are labeled X_0 (control), X_1, X_2, and so on; X_P indicates that a placebo has been given to control subjects (in designs incorporating parallel treatment arms) or during the control condition (in time-series or crossover design) to control for expectancy.
- Y indicates that a secondary treatment has been coadministered, concomitant with the primary treatment. Variations in levels of the secondary treatment, if any, may be distinguished by subscripts in a similar manner as for X. Absence of Y indicates absence of co-treatment.
- O is the observation (or measurement of the dependent variable) in the study. O may represent a test result, a record, or other data; when

more than one observation is involved over time, they are variously labeled as O_1, O_2, etc., to distinguish them.

- An arrow represents the experimental order (sequence of events during the study period).
- A dashed line indicates that intact groups (e.g., hospitals, clinics, or wards) have been compared (in other words, that subjects have *not* been allocated to treatment on a random basis).
- R indicates that study subjects have been allocated to treatment groups on a random basis. (Thus, a dashed line and R generally will not appear in the same design as these represent alternative methods of subject allocation to treatment.)

Alternative Research Designs

Several alternative research designs have been used to evaluate the effects of an intervention on some specified outcome. Each of these differs according to its adequacy in ensuring that valid inferences are made about the effects and generalizability of an intervention.

Pre-experimental Research Designs

The literature regrettably includes many studies that use designs which fail to control for most threats to internal validity. These are most properly termed "pre-experimental" designs because they contain only few of the essential structural elements needed to draw unambiguous inferences about the impact of an intervention. They are presented below to heighten the reader's awareness of their glaring deficiencies. The three most common are the following:

1. The one-shot case study
2. The pretest-posttest only design
3. The static-group comparison

Pre-Experimental Research Design # 1: The One-Shot Case Study

$$X \rightarrow O$$

Some studies in medicine utilize a design in which a single patient (or series of patients) is studied only once, following the administration an intervention. No pre- to post-intervention comparisons are made, and no concurrent control groups are used. Instead, inferences about causality are predicated on expectations of what would have been observed in the absence of the intervention, usually based on implicit comparison with past information. This most rudimentary pre-experimental design is termed the *one-shot case study* and is diagrammed as follows: X for the intervention, followed by an arrow, and O for the observation. Consider an example from the literature by R.F. Visser, published in the journal *Clinical Cardiology* [10] (summary and design structure are given in Fig. 5.1).

$$X \rightarrow O$$

Visser RF. Angiographic assessment of patency and reocclusion: Preliminary results of the Dutch APSAC Reocclusion Multicenter Study (ARMS). Clin Cardiol 1990;13:45-47.

In a multicenter study, 156 patients were treated with the thrombolytic drug anistreplase, within 4 hours of the onset of pain from an acute myocardial infarction (AMI), followed by continuous administration of heparin after 3-4 hours. Patency of the infarct-related vessel was defined by coronary angiography 90 minutes after anistreplase administration; angiography was repeated at 24 hours, among patients with a patent infarct-related vessel, to assess re-occlusion. Two cardiologists independently evaluated the angiograms and perfusion rates, using Thrombolysis in Myocardial Infarction (TIMI) criteria. Patency at 90 minutes was 73-75%; re-occlusion rate at 24 hours was 4%. The authors concluded that "...this patency rate corresponds with previous studies" and "...the low re-occlusion rate is noteworthy and probably reflects the prolonged action of anistreplase" [10].

Fig. 5.1 Example of a one-shot case study

In this study, the X represents the anistreplase, and the O represents the patency of the infarct-related vessels, as measured by TIMI criteria for perfusion. The authors contend that the X probably caused O, but have they presented convincing evidence of that association and protected the internal validity of their study?

The answer is that studies such have almost no value for determining cause and effect because, as Campbell and Stanley have noted, securing evidence of this nature involves, at minimum, making at least one direct comparison. Although the authors allude to the results of previous studies of patency following an AMI, no explicit data are presented against which patency in this investigation is compared; the absence of such control is even more striking for reocclusion rates. Even if data from historical controls were given, there is no assurance that previous patient characteristics and ancillary medical management were equivalent; in fact, they usually are not, due to differences in the health of a given population and alterations in medical technology over time. In addition, while standardized methodology (TIMI criteria) was used to determine initial patency and reocclusion, those reading the angiograms were aware of (and may have been influenced by) the intervention. Thus, *history*, *maturation*, *selection*, *experimental mortality*, and *expectancy* (*experimenter bias*) potentially threaten the internal validity of this study because each could explain the outcome. Furthermore, the external validity of this study also is threatened by the *interaction of selection and treatment* (due to small numbers of highly selected patients who may not be representative of the general population of patients with AMI), as well as by *multiple treatment interference* (note: heparin also was given to all subjects). As noted earlier, importance usually is not attached to the generalizability of a study that cannot be shown to be internally valid.

Pre-Experimental Research Design # 2 The One-group Pretest-Posttest Only Desig

$$O_1 \rightarrow X \rightarrow O_2$$

The *one-group pretest-posttest only design* represents a very slight improvement over the one-shot case study; it is a second pre-experimental design which also is commonly found in the medical literature. This design differs from the one-shot case study in that it collects baseline observations on study subjects that can be compared to observations made after the intervention. (The terms "pretest" and "posttest" are used generically in this chapter to refer to assessments of the dependent variable made, respectively, before and after the intervention.) Because study subjects are observed under more than one treatment condition, the one-group pretest-posttest study is considered one of the simplest versions of repeated measurement designs, described later in this chapter. Like the one-shot case study, this design contains no parallel comparison groups and is diagrammed as an O_1, for the pre-intervention observation; followed by an X, for the intervention; and followed by O_2, denoting the post-intervention observation, with arrows between. An example of a study employing this design was published by Wender and Reimmer in the *American Journal of Psychiatry* [11] (summary and design structure are given in Fig. 5.2).

In this study, O_1 represents the baseline attention deficit hyperactive disorder (ADHD) score, X is the bupropion treatment, and O_2 is the post-treatment ADHD score (Fig. 5.2). In the opinion of the authors, the improvement in O_2 relative to O_1 is the result of X. Can the authors' primary conclusion withstand scrutiny?

Again, we first consider internal validity. As in any repeated measures design, study subjects served as their own controls, effectively eliminating the threat of selection (allocation) bias. However, this design fails completely to control for the following other factors that also could account for the results. First, *history effects* are a potential threat to the internal validity of this study because it is possible that patients may have experienced an event external to the intervention, and that this event, not the intervention, may have improved their ability to focus. A second potential threat is *maturation* because, as in any longitudinal study, the conditions of the study subjects may have changed on their own. Yet another threat to internal validity is *testing*, since exposure to the pretest may have improved performance on the posttest. There is also the threat of *instrumentation effects* as the tests may not

$$O_1 \rightarrow X \rightarrow O_2$$

Wender P, Reimherr F. Buproprion treatment of attention deficit hyperactivity disorders in adults. Am J Psych 1990;147:1018-1020.

Nineteen adults with attention deficit hyperactivity disorder (ADHD) were treated for 6-8 weeks with buproprion, after discontinuing prior medication. Severity of ADHD was rated before and after treatment using the Clinical Global Impression (CGI), and Targeted Attention Deficit Symptoms (TADDS) scales. Fourteen patients responded to bupropion: 8 had CGI scores indicating marked response and 6 had scores suggesting moderate response. TADDS scores before and after treatment differed significantly ($p<.0005$). The investigators concluded that bupropion appeared to be effective in the treatment of ADHD, though they noted that the study suffered "...from all the limitations of any open trial" [11].

Fig. 5.2 Example of the one-group pretest-posttest only design

have been well standardized. (Indeed, the authors are silent about the test-retest reliability of their instruments.) *Statistical regression* poses another possible threat, if the study subjects had been chosen on the basis of extremely poor scores on the initial test. In the final analysis, because so many potential individual biases are uncontrolled in this study, there is also the strong likelihood that interaction of these factors could undermine its internal validity and the conclusions drawn from it. Indeed, Campbell and Stanley argued that this type of design should be used only when nothing else can be done.

The study also suffers from several threats to external validity, namely, the potential for *selection-treatment interaction*. First of all, very few subjects were studied, and it is highly unlikely that they were representative of all patients being treated for ADHD (selection-treatment interaction). Second, the subjects (as well as their doctors) were unblinded, and subjects may have "improved" due to the effects of their participation in the study (*reactive effects of experimental arrangements*). These issues are noted only for completeness. As noted above, this study fails to meet criteria for internal validity; thus, its generalizability is unimportant.

Pre-Experimental Research Design # 3
The Static-Group Comparison

$$X \rightarrow O_1$$
- - - - - -
$$O_2$$

A third pre-experimental design also found in the literature is the *static-group comparison*. This design incorporates two groups: one that receives an intervention (again denoted as X) and a second that does not receive an intervention and which serves a control (denoted by the absence of X). Groups one and two typically are observed concurrently after the intervention has been applied in one of the groups, and the observations made in these groups are denoted by the Os. This design includes no pretesting or baseline measurements. Note that both intervention and control groups are separated, schematically, by a dashed line to indicate that study subjects were assigned to treatment as intact groups, that is, they were not randomly allocated to treatment. A study, published by Bolland et al. in the *Journal of the American Dietetic Association* [12], employed a variant of this design which tested for effects extended over time (summary and design structure are given in Fig. 5.3).

Are these conclusions credible? A review of the structure of this design will be revealing. In this study, X represents the food quantity estimation intervention, and the O represents the post-intervention assessments of knowledge of food quantities in the experimental (trained) and control (untrained) groups, assessed at three different times among trained subjects. (The reader should note that the use of deferred assessments is not typical of the static-group comparison design but was used in this study in an attempt to define persistence of treatment effects.) The broken line

$$X \rightarrow O_1$$
- - - - - - - - -
$$O_2$$

Bolland J et al. Improved accuracy of estimating food quantities up to 4 weeks after treatment. J Am Dietetic Assn 1990;90:1402-1407.

Two hundred and eight student volunteers from an introductory nutrition series were divided into two groups. One group received training in estimating food quantities, the other no training. Training comprised a single 10-minute session during which subjects watched an investigator display and explain the portion sizes of 10 different food models which then were disseminated to the students for closer observation. To assess learning, the trained subjects estimated quantities of 6 real foods immediately after training, a week later or 4 weeks later; the untrained study subjects performed their assessments immediately after the training. The investigators found that estimates made by subjects immediately and a week after their training were comparable (NS) and were significantly better ($p<.05$) than those at 4 weeks and vs. untrained subjects. They concluded that "These results support the use of training, with food models, to improve an individual's ability to estimate food quantities accurately, and indicate that the impact of such training lasts for at least one week, and can last up to four weeks". They also claimed that the findings from their study "imply that training with periodic reviews may be necessary in a clinical setting to ensure that patients estimate their food consumption accurately" [12].

Fig. 5.3 Example of the static-group comparison design

between the experimental and control groups indicates the intact nature of the comparison groups, signifying that subject assignment to the intervention or control comparison group was not random.

The static-group comparison design represents an improvement over the one-shot case study because the inclusion of a contemporaneous control group permits comparison of the results of the trained study subjects with the other, untrained study subjects, evaluated approximately in parallel, thereby avoiding the obvious biases inherent in the use of external or historical controls (or, in the worst-case scenario, no controls). Moreover, the fact that study subjects in both groups are being evaluated in the same way during a relatively short interval decreases the potential for maturation and instrumentation effects (assuming uniform data collection). Finally, this design also represents an improvement over the one-group pretest-posttest only design because the absence of pretesting and subject selection based on extreme pretest scores obviates the threat of testing effects and statistical regression.

Nonetheless, there are two potential threats to internal validity for which this design affords absolutely no protection. The first threat is *selection* (or *allocation bias*). The authors do not tell us how the study subjects were divided into treatment groups. Was it by instructor preference or self-selection by the study subjects? Either of these scenarios would be equally flawed because without baseline (pre-intervention) assessments, there is no way to determine whether the observed outcomes were due to the training or to pre-intervention differences in the subjects' knowledge about estimating food quantities. Even if the investigators had attempted to match the groups on other variables, such matching would be ineffective in achieving true baseline parity among trained versus untrained subjects, especially if subjects had, indeed, self-selected participation in the intervention. In addition, even though the study was relatively short in duration, the validity of the conclusions, nonetheless, is threatened by the potential for *experimental mortality* (*attrition bias*) as no information is given about whether *all* subjects who began this study actually completed it or whether attrition (if it did occur) differed systematically between the two groups. Thus, even if subjects were comparable on average before training, the apparent superiority of the trained group (relative to the untrained group) on the outcome measure possibly could have been due to several of the less knowledgeable students dropping from the former group (or, conversely, due to some of the more knowledgeable students dropping from the latter group) prior to testing.

The primary threat to external validity is the *interaction of selection and treatment.* (After all, how representative is one class of introductory nutrition students of the larger relevant population?) However, since the internal validity of the study is severely compromised, this threat to external validity has little if any importance.

True-Experimental Research Designs

The most prominent characteristic of true-experimental designs is random allocation of study subjects, drawn from a common population, to alternative treatment conditions. When this approach is employed, participants' baseline characteristics can be expected to be equally distributed across the various comparisons according to the "laws" of probability, especially when sample size is large. Even when randomization does not result in perfect equivalence, most workers in the field believe that this form of treatment allocation is the best way to reduce the threat of selection bias. The theoretical underpinnings of randomized designs can be traced to Fisher and Mackenzie's agricultural experiments in the 1920s [13]; however, it was not until the late 1940s that they made their appearance in the medical literature, when the RCT was first used to demonstrate the efficacy of streptomycin in the treatment of tuberculosis [14]. Since that time, the RCT has been considered the standard to be met for clinical research, even though investigations of this type comprise only a minority of the clinical research ever conducted or published. Randomization also is important in many preclinical/basic science research protocols, though other considerations may minimize application of this approach in the nonclinical setting.

Most commonly randomization is *fixed*, less commonly it is *adaptive*. With fixed random allocation, each subject has an equal probability of assignment to the alternative study arms, and that probability remains constant throughout the study. The randomization process can be performed according to a coin toss or a table of random numbers or special computer software can be used. This type of randomization is known as *simple randomization* and works best when sample size is relatively large. However, when sample size is small, simple randomization may result in statistically unequal groupings. Under these circumstances, restrictive randomization methods (e.g., *blocked randomized designs* or *stratified random allocation)* can be employed. With *blocked randomization,* subjects are assigned to treatment in groups (blocks) that are similar to one another with regard to a source (or several important sources) of variability that is (are) not of primary interest to the experimenter (e.g., a potential confounding variable such as gender, geographic area). *Stratified randomization* is performed by conducting separate randomization procedures within each of two or more subgroups of subjects that are defined according to prespecified patient characteristics (usually important prognostic risk factors) and increases the likelihood that allocation to treatment is well balanced within each stratum. With *adaptive methods* (a Bayesian approach increasingly used in contemporary clinical trials) [15], the probability of allocation changes in response to accumulating information during the study about the composition of, or outcomes associated with, the alternative treatment arms. (For a comprehensive discussion of the theory and techniques of adaptive randomization, the reader is referred to Hu and Rosenberger, 2006 [16].)

As noted, the purpose of randomization is to render the comparison groups as similar as possible at study entry to permit valid inferences to be drawn about the effects of an intervention. However, during the course of the trial, some patients may not initially receive the intended intervention or, during the course of the study, may drop out or cross over to the alternate treatment for a variety of reasons. One widely used solution to circumvent these problems is *intention-to-treat analysis* (ITT), which defines the comparison groups according to initial assigned treatment rather than to the treatment actually received or completed (i.e., "once randomized, always analyzed"). Many workers in the field consider ITT analysis to be the gold standard method of analysis for clinical trials [17], describing it as the least biased for drawing inferences about trial results [17, 18], and it is considered the pivotal analysis by major regulatory bodies in Europe and in the USA for approval of new therapeutics. However, the reader should note that ITT analysis provides only a pragmatic estimate of the benefit of a new treatment policy rather than an estimate of potential benefit in patients "who receive treatment exactly as planned"; moreover, full application of this method "is possible only when complete outcome data are available for all randomized subjects" [19]. Thus, The ITT approach is not without its critics [20]. Some clinical trialists argue that efficacy is best demonstrated when analysis focuses on subjects who actually received the treatment of interest (sometimes termed "efficacy subset analysis"), arguing that ITT approaches provide an overly conservative estimate of the magnitude of treatment effects principally due to dilution of effects by nonadherence. In addition, ITT analysis creates difficulty in interpretation of findings if numerous participants cross over to opposite treatment arms. Finally, it is suboptimal for studies of equivalence, generally increasing the likelihood of erroneously concluding that no difference exists between two test articles [21]. A common solution is to employ both methods of analysis in the same study, using ITT and "on-treatment" approaches as primary and secondary analysis, respectively.

Four of the most common true-experimental designs found in the biomedical literature are the following:

1. The pretest-posttest control group design
2. The posttest only control group design
3. The true-experimental 2×2 factorial design
4. The crossover study (two-period design)

The first two designs can be used to evaluate the impact of a single intervention (vs. control or an alternate intervention), and the third and fourth permit the investigator to examine the separate effects of two interventions (again, vs. control or an alternate intervention) applied within the same study. All provide much better protection than do pre-experimental designs against most threats to internal validity.

True Experimental Design # 1
The Pretest-Posttest Control Group Design

$$\begin{array}{l} R \rightarrow O_1 \rightarrow X \rightarrow O_2 \\ R \rightarrow O_3 \qquad\quad\ \ \rightarrow O_4 \end{array}$$

In the most common form of the *pretest-posttest control group design*, study subjects are randomly allocated to two comparison groups or treatment arms. One group receives the experimental intervention and the second, no intervention, a placebo, or an alternate intervention. Both groups are observed, in parallel, before and after the intervention on the same outcome measure(s) to determine whether change varied as a function of the treatment. The structure of this design is represented symbolically above: R denotes that subjects have been randomly allocated to the comparison groups; X denotes that a treatment has been given to the first group; absence of X in the second group indicates that this is a control group (the control group also could have been denoted by X_0 [or X_p if a placebo had been given]). O and its positioning indicate the observations made in both groups before and after the intervention. An example of a study incorporating this design was published by Gorbach et al. in the *Journal of the American Dietetic Association* [22] (summary and design structure are given in Fig. 5.4).

The structural representation of this study is a clue to the strength of its internal validity. Here, X represents fat reduction dietary intervention; the absence of X represents no dietary intervention, the control group; O_1 and O_3 represent baseline fat intake in the experimental and control groups; O_2 and O_4 represent post-intervention fat intake in both groups; R signifies that the study is randomized.

Because study subjects have been randomly allocated to comparison groups from a common subject pool, selection bias has been removed as a serious threat to internal validity, assuming that the randomization was effective. Having baseline measures of the dependent variable (and other

$$R \rightarrow O_1 \rightarrow X \rightarrow O_2$$
$$R \rightarrow O_3 \qquad \rightarrow O_4$$

Gorbach SL et al. Changes in food patterns during a low-fat dietary intervention in women. J Am Diet Assoc 1990;90:802-809.

Three hundred and three women at high risk for breast cancer (including 65% with advanced educations and 25% with annual household incomes >$50,000) were recruited from 3 clinical units. Of these, 184 were randomized into a 12 month-long dietary intervention group that encouraged reduction of fat intake to 20% of total calories and 119 were randomized into a control group in which customary diets were followed. The intervention employed group sessions to teach the nutrition information and behaviors to promote healthy life-style dietary changes. Four-day food records were collected from study subjects at the beginning of the study and again at 12 months, and compared by t-test. To enhance validity and reliability of data collection, a standardized protocol was followed for gathering and documenting food records, and data additionally were blind-coded to enhance experimenter objectivity. The results showed a 60% reduction in daily fat intake (76 to 31 gm for the experimental group, $p<.001$). In contrast, a far smaller decrease (74 to 66 gm, $p<.01$) was observed in the control group. The authors found that not only was the intervention successful in reducing fat intake, but it promoted other beneficial dietary changes and led to weight loss (an unintended benefit). The authors, therefore, concluded that the principles and strategies of this intervention hold promise for future public health programs, including diet and life-style changes [22].

Fig. 5.4 Example of the pretest-posttest control group design

key variables that potentially could influence it) and comparing them between groups permits us to confirm or reject this assumption; these comparisons typically are expressed in tabular form in most published RCTs. History effects are controlled because if a potentially confounding general external event had occurred, it should have affected the comparison groups equally since they are studied in parallel; nonetheless, as noted earlier in this chapter, the investigator must be vigilant and attempt to control for differences between comparison groups that might occur on a more "micro" level (i.e., within group variations in temperature, time of day, season, etc.). For similar reasons, the use of a parallel design also protects against the threats of maturation, testing, and instrumentation effects because natural variations in these factors should impact comparison groups equally; instrumentation effects also are minimized here because all data were collected using standardized techniques. In this study, subjects were selected on the basis of high risk for breast cancer, *not* on the basis of extremes in pre-intervention fat and energy intake. However, even if they had been chosen according to the latter criterion, average regression effects would not confound interpretation of the results because if they had occurred, they should have been equivalent in the comparison groups, given that the subjects were randomly allocated from a common subject pool. Thus, this design also protects against statistical regression. Finally, while treatment assignment could not be fully blinded (as noted earlier, a common characteristic of studies evaluating impact of lifestyle interventions) to entirely eliminate the threat of expectancy effects, the investigators endeavored to reduce them by standardizing their methodology for outcome ascertainment and by blind-coding data to ensure that subjects in the control group and those receiving the intervention were evaluated uniformly and impartially. The one error made in this study was the use of an incorrect test of statistical significance (i.e., computing two sets of t-tests, one for the experimental group and one for the control group, rather than conducting direct statistical comparisons of the changes between the groups). With this single exception (which Campbell identified as "a wrong statistic in common use" among investigators employing these designs [1]), the use of random allocation to parallel treatment groups afforded by the application of the pretest-posttest parallel group design, coupled with standardized data collection methodology, protected this study very well from most factors that could have undermined its internal validity, thus maximizing the likelihood that the intervention, rather than other factors, was responsible for the observed outcomes.

However, the external validity of this study is open to question. The reason is that randomized designs, including this model, may lead to conclusions that, while internally valid for the study, may not generalize to the reference population for the following three reasons.

First of all, in this study, pretests were used to assess relative change in fat and energy intake in the comparison groups. Their use may have sensitized study subjects to the intervention, with the possibility that results might not generalize when the intervention is applied without pretesting. This threat to external validity, known as the *interactive effect of testing and treatment* and described earlier, is a potential problem for any pretest-posttest comparison design, randomized or not, unless the testing itself is considered a component of the intervention being studied.

Another potential threat to external validity is the *interaction of selection and treatment*. Since the purpose of hypothesis testing is to make inferences about the reference population from which study subjects are drawn, the representativeness of the study group must be ascertained for the general population of women at high risk for breast cancer. As noted, the majority of subjects in this study were well educated, and a quarter had annual household incomes that were relatively high for the time (1990). It is also relevant that patients were excluded from the study for a number of reasons including, but not limited to, their unwillingness to sign an informed consent form, or because they were judged by the study nutritionist to be potentially unreliable in complying with the study protocol. Unfortunately, as is the case for many published RCTs, the authors fail to state how many patients were excluded for these reasons, making it difficult to evaluate the potential adverse impact of the selection-treatment interaction, which must be considered, even though hundreds of subjects were enrolled in the trial.

A third potential threat to the external validity is *the reactive effects of the experimental arrangements*. Because the intervention was not part of the routine care of this population and informed consent was required, subjects certainly were aware of their participation in an "experiment." All subjects would have been exposed to the novelty associated with random allocation techniques and new ways of keeping food records. Subjects in the intervention group would have been exposed to new health-care providers (in this study, the nutritionists) and, as a part of such intervention, may well have received more attention from project personnel than those told to follow customary diets (i.e., the control group), unless a "Hawthorne control" had been built into the study (which it had not). Any of these factors might have led to changes that were due to reactivity to the experiment (a possibility that is supported by changes in fat and energy consumption, albeit of a lesser magnitude, among control group participants), raising the concern that the effects of the intervention might not be replicated when applied nonexperimentally.

True-Experimental Design # 2
The Posttest Only Control Group Design

$$\begin{array}{lll} R \rightarrow X \rightarrow & O_1 \\ R \rightarrow \quad\;\; \rightarrow & O_2 \end{array}$$

The next approach, called a *posttest only control group design*, again utilizes two groups: each has been randomly allocated to treatment; as before, one group receives the intervention, represented by X, and the second group either receives no intervention, an alternate intervention, or—if it is a drug study—sometimes a placebo (designated as X_p). Both are observed after the intervention only, as shown by the positioning of O. The major distinction between this design and the preceding one is that, here, study subjects are *not* assessed on the dependent (outcome) variable at baseline. Instead, they are compared only *after* the intervention. Unless knowledge of relative *change* on an

$$R \rightarrow X \rightarrow O_1$$
$$R \rightarrow X_p \rightarrow O_2$$

β-Blocker Heart Attack Research Group. A randomized trial of propranolol in patients with acute myocardial infarction. JAMA 1982;247:1707-1714.

A multicenter placebo-controlled randomized study was used to test the hypothesis that regular administration of the β-blocker, propranolol, would reduce mortality among patients who had suffered a recent myocardial infarction (MI). Approximately 4,000 patients, 30- 69 years of age, were randomized to either propranolol or placebo, 5-21 days after the MI, and were followed 2-4 event-free years (avg. 25 months). Dosage assignments were made through a coordinating center, and were blinded both to patients and physicians. Mortality (all causes) was approximately 7% in the propranolol group and 10% in the placebo group (p<.005). Deaths due to arteriosclerotic heart disease were approximately 6% and 9%, respectively, in the propranolol and placebo groups (p<.01); sudden cardiac deaths also were less frequent among patients taking propranolol (3.3% vs. 4.6% among controls [p<.05]). Side effects were rare. Based on these findings, the authors concluded that propranolol is recommended for at least 3 years among patients who have had a recent MI and no contraindications to β-blockade [23].

Fig. 5.5 Example of the posttest only control group design

outcome is required, baseline assessments of the dependent variable are not necessary for establishing comparability of the comparison groups in true-experimental designs, since random allocation to treatment should eliminate the threat of selection bias. As noted earlier, this is especially true if the number of study subjects is large and the randomization strategy is properly executed. Nevertheless, baseline data on relevant demographic and clinical variables other than study outcomes typically are collected to permit examination of this assumption.

The posttest only control group design is especially appropriate in situations where within-subject outcomes logically cannot be defined before application of the intervention (e.g., in studies relating impact of the intervention on survival). A classic example was published by the β-Blocker Heart Attack Research Group in the *Journal of the American Medical Association* [23] (summary and design structure are given in Fig. 5.5).

In this study design, X represents the experimental drug, in this case propranolol, and X_p is the placebo. O_1 and O_2, respectively, represent the percent mortality for the propranolol and placebo groups. As before, the symbol R denotes the use of randomized allocation to treatment group.

How well does this study design protect against threats to internal validity? The answer is very well. Again, as for pretest-posttest parallel control group design, the use of random allocation of almost 4,000 patients to treatment assignment controls for selection bias (the comparability of the distributions of baseline clinical variables, electrocardiographic abnormalities, age, gender, and other descriptors between the propranolol and placebo groups noted in their manuscript illustrates this point). In addition, the use of parallel comparison group post-intervention comparisons, rather than sole reliance on within-group changes without controls, effectively rules out history, maturation, testing, mortality, regression, and instrumentation effects and their interactions as competing explanations for the outcomes. In addition, because the study was double blinded, both subject expectancy and experimenter bias also are eliminated as potential threats to validity.

The study also is superior to that of Gorbach et al. with regard to external validity. The reason is that the posttest only comparison group design does not require pre-intervention assessments as a benchmark against which to establish intervention effects. Thus, by definition, it controls for the reactive effects of testing. Indeed, this is the primary advantage of this design versus the pretest-posttest parallel group design. In this study, the outcomes of the intervention were all "hard" events rather than behavioral or educational outcomes, and the intervention, itself, involved medication rather than promotion of lifestyle change. Therefore, the reactive effects of experimental arrangements, if any, should be minimal, provided that the investigators took care to minimize the obtrusiveness of the experimental manipulations and measurements. Nonetheless, while the study was large and multicentered, the authors reported that 77% of those patients invited to participate did not do so. Therefore, despite the many thousands of patients enrolled, there is still a question of how representative the sample was of the general population after a recent MI. Consequently, the external validity of this study potentially is threatened by the *selection-treatment interaction* which, as noted earlier, is a common problem in many RCTs.

True-Experimental Design # 3
The 2 X 2 Factorial Study

R→	**X**	**Y → O_1**
R→		**Y → O_2**
R→	**X**	**→ O_3**
R→		**→ O_4**

The first two true-experimental designs permitted the investigator to evaluate the impact of a primary treatment versus an alternative primary treatment or control. True-experimental factorial designs are modifications that include a secondary treatment administered concurrently with the primary treatment to permit examination of the modification of the main and interactive effects of each. They can be designed with and without pretests (as above) and with or without blinding, if the latter is not practical or possible.

An example of these designs is diagramed above. This exemplar is termed a *2×2 factorial true-experimental design* and includes four concurrent parallel groups: the first two groups receive a primary treatment, denoted by X, and the second two receive no primary treatment, denoted by the absence of X (or, alternatively, X_0) or X_p if placebos are given to the nontreatment controls. In a variation of this design (for evaluation of comparative effectiveness), the second group might receive an alternative primary treatment (in this case, these treatments would be designated X_1 and X_2 to differentiate them). One group receiving the primary treatment and one receiving an alternate treatment, or no primary treatment, also receive a secondary treatment, denoted here as Y. The remaining two groups do not or may receive a placebo. The groups are observed in parallel after application of the intervention, as denoted by O. A 2×2 true-experimental design, published by the International Study Group in *The Lancet* [24], was employed to evaluate the relative effectiveness and safety of two thrombolytic drugs administered with or without heparin (summary and design structure denoted are given in Fig. 5.6).

In this study, X_1 represents streptokinase, and X_2 represents alteplase. Y indicates concomitant administration of heparin; the absence of Y indicates that *no* heparin was given. O_1–O_4 denote the percentages of in-hospital deaths in each of the comparison groups (Fig. 5.6).

Because this study (like those using true-experimental designs #1 and #2) employed a design that randomly allocated subjects to four large parallel treatment arms, selection bias is controlled as are history effects, maturation, instrumentation, testing, experimental mortality, and regression. Unfortunately, neither patients nor investigators were blinded to the former's treatment assignment. Thus, the study did not control for the potential effects of *expectancy*. This omission is important because even though the dependent variable clearly was an "objective outcome" (i.e., death) and randomization led to groups that appeared to be well balanced at study entry, knowledge of the treatment assignment still could have resulted in unintended differences between the treatment arms in the use of nonprotocol-mandated co-interventions (e.g., percutaneous coronary angioplasty or coronary bypass grafting) that, themselves, could have influenced study outcomes. This design flaw, of course, is not a limitation of the true-experimental factorial design (which, otherwise, controls very well for major threats to internal validity) but, as noted earlier, is a problem associated with any "open" (unblinded) study. Had the study been blinded,

$$\begin{array}{lll} R\rightarrow & X_1 & Y\rightarrow O_1 \\ R\rightarrow & X_2 & Y\rightarrow O_2 \\ R\rightarrow & X_1 & \;\;\rightarrow O_3 \\ R\rightarrow & X_2 & \;\;\rightarrow O_4 \end{array}$$

The International Study Group. In-hospital mortality and clinical course of 20,891 patients with suspected acute myocardial infarction randomized between alteplase and streptokinase with or without heparin. The Lancet 1990;336:71-74.

In an unblinded clinical trial, approximately 21,000 patients with a suspected acute myocardial infarction of <6-hrs duration were randomly allocated to receive one of two thrombolytic drugs: alteplase (t-PA) or streptokinase (SK). In addition, half of the study subjects in each treatment arm were randomly assigned to receive heparin <12 hrs after the start of thrombolytic therapy. Co-administration of aspirin and intravenous β-blockade was recommended, by protocol, for all subjects in the absence of contraindications to either. The results indicated that the overall fatality rate was low for all groups, and no significant differences in hospital mortality – the primary endpoint – were found between patients who had been allocated to alteplase or streptokinase, or between those given heparin vs. no heparin. An interaction was found between heparin and the type of thrombolytic therapy, with lower mortality rates evidenced when heparin was added to streptokinase; however, no thrombolytic therapy-heparin interaction was noted with respect to other clinical outcomes. Due to the low mortality rates in all groups the authors concluded that SK, t-PA, and heparin are each relatively safe. However, because mortality was not consistently lower with heparin, it was concluded that further clinical trials were needed to establish a possible beneficial effect of similar administration of heparin and thrombolytic therapy [24].

Fig. 5.6 Example of a 2×2 factorial true-experimental design

this true-experimental factorial design, like the two preceding true-experimental designs, would, in theory, have afforded full protection against most, if not all, serious threats to internal validity.

The chief advantage of this study design for external validity (vs. the crossover study, discussed below) lies in fact that its structure permits a purposive and systematic evaluation of the separate and combined (i.e., interactive) effects of concomitant investigational therapies, thereby avoiding unplanned carryover effects and precluding the threat of multiple treatment interference. Though this design can increase the efficiency of interventional trials by permitting simultaneous tests of several hypotheses, the reader should be aware that if interactions are severe, loss of statistical power is possible [25]. A limitation to the external validity of this particular study (but not to factorial designs in general) is the coadministration of noninvestigational drugs (i.e., β-blockade and aspirin) among all patients without contraindications to these therapies, which prevents us from generalizing the mortality findings to similar patients in whom these therapies are not given.

True Experimental Design # 4
The Two-Period Crossover (Change-Over) Design

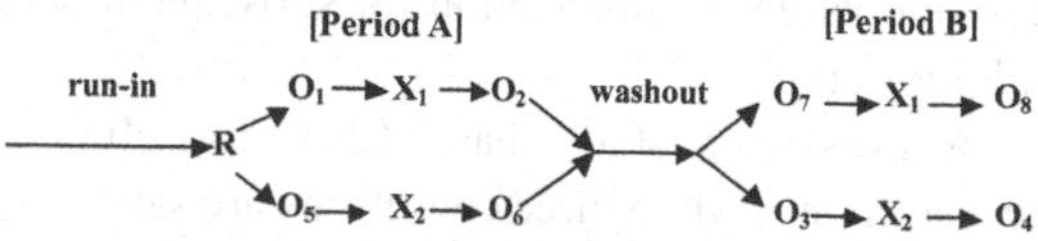

In the previous example, the main and interactive effects of two treatments were evaluated. To accomplish this, a factorial parallel (between-subjects) design was used that required allocation of large numbers of subjects into four different treatment arms, resulting in one protocol-mandated exposure per subject during the course of the study. In contrast, if the study objectives were to determine only the main (isolated) effects of two treatments, rather than their interactions, this objective could be accomplished more efficiently (i.e., with fewer subjects producing equivalent statistical power or precision) using the *true-experimental crossover* (or *changeover*) *design*. A crossover design is a type of repeated measures design in which each subject is exposed to different treatments during the study (but they "cross" or "change" over from one treatment to another). The order of treatment administration (determined à priori via randomization) is termed a "sequence," and the time of the treatment administration is called a "period." The statistical efficiency of the design results from the fact that each subject acts as his or her own control, thereby minimizing error due to (and sample size needed to overcome) the effects of between-subject variability. Crossover designs have enjoyed popularity in many disciplines including medicine, psychology, and agriculture. They are commonly used in the early stages of clinical trials to assess the efficacy and safety of pharmacological agents and constitute the preferred methodological approach for establishing bioequivalence.

A variant that can be used for these purposes is the "n-of-1" study, a mini-RCT in which a single patient is observed during exposure to randomly ordered sequences of treatment (frequently given in varying doses) and placebo. Both the patient and clinician are blinded as to treatment allocation, and the codes are broken after the trial. Responses, such as reported side effects, are graphed or analyzed through a variety of parametric and nonparametric statistical techniques. When performed in series, the "n-of-1" study can provide valuable information for subsequent parallel group trials.

A crossover study has utility for clinical research only when three conditions are satisfied: (1) subjects must have a chronic stable disease that is not likely to progress during the study; (2) study endpoints must be transitory, that is, must reflect temporary physiological changes (e.g., blood pressure) or relief of pain, rather than cure (or death); and (3) the investigational treatments must be able to deliver relatively rapid effects that are quickly reversible after their withdrawal. The latter point is especially critical. If the effects of the investigational interventions are permanent or more long lasting than anticipated, their carryover effects could compromise the validity of data obtained after the initial period (e.g., cause under- or overestimation of the efficacy of the second treatment) and undermine the efficiency of the study.

Although crossover studies can involve multiple periods and sequences, the most common is true-experimental design #4, the two-period crossover design, illustrated symbolically above. When this approach is used to test the efficacy and safety of different investigational drugs, subjects normally will undergo a run-in period during which noninvestigational medications are discontinued and a suitably long washout interval between the two active treatment periods, A and B, (the latter guided by the bioavailability of the drugs) so as to minimize the likelihood of carryover effects. Typically, half of the sample initially receives the first drug, denoted by X_1, and the other half initially receives the second drug, denoted by X_2. Following the washout, study subjects who received the first drug are given the second drug, and vice versa, resulting in a fully counterbalanced design. Observations are recorded pre- and postdrug administration in the two treatment periods, denoted by O. The symbol R to the left of the diagram indicates that the order of initial treatment assignment is allocated at random to counter possible order effects. An example of a study employing a crossover design was conducted by Seabra-Gomes et al. [26] who evaluated the relative effects of two antianginal drugs on exercise performance in men with stable angina (summary and design structure are given in Fig. 5.7).

In this study, X_1 denotes isosorbide-5-mononitrate and X_2 stands for isosorbide dinitrate. O_1–O_3 are the outcome variables measured among patients receiving X_1 during period A; O_4–O_6 are the same variables measured during period B. O_7–O_{12} are the outcome variables measured among patients initially receiving X_2. R indicates that the order of the initial drug assignments was randomly allocated.

As with all other true-experimental models, internal validity is very well controlled with this design. Selection bias is eliminated because study subjects are their own controls and comparisons of outcomes are made within rather than between

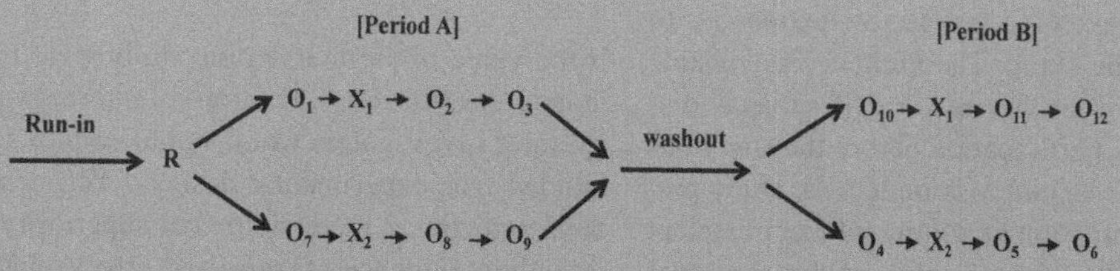

Seabra-Gomes R, et al. Comparison of the effects of a controlled-release formulation of isosorbide-5-mononitrate and conventional isosorbide dinitrate on exercise performance in men with stable angina pectoris. Am J Cardiol 1990;65:1308-1312.

Thirty-three men with stable exertional angina took part in a crossover study comparing impact of isosorbide-5-mononitrate (IS-5-MN) vs. conventional isosorbide dinitrate (ISDN) on exercise performance. The 2-week administration of both drugs (IS-5-MN 60 mg once daily; ISDN 20 mg 3 times daily) was preceded by a 1-week single-blind placebo run-in before Period A during which cardioactive drugs were discontinued, followed by a 1-week single-blind washout before Period B. Outcome assessments, based on the results of exercise treadmill testing and blood pressure and heart rate monitoring, were performed 6 times per subject: before, during and after Periods A and B. Outcome variables included time to onset of angina, total exercise duration, heart rates and systolic blood pressures. Statistical analyses were conducted to answer 3 questions: (1) Were there any treatment effects 6 hours after a single dose or after 2 weeks of continuous drug treatment? (2) Did treatment effects differ by drug type and (3) Was there any difference between the effect after a single dose and after 2 weeks of continuous treatment? The results (defined among 28 subjects who completed the study) showed that controlled release IS-5MN, when compared with the preceding placebo, prolonged total exercise time and duration of exercise before angina and reduced the frequency of ischemic systems. These effects were found after a single dose and after 2 weeks of continuous treatment. ISDN produced similar improvement, but was significantly less effective in reducing myocardial ischemia defined as maximal ST depression. Resting and exercise hemodynamic variables showed few significant differences as a function of drug type. The authors concluded that "once-daily, controlled-release isosorbide-5-mononitrate appears as effective as conventional isosorbide dinitrate 3 times daily in patients with stable angina pectoris" [26].

Fig. 5.7 Example of a true-experimental two-period crossover study

individuals. As for true-experimental designs #1–3, the use of parallel comparison groups studied within a relatively short time interval generally affords good control of history, maturation, and similar effects. In addition, the use of double blinding (specific to this study, though not necessarily to this design) eliminates the threat of expectancy on the part of the investigator and subject.

There are, however, a number of potential threats to the external validity of any crossover study. Most prominent are the *interactive effects of testing and treatment* which could limit generalizability due to the potential sensitization (or desensitization) effects of multiple pre-intervention assessments. Of course, here again, the less obtrusive the measures, the less worrisome the threat. Second, a study of this nature is vulnerable to the threat of a *selection-treatment interaction.* The reason is that the number of study subjects in this study is relatively small, as is commonly the case in crossover studies (indeed, as noted previously, this is an advantage of these studies compared with parallel designs without crossover, which require larger numbers of subjects for equivalent power). This reduces the number of comparisons that can be made and amplifies the impact on outcome of the choice to participate or not to participate based on factors extraneous to the aims of the study. The number of available comparisons is further reduced if subjects discontinue their participation before the study has ended because failure to complete the study precludes determination of within-subject treatment differences—the underpinning of the crossover study. If the number of dropouts were high, the study could be underpowered despite initial planning to avoid this. (The reader should note that in the Seabra-Gomes study, 15% of subjects initially participating failed to complete it; their data could not be used.) In addition, unless the experimenter took care to reduce the obtrusiveness of the study, the inherently novel aspects of the crossover design (alternating treatments, coupled with multiple observations) could cause reactive effects that might not appear in a more natural setting (*reactive effects of experimental arrangements*). Perhaps the greatest potential threat to the external validity of a crossover study lies in the potential for *multiple treatment interference* because, as noted above, there may be carryover effects between treatments that may not be generalized to the single treatments under investigation. This may occur when the alternative treatments being compared are not adequately separated in time ("washed out") or, unbeknownst to the investigator when designing the trial, lead to permanent change (e.g., cause liver or kidney damage). Under these circumstances, the response to treatment in period B may be importantly influenced by a residual effect from the treatment given during period A, producing an under- or overestimation of the efficacy of the second treatment. Because of this potential limitation, crossover studies generally are less favored than parallel designs for definition of treatment efficacy. Indeed, as a practical matter, when such studies are undertaken to obtain regulatory approval or labeling elements for a treatment, investigators should consult with the appropriate regulatory body (in the United States, the Food and Drug Administration [FDA]) as to the acceptability of the design for the particular purpose.

Quasi-experimental Designs

If the value of an intervention study were to be judged solely on considerations of internal validity, most investigators would opt to employ fully blinded true-experimental designs. Yet, despite their undisputed methodological superiority for providing evidence of cause and effect relationships, these designs only are employed in a minority of published studies that have evaluated the impact of interventions on outcomes of interest. As noted above, even well-constructed, true-experimental designs are subject to limitations in external validity. They also can be difficult, if not impossible, to apply within the constraints of many research environments. Such constraints may include the lack of concurrently available comparison groups (commonly due to ethical problems caused by withholding a preferred treatment from control subjects) and, especially, to the inability to randomly allocate study subjects into different treatment groups in order to minimize the threat of selection bias, (in clinical research, commonly due to physician or patient refusal based on assumptions about outcome or to more complex psychological factors). To compensate for these deficiencies, and to render research feasible in constrained situations, Campbell and Stanley popularized a concept known as "quasi-experimental" design. This approach can be applied to individual subjects or to populations and to evaluations conducted in practice-based and field settings. It can help the investigator to control some threats to internal validity that would be uncontrolled with "pre-experimental" designs or externally controlled studies and can be very useful in the evaluation of therapies, educational programs, and policy changes in many disciplines.

Like true-experimental designs, all quasi-experimental designs involve the application of an intervention and observations of at least one outcome that is related to the intervention. However, quasi-experimental designs typically lack the hallmark of the true experiment, that is, random allocation to treatment group. Of these, the most widely used for evaluating the impact of clinical and other health-related interventions on group outcomes are the following:

1. The nonequivalent control group design
2. The time-series design
3. The multiple time-series design

The first design can be used to evaluate the impact of an intervention using a single "before and after" assessment of the dependent variables in two or more comparison groups. The second uses multiple assessments, conducted over time, of the dependent variable in a single group of subjects. The third (a combination of quasi-experimental designs #1 and #2) includes multiple assessments, again over time, but in two or more parallel groups. Because the observations in designs #2 and #3 are "broken up" by the imposition of the intervention, both also are termed "interrupted time-series designs." (The reader is referred to Kazdin [27] or to Janosky et al. [28], for a detailed discussion of other quasi-experimental designs used for research with single or small groups of subjects, and to Stanley and Campbell [1], Cook and Campbell [2], and Shadish, Cook, and Campbell [29], for additional quasi-experimental designs used with larger groups or populations).

Quasi-Experimental Design # 1 The Nonequivalent Control Group Desigı

$O_2 \rightarrow X \rightarrow O_2$

O_3-------> O_4

The *nonequivalent control group design* (also termed the *nonequivalent comparison design*) compares outcomes among two or more intact groups, at least one of which receives the intervention; another serves as the control. This design is most useful when concurrent comparison groups are available, when random allocation to treatment condition is not possible, and when pretesting of the dependent variable can be performed so that baseline similarity of the comparison groups can be evaluated. It is commonly used when comparison groups are spontaneously or previously assembled entities (e.g., different clinics, wards, schools, or geographic areas) or when logistic difficulties preclude random allocation to treatment within the same entity.

The basic structure of this design is symbolized above. It is almost identical to the pretest-posttest true-experimental control group design except that study subjects are not randomly assigned to treatment groups; therefore, the groups cannot be assumed to be equivalent before the intervention. As before, X symbolizes the intervention, O denotes the pre- and post-intervention assessments in each of the comparison groups, and the dashed line (and absence of R) indicates that intervention was applied to an intact group (i.e., allocation was not random).

Steyn et al. [30] used a nonequivalent control group design to examine the intervention effects of a community-based hypertension control program (the Coronary Risk Factor Study [CORIS]) that was introduced for 4 years among white hypertensive residents in two rural South African towns (summary and design structure are given in Fig. 5.8).

In this study, O_1, O_3, and O_5 represent baseline systolic blood pressure and diastolic blood pressure in the intervention and control towns; O_2, O_4, and O_6 represent post-intervention blood pressures in these towns. X_1 represents the low-intensity hypertension reduction intervention, X_2 represents the high-intensity intervention, and the absence of X denotes the lack of intervention (the control). The dashed line indicates intact (nonrandom) treatment assignment.

Because allocation to the intervention was not performed randomly, confounding variables may have influenced the observed outcomes. Therefore, internal validity is not as well protected as it is with true-experimental design #4 (the "pretest-posttest control group design"), which has a similar structure but includes random allocation. The greatest potential threat to internal validity with this design is differential *selection*, which could cause the comparison groups to vary on key factors related to the dependent variable; if present, selection bias could interact with other potential biases such maturation (e.g., a sicker group could have disease that might progress more rapidly) or regression (if one of the two groups were chosen on the basis of extreme values). Selection bias can occur if the investigator evaluates the intervention in two intrinsically

$$O_1 \rightarrow X_1 \rightarrow O_2$$

$$O_3 \rightarrow X_2 \rightarrow O_4$$

$$O_5 \quad \rightarrow \quad O_6$$

Steyn K. et al. The intervention effects of a community-based hypertension programme in two rural South African towns: the CORIS Study. S Afr Med J 1993;83:885-891.

Two levels of an intervention were implemented in two South African towns to improve hypertension control. In one town, intervention was primarily communication via mass media, e.g., billboards, posters, postal mailings ("low intensity intervention"); in the second town, intervention comprised similar mass media communication plus targeted management including active follow-up of identified hypertensives ("high intensity" intervention). A third town served as a control. The number of study subjects in each town was just greater than 2,000. Assessments of systolic and diastolic blood pressures were conducted for all three comparison groups prior to and following introduction of the intervention. The investigators found that while blood pressures were comparable at baseline among all subjects, magnitude of change in the low and high intensity intervention towns was greater than that observed among controls, though no clear differences were found when low and high intensity interventions were compared. Progressive decreases in blood pressures were accompanied by parallel increases in the proportion of hypertensive subjects on drug treatment and under control. The investigators concluded that the intervention was successful in reducing this cardiovascular disease risk factor in the intervention towns vs. the control towns [30].

Fig. 5.8 Example of a nonequivalent control group study

dissimilar populations or uses a nonuniform subject recruitment approach (e.g., permits subjects to self-select their treatment assignment). However, if care is taken to avoid these practices, the availability of baseline measures of the dependent variable, a critical component of the nonequivalent control group design, permits the investigator to evaluate the extent and direction of a potential selection bias and to minimize it, as appropriate, through covariance analysis. Therefore, this design affords much greater control for this selection bias than pre-experimental design #3 ("the static-group comparison") which also contrasts outcomes across intact groups, but which lacks critical baseline data needed to establish initial comparability. Where pre-intervention data show relative comparability between groups on relevant variables, the nonequivalent control group design generally is appropriate; when pre-intervention comparability is not present, an alternative design should be used. In the CORIS study, the authors state that the groups had similar blood pressures prior to the intervention. Thus, it is not likely (though, certainly, it is not impossible) that the differences found after the intervention were attributable to selection bias. The inclusion of baseline measures also permits the investigator to evaluate the potential threat of experimental mortality (attrition bias). If there were losses to follow-up among the comparison groups, their potential impact could be evaluated by comparing baseline characteristics of those who withdrew with those who completed the study. The authors of CORIS, who performed this analysis, found that those who withdrew were similar to those who remained with regard to age, gender, initial cholesterol levels, blood pressure, body mass index, and smoking behavior. Thus, the potential threat of experimental mortality was effectively ruled out.

In the absence of differential selection and a hypothesized interaction between selection and the day-to-day experiences of the subjects, history effects are not plausible as an alternative (rival) explanation for the observed outcomes and, thus, also can be ruled out as a major potential threat to internal validity when using the nonequivalent control group design. The reason is that, barring evidence to the contrary, external events occurring in one comparison group should be just as likely to occur in the other when subjects are evaluated in parallel. However, as with true-experimental designs, the burden remains with the investigator to ascertain the degree to which other relevant events may be occurring in the intact group settings that might also affect outcomes; this is especially important when comparators are geographically separated, as in this study. Also, because groups are studied in parallel, internal validity threats such as maturation, testing, instrumentation, and regression effects are fairly well controlled (again, assuming the groups share common baseline characteristics). Finally, any potential biases associated with expectancy are not inherently greater than those found with true-experimental designs and may be reduced, at least in part, by uniform standards for data collection and analysis (as was done in CORIS).

As with true-experimental design #2, the use of *pre-intervention testing* (essential with this design for establishing baseline comparability of the comparison groups) may pose a threat to external validity unless the testing itself were deemed to be part of the intervention, as it would appear to be in the CORIS study. Additionally, as with *any* design, a *selection-treatment interaction* can occur if the study subjects are not representative of all subjects who potentially could be studied. Indeed, the authors of CORIS recognized that their findings did not necessarily apply to individuals of ethnic backgrounds and socioeconomic statuses not included in CORIS. In general, however, the nonequivalent control group design places far fewer restrictions on sampling and, therefore, tends to be more generalizable than the typical randomized parallel group trial. Lastly, the *reactive effects of experimental arrangements* potentially could limit the external validity of studies using this design, but because they entail comparisons of interventions applied to naturally occurring groupings, they tend to be less reactive and, thus, have better external validity than most true experiments.

Quasi-Experimental Design # 2
The Time-Series Design

$$O_1 \rightarrow O_2 \rightarrow O_3 \rightarrow O_4 \rightarrow X \rightarrow O_5 \rightarrow O_6 \rightarrow O_7 \rightarrow O_8$$

The previous example compared the impact of an intervention on outcomes using several intact groups. Occasionally, an investigator planning to evaluate an intervention may be unable to identify a suitable (or any) comparison group. This might occur when patients are candidates for a treatment, the effectiveness of which is to be tested, but an alternate treatment is not available, or if available, is viewed as unacceptable by the patients or their physicians; a similar problem frequently occurs when a specific treatment cannot be withheld for what are considered ethical reasons. Thus, sometimes, interventions must be presented to entire groups, for example, all patients potentially at risk. In these cases, an investigator might opt for a pre-experimental design without a control group (e.g., the pretest-posttest only design), in which a single group of study subjects is observed on just one occasion before and after the intervention, or might compare results obtained in study subjects with external or historical controls. The literature reflects many such examples. Unfortunately, as noted earlier, pre-experimental designs provide very poor control against important threats to internal validity, and comparing results from a current treatment group with those obtained among historical controls is almost always biased in favor of the former, principally due to improvement in the general health of the population over time.

The *time-series design* (sometimes called an *interrupted* time-series) represents an improvement over both of these pre-experimental approaches. In its simplest form, multiple observations (the number depending on the stability of the data) are generated for a single group of subjects both before and after application of an intervention. The objective of any study using such a design is to provide evidence that observations made before (and sometimes after) imposition of the intervention differ in a *consistent* manner from

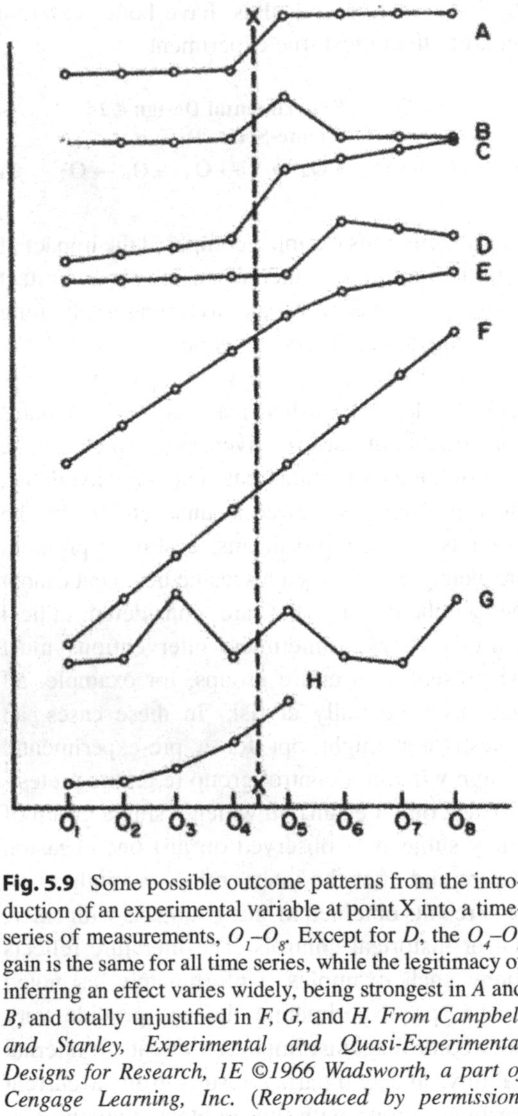

Fig. 5.9 Some possible outcome patterns from the introduction of an experimental variable at point X into a time-series of measurements, O_1–O_8. Except for *D*, the O_4–O_5 gain is the same for all time series, while the legitimacy of inferring an effect varies widely, being strongest in *A* and *B*, and totally unjustified in *F, G*, and *H. From Campbell and Stanley, Experimental and Quasi-Experimental Designs for Research, 1E ©1966 Wadsworth, a part of Cengage Learning, Inc.* (*Reproduced by permission*, www.cengage.com/permissions)

observations made during the intervention. While special autoregressive statistical procedures often are used for analysis, the hallmark of this and other types of time-series designs is visual analysis of temporal outcome changes in relation to the intervention. Shown below are examples of hypothetical data, reflecting various levels of evidence for inferring cause and effect that, theoretically, can be produced with a time-series design. The reader should note that patterns reflected by lines A and B provide the strongest evidence for inferring intervention effects (note that both show sharp increases in slope concomitant with the intervention, following a stable baseline), those reflected by lines C–E are equivocal, whereas those shown by lines F–H provide no justification for such an inference (Fig. 5.9).

Time-series designs can be used to evaluate continuous or temporary interventions and can incorporate retrospectively or prospectively acquired data. They are especially useful and appropriate for modeling temporal changes in response to programmatic interventions or health policy changes in otherwise stable populations. A time-series design was used by Delate et al. [31] to evaluate economic outcomes of a cost-containment policy for Medicaid recipients that was applied continuously throughout their study (summary and design structure are given in Fig. 5.10).

In this study, O represents the number of antisecretory drug claims and expenditures per member per month (PPIs and H_2As) before and during the post-policy period (24 such outcomes were measured in total, though only eight observations are shown here for ease of interpretation). X is the prior authorization policy; the ∞ symbol indicates that the intervention is applied continuously. The pattern of the observed H_2A data (which emulates line A of Fig. 5.9) and the obverse pattern of the PPI data are used to buttress the investigators' conclusions that the observed changes in the number of claims filed for, and expenses associated with, antisecretory drugs are due to the imposition of the policy.

An example of a time-series design evaluating a temporary intervention can be found in the work of Reding and Raphelson [32] who evaluated the impact of an addition of a psychiatrist to a mobile psychiatric crisis team on psychiatric hospitalization admission rates in Kalamazoo County, Michigan (summary and design structure are given in Fig. 5.11).

In this study, X denotes the "mobile psychiatrist" intervention and O, the number of state hospitalizations during each of the monthly assessments before, during, and after the intervention (again, 30 outcome assessments actually were performed, reduced to eight for ease of presentation here). The authors' conclusion that the intervention caused the changes in the pattern of

$$O_1 \rightarrow O_2 \rightarrow O_3 \rightarrow O_4 \rightarrow X_\infty \rightarrow O_6 \rightarrow O_7 \rightarrow O_8$$

Delate T, Mager DE, Sheth J, Motheral BR. Clinical and financial outcomes associated with a proton pump inhibitor prior-authorization program in a Medicaid population. Am J Manag Care 2005;11:29-36.

Clinical and financial data were compared 12 months before and after imposition of a prior-authorization policy for proton inhibitors (PPIs) among 5965 Medicare enrollees with a least one gastrointestinal disorder treatable by an antisecretory drug. During the pre-policy period, there were 377,574 PPI claims vs. 105,745 PPI claims during the post-policy period whereas less-costly histamine2-receptor antagonist (H2A) claims rose from 238,157 to 467,047 over the same interval. In the month following policy implementation, there was a corresponding 91% decrease in PPI expenditures per member and a 223% increase in H2A expenditures per member ($p<.001$, both); these patterns intensified modestly over time and did not result in differential use of ambulatory or inpatient medical services between patients using PPIs vs. H2As. The investigators concluded that prior authorization for PPIs reduced use of relatively high-cost PPIs and encouraged use of lower-cost H2As without adverse clinical consequences [31].

Fig. 5.10 Example of a time-series design (continuous intervention)

$$O_1 \rightarrow O_2 \rightarrow O_3 \rightarrow O_4 \rightarrow X \rightarrow O_6 \rightarrow O_7 \rightarrow O_8$$

Reding GR, Raphelson M. Around–the-clock mobile psychiatric crisis intervention: another effective alternative to psychiatric hospitalization. Community Mental Health J 1995;31:179-87.

To increase its impact, a psychiatrist was added to a mobile 24-hour psychiatric crisis intervention team that had been operating in the Kalamazoo County community for 10 years. His period of service was 6 months ("the program period") after which it was terminated. The number of state psychiatric hospital admissions during the program period was compared to those 12 months before and 18 months after the program was terminated. The investigators found a sharp sustained drop in state psychiatric hospitalization rates during the program period that was not offset by admissions to the local private clinic during the same interval. This reduction was largely reversed following termination of the program. The investigators concluded that the addition of a "mobile psychiatrist" to an "around-the-clock" mobile intensive crisis team represents an effective community-based alternative to hospitalization [32].

Fig. 5.11 Example of a time-series design (temporary intervention)

hospitalizations is based on data patterns that conform to the inverse of those shown in Fig. 5.9, line B (i.e., changes on the dependent variable contemporaneous with the intervention that return to baseline after termination).

In both of these studies, the threats of selection bias and experimental mortality are controlled, provided that the same subjects participate in each of the pre- and post-intervention assessments. Since this is rarely the case in community-based studies, the investigators must take steps to evaluate natural migratory patterns within the community to ensure that these do not confound their results. Dynamic changes within subjects or populations (i.e., maturation effects), if any, usually are well controlled with time-series designs because they (like regression effects) are unlikely to cause variations that occur only when the intervention is applied. For similar reasons, the time-series design controls for testing effects even in cases in which the measurement process is more obtrusive than that used in the Delate and Reding studies.

The chief potential threat to internal validity of studies using time-series designs is *history*. Because human subjects rarely are studied in a vacuum, the investigator must be on the alert for outside influences (e.g., programs, policy changes, or even seasonal fluctuations) occurring coincident with the intervention that also might affect study outcomes. For example, to accept Delate's conclusions, one would have to believe that there were no other factors (e.g., changes in physician prescribing patterns, advertising campaigns) to which the subjects were exposed that would have caused them to use fewer PPIs during the post-program period. Similarly, the Reding conclusions are tenable only if one accepts that nothing else (such as another psychiatric intervention or availability of new treatments, etc.) occurred in Kalamazoo County specifically during the tenure of the mobile psychiatrist that also might have reduced admissions to state hospitals. If careful documentation by the investigator rules this out, then history effects become a less plausible alternative hypothesis for the observed changes. A second internal validity threat is *instrumentation*. If the calibration of an objective measure (or the instrument itself) changes during the study, and if this change occurs when the intervention is applied, then it is difficult to know whether the observations made after the intervention are due to it or to changes in the instrument. The same problem may occur when measurement criteria or outcome adjudicators change in parallel with the intervention, especially when the latter are aware of the study hypothesis. With administrative data, there is always a chance that the methodology used for record keeping might spuriously influence outcomes. For example, a change in the coding of diagnostic rating groups (DRGs) during an intervention might lead the investigator to conclude incorrectly that there were more (or less) hospitalizations for a given disease during this interval. To minimize these potential effects, the investigator should endeavor to standardize measures and educate research personnel about such issues. Finally, whenever possible, steps should be taken to blind those interpreting outcomes to knowledge of the treatment period to reduce the influence of expectancy on these assessments.

As with all designs that evaluate change over time, the use of multiple observations, if obtrusive, could compromise external validity by sensitizing subjects to their treatments. The potential for a testing-treatment interaction (or testing reactivity) is heightened with a time-series design because multiple pre-intervention assessments are required to establish the stable pre-intervention pattern against which changes in slope and/or intercept of the post-intervention assessments are compared. For this reason, studies using these designs generalize best when performed in settings in which data are collected as part of routine practice. Additionally, when based on "natural experiments," like those reported by Delate and Reding, they cause few, if any, reactive effects because the interventions are experienced as part of the subject's normal environment. As with any design, however, the ability to generalize outcomes depends on the similarity of the study group to the reference population.

Readers with clinical experience may recognize a variant of the time-series design in which an intervention is reintroduced after one or more intervals of withdrawal. In behavioral research with single subjects or with series of subjects (e.g., studies designed to extinguish inappropriate actions among children with autism or adult schizophrenics or to improve task performance in the setting of attention deficit hyperactivity disorder), this approach is termed an *ABAB Design*, where A and B respectively denote alternating control and intervention periods. (It is called a *BABA Design* when the sequence begins with the intervention, followed by its withdrawal and reintroduction, etc.) In other specialties, it is more commonly termed an *equivalent time samples design* or a *repeated treatment design*. This general approach has greater control of history and instrumentation effects than the classic time-series design because the probability of some external event or unintentional instrument or observer change tracking with (and accounting for) the effects of intermittent applications of the intervention is arguably lower than it would be when only one application of the intervention is involved. It can be particularly useful as the basis for relatively rigorous determination of the effects of pharmacological therapies (particularly adverse outcomes of chronically employed drugs), when such effects are predictably transient or reversible in nature. For example, with age, individuals tend to perceive arthralgias and myalgias with relative frequency. Hypercholesterolemia is fairly widespread according to current epidemiological definitions, and the prescription of HMG-CoA reductase inhibitors (statins) to control cholesterol is quite common. The drugs have been well demonstrated in RCTs to reduce coronary disease events and, specifically, mortality, among patients so treated. In some patients (the minority), statins also can cause myalgias and, in fewer still, polyserositis with arthralgias. Most patients are aware of these potential problems from constant reference to them in the news media and often ascribe their symptoms to the statins because of expectancy. Thus, when patients complain of myalgias and/or arthralgias while taking statins, it is incumbent upon the physician to determine whether the association truly is cause and effect. The best approach is to employ an equivalent time samples design, beginning with a careful history of current symptoms on drug (O) followed by withdrawal of sufficient duration to allow drug effects to dissipate, another careful history, and then reinstitution ("rechallenge") with the drug, with another O after some period of use. If the result is unclear, the series can be repeated. Unfortunately, in the real world, patients tend to confound outcome by interposing anti-inflammatory drug use concomitantly with cessation of the statin and often refuse the rechallenge. Nonetheless, this example illustrates the importance of understanding and applying the principles of study design in the course of clinical practice. (For further details about the pros and cons of this design as a tool for research and methods for implementing it in clinical populations, the reader again is referred to the works of Campbell and Stanley [1], Cook and Campbell [2], Kazdin [27], Janosky et al. [28], and to Haukoos et al. [33].)

Quasi-Experimental Design # 3
The Multiple Time-Series Design

$$O_1 \rightarrow O_2 \rightarrow O_3 \rightarrow O_4 \rightarrow X \rightarrow O_5 \rightarrow O_6 \rightarrow O_7 \rightarrow O_8$$

$$O_1 \rightarrow O_2 \rightarrow O_3 \rightarrow O_4 \rightarrow \quad \rightarrow O_5 \rightarrow O_6 \rightarrow O_7 \rightarrow O_8$$

The *multiple time-series design* combines the unique features of nonequivalent control group and time-series designs to maximize internal validity. It evaluates relative change over time on one or more dependent variables in two or more intact comparison groups (again, usually preexisting groups assembled for other purposes) at least one of which receives an intervention and one of which does not (the control). Thus, this design creates two experiments, one in which the intervention is compared against a no-intervention control and the second in which pre-intervention time-series data are compared with those obtained after the intervention, thereby increasing the amount of available evidence to buttress a claim of an intervention effect. In its most general design structure, shown above, X symbolizes the intervention (applied within one of the groups), O is the pre- and post-intervention assessment of the dependent variable(s), and the dashed line denotes the intact nature of the comparators. The design is most appropriate when it is not possible to randomly allocate subjects to an intervention, when a concurrent "no-intervention" group is available for comparison, and when serial data can be (or have been) generated for both groups during the pre- and post-intervention periods. As for the nonequivalent control group design, the availability of baseline data is necessary to evaluate initial comparability of the intervention and control groups. The multiple time samples design was used by Holder et al. [34] to evaluate the effects of a community-based intervention on high-risk drinking and alcohol-related injuries (summary and design structure are given in Fig. 5.12).

In this study, X represents the community-based alcohol deterrence intervention; O (made approximately monthly over a 5-year interval) denotes average (1) frequency of drinking, (2) number of alcoholic drinks consumed per drinking occasion, (3) instances of driving while intoxicated, (4) motor vehicle crashes (daytime, DUI-related, nighttime injury-associated), and proportion of (5) emergency room and (6) hospital admissions for violent assault among the

$$O_1 \rightarrow O_2 \rightarrow O_3 \rightarrow O_4 \rightarrow X \rightarrow O_6 \rightarrow O_7 \rightarrow O_8$$

$$O_1 \rightarrow O_2 \rightarrow O_3 \rightarrow O_4 \rightarrow \quad \rightarrow O_6 \rightarrow O_7 \rightarrow O_8$$

Holder HD, Gruenewald PJ, Ponicki WR, Treno AJ, Grube JW, Saltz RF, Voas RB, Reynolds R, Davis J, Sanchez L, Gaumont G, Roeper PR. Effect of community-based interventions on high risk drinking and alcohol-related injuries. JAMA 2000;284:2341-2347.

To reduce high-risk alcohol consumption patterns, a 5-year community-based intervention, including initiatives to limit access to alcohol and heightened law enforcement, was implemented in 3 large demographically-diverse communities in California and South Carolina. Primary outcomes (self-reported drinking patterns [by population surveys] and documented motor vehicle crashes [from traffic records]) were assessed monthly before and after initiation of the intervention and compared with data obtained during the same interval from 3-matched control communities; secondary outcomes (emergency room [ER] and hospital admissions for violent assault) were compared within one intervention-comparison pair and one additional intervention site. Regression analysis (examining temporal changes in the relative ratios of the outcome measures in the intervention and control communities, corrected for changing demographics and population size), revealed consistent reductions from before to after the intervention in the number of alcoholic drinks consumed per occasion (though not in the total quantity of alcohol consumed), instances of driving while intoxicated (DUI), and rates of nighttime (but not daytime) and DUI-related motor vehicle crashes in the intervention vs. the control communities. Intervention-associated reductions in ER and hospital admissions for violent assault also were observed over time, though the latter were less marked. The investigators concluded that a comprehensive community-based alcohol deterrence intervention can reduce high-risk alcohol consumption patterns and associated motor-vehicle injuries and assaults, though a "test of the full generalizability… will require much larger effectiveness trials" [34].

Fig. 5.12 Example of a multiple time-series design

intervention versus comparison communities. The investigators' conclusion that the intervention caused reductions in high-risk drinking behavior and associated motor vehicle accidents and assaults is based on sustained differential trends in post-versus pre-intervention outcomes among the intervention versus matched control communities.

All of the potential threats to internal validity protected by the time-series design also are protected by the multiple time-series design. However, with the addition of a parallel comparison group, there is better control for the potential threat of history unless, as with the non-equivalent control group design, the comparison groups are so poorly selected as to have different external experiences. Similarly, as previously noted, the use of a parallel control group generally affords good protection against threats to validity potentially caused by instrumentation, maturation, and testing because if pre- to post-intervention differences were influenced by these factors, they should be just as likely to impact both the experimental and control groups (again, assuming reasonable baseline equivalence between comparators). Indeed, when properly executed, the multiple time-series design essentially is free from the most important threats to internal validity of an intervention study and, for this reason, generally is considered to be among the most rigorous of the various quasi-experimental designs. The threats to the external validity of a multiple time-series design are similar to those of the non-equivalent control group and time-series designs and, as for these designs, are minimized by the use of unobtrusive measures, naturalistic interventions, and careful selection of comparators.

Summary

This chapter has reviewed a variety of alternative research designs commonly used to evaluate the impact of interventions. The examples of their application have been drawn from clinical research. However, the reader should be aware that, to achieve optimal rigor and strength of conclusions, the same design principles can and should be applied in preclinical, cellular, and molecular studies though, because of the relative homogeneity (and nonhuman characteristics) of test material in basic science studies, issues of randomization, blinding, sample sizes, etc., may be handled somewhat differently than in clinical research. Nonetheless, it should be clear from a comparison of the relative strengths and weaknesses of the various study designs reviewed in this chapter that there is no perfect study. The pre-experimental designs offer the least protection against major potential threats to internal validity, providing weakest evidence to support a claim of cause and effect. The true-experimental designs offer the best control over most internal validity threats, providing strongest evidence to support intervention effects, but their generalizability may be compromised by highly restrictive inclusion criteria, patient reluctance to participate in a randomized study, or reactivity caused by pre-intervention testing or the experimental arrangements. The quasi-experimental designs fall somewhere in the middle, providing more protection against internal validity threats than pre-experimental designs but less than that afforded by true-experimental designs. Because most quasi-experimental designs lend themselves to "real-world" studies of "typical" (rather than the "ideal") subjects or populations, they also offer certain advantages in external validity. Therefore, in many situations, they represent a good compromise for the researcher, particularly when their strengths and limitations are recognized.

Take-Home Points

- The ability to draw valid inferences from data is the cornerstone of research and provides the basis for understanding the new knowledge that research results represent.
- Internal validity reflects the extent to which a manipulated variable can be shown to account for changes in a dependent variable. It is indispensable for interpreting the experiment.
- Ten common threats to internal validity include selection bias, history effects, maturation effects, testing effects, instrumentation effects, statistical regression, experimental mortality, interaction of these factors, experimenter bias, and subject expectancy effects.
- Four threats to external validity (generalizability) are reactive effects of testing, interactive effects of selection and treatment, reactive effects of experimental arrangements, and multiple treatment interference.
- A variety of research designs can be used to evaluate interventions. Each differs in its adequacy for ensuring that valid inferences are made about effects and generalizability.
- The poorest for controlling threats to internal validity are termed "pre-experimental designs." These lack adequate control groups.
- The strongest are termed "true-experimental designs." They incorporate control groups to which subjects have been randomly allocated but may suffer from lack of generalizability.
- Quasi-experimental designs represent a good compromise when randomization is not possible.

References

1. Campbell DT, Stanley JC. Experimental and quasi-experimental designs for research. Boston: Houghton Mifflin Company; 1963.
2. Cook TD, Campbell DT. Quasi-experimentation: design and analysis for field settings. Chicago: Rand McNally; 1979.
3. Kim SYH, Holloway RG, Frank S, Beck CA, Zimmerman C, Wilson MA, Kieburtz K. Volunteering for early phase gene transfer research in Parkinson disease. Neurology. 2006;66:1010–5.
4. Woodward SH, Stegman WK, Pavao JR, Arsenault NJ, Hartl TL, Drescher KD, Weaver C. Self-selection bias in sleep and psychophysiological studies of posttraumatic stress disorder. J Trauma Stress. 2007;20: 619–23.
5. Lanfear DE, Jones PG, Cresci S, Tang F, Rathore SS, Spertus JA. Factors influencing patient willingness to participate in genetic research after a myocardial infarction. Genome Med. 2011;3:39.
6. McCuen RH. The elements of academic research. New York: ASCE Publications; 1996.
7. Rosenthal R. The effect of the experimenter on the results of psychological research. In: Maher BA, editor. Progress in experimental personality research. New York: Academic; 1964.
8. Mayo E. The human problems of an industrial civilization. New York: Macmillan; 1933.
9. Saretsky G. The OEO P.C. experiment and the John Henry effect. Phi Delta Kappan. 1972;53:579–81.
10. Visser RF. Angiographic assessment of patency and reocclusion: preliminary results of the dutch APSAC reocclusion multicenter study (ARMS). Clin Cardiol. 1990;13:45–7.
11. Wender P, Reimherr F. Buproprion treatment of attention deficit hyperactivity disorders in adults. Am J Psychol. 1990;147:1018–20.
12. Bolland J, Ward J, Bolland T. Improved accuracy of estimating food quantities up to 4 weeks after treatment. J Am Diet Assoc. 1990;90:1402–7.
13. Fisher RA. The arrangement of field experiments. J Min Agric. 1926;33:503–13.
14. Medical Research Council. Streptomycin treatment of pulmonary tuberculosis. BMJ. 1948;2:769–82.
15. Berry DA. Adaptive designs: the promise and the caution. J Clin Oncol. 2011;29:606–9.
16. Hu F, Rosenberger WF. The theory of response adaptation in clinical trials. Hoboken: Wiley; 2006.
17. Heritier SR, Gebski VJ, Keech AC. Inclusion of patients in clinical trial analysis: the intention-to-treat principle. MJA. 2003;179:438–40.
18. Montori VM, Guyatt GH. Intention-to-treat principle. CMAJ. 2001;165:1339–41.
19. Hollis S, Campbell F. What is meant by intention to treat analysis? Survey of published randomised controlled trials. BMJ. 1999;319:670–4.
20. Sackett DL, Gent M. Controversy in counting and attributing events in clinical trials. N Engl J Med. 1979;301:1410–2.
21. Lewis JA, Machin D. Intention to treat—who should use ITT? Br J Cancer. 1993;68:647–50.
22. Gorbach SL, Morrill-LaBrode A, Woods MN, Dwyer JT, Selles WD, Henderson M, Insull Jr W, Goldman S, Thompson D, Clifford C. Changes in food patterns during a low-fat dietary intervention in women. J Am Diet Assoc. 1990;90:802–9.
23. B-Blocker Heart Attack Research Group. A randomized trial of propranolol in patients with acute myocardial infarction. JAMA. 1982;247:1707–14.
24. The International Study Group. In-hospital mortality and clinical course of 20,891 patients with suspected acute myocardial infarction randomized between alteplase and streptokinase with or without heparin. Lancet. 1990;336:71–4.
25. Stampfer MJ, Buring JE, Willett W, Rosner B, Eberlein K, Hennekens CH. The 2 × 2 factorial design: its application to a randomized trial of aspirin and carotene in U.S. physicians. Stat Med. 1985;4:111–6.
26. Seabra-Gomes R, Aleixo AM, Adao M, Machado FP, Mendes M, Bruges G, Palos JL. Comparison of the effects of a controlled-release formulation of isosorbide-5-mononitrate and conventional isosorbide dinitrate on exercise performance in men with stable angina pectoris. Am J Cardiol. 1990;65:1308–12.
27. Kazdin AE. Single case research designs. New York: Oxford University Press; 1982.
28. Janosky JE, Leininger SL, Hoerger MP, Libkuman TM. Single subject designs in biomedicine. New York: Springer; 2009.
29. Shadish WR, Cook TD, Campbell DT. Experimental and quasi-experimental designs for generalized causal inference. Boston: Houghton Mifflin Company; 2002.
30. Steyn K, Rossouw JE, Jooste PL, Chalton DO, Jordaan ER, Jordaan PC, Steyn M, Swanepoel AS. The intervention effects of a community-based hypertension programme in two rural South African towns: the CORIS Study. S Afr Med J. 1993;83:885–91.
31. Delate T, Mager DE, Sheth J, Motheral BR. Clinical and financial outcomes associated with a proton pump inhibitor prior-authorization program in a Medicaid population. Am J Manag Care. 2005;11:29–36.
32. Reding GR, Raphelson M. Around–the-clock mobile psychiatric crisis intervention: another effective alternative to psychiatric hospitalization. Commun Ment Health J. 1995;31:179–87.
33. Haukoos JS, Hopkins E, Byyny RL, Conroy AA, Silverman M, Eisert S, Thrun M, Wilson M, Boyer B, Heffelfinger JD, Denver ED HIV Opt-Out Study Group. Design and implementation of a controlled clinical trial to evaluate the effectiveness and efficiency of routine opt-out rapid human immunodeficiency virus screening in the emergency department. Acad Emerg Med. 2009;16:800–8.
34. Holder HD, Gruenewald PJ, Ponicki WR, Treno AJ, Grube JW, Saltz RF, Voas RB, Reynolds R, Davis J, Sanchez L, Gaumont G, Roeper PR. Effect of community-based interventions on high risk drinking and alcohol-related injuries. JAMA. 2000;284: 2341–7.

Protocol Development and Preparation for a Clinical Trial

6

Joseph A. Franciosa

Introduction

A clinical trial protocol is a written document that provides a detailed description of the rationale for the trial, the hypothesis to be tested, the overall design, and the methods to be used in carrying out the trial and in analyzing its results. The protocol represents the means by which a hypothesis will be tested. As such, it must be written in its entirety before the study is performed to help assure the credibility of the results. In addition, it must be prepared in as detailed a manner as possible in order that the elements of the trial can be subjected to constructive critique and that others can replicate it in the future with the expectation of obtaining essentially the same results.

A protocol has a structure and organization made up of elements that follow the conception, development, and conduct of a clinical trial in a chronological fashion. Although these elements vary from protocol to protocol, they typically include the following, in this suggested order: a statement of the background and rationale for the trial; a brief overview of the study design, including the purpose of the study or statement of the hypothesis being tested and the significance of its possible results; a detailed description of the study population, including patient eligibility criteria; implementation of the intervention, study specific visits, and observations made; a plan for safety monitoring, including reporting of adverse events; ethical considerations; a description of data management plans, including methods of data generation, recording and processing; and statistical considerations, including a detailed description of the study design.

The purposes of this chapter are to briefly describe the clinical trial and to discuss, in depth, the various stepwise components of the protocol structure and organization that guide it. This chapter will focus primarily on protocols for conducting trials in human subjects or patients, with special emphasis on randomized controlled clinical trials that test specific hypotheses. Protocols for other types of clinical research (e.g., epidemiological studies) or for preclinical research (e.g., animal or laboratory bench studies) will not be specifically addressed here, though many of the principles of clinical trials generally are applicable. Though there is ample published in formation available about protocol development for clinical trials, much of this is dispersed throughout websites, institutional guidelines, proceedings, literature, books, and software and may be difficult to locate [1, 2].

J.A. Franciosa, MD (✉)
Department of Medicine, State University of New York Downstate Medical Center, Brooklyn, NY, USA
e-mail: josephafranciosa@gmail.com

P.G. Supino and J.S. Borer (eds.), *Principles of Research Methodology: A Guide for Clinical Investigators*, DOI 10.1007/978-1-4614-3360-6_6, © Phyllis G. Supino and Jeffrey S. Borer 2012

Background, Rationale, and Overview of Study Design

Background and Rationale

The background and rationale section of a protocol is a brief but comprehensive introductory section that should provide a compelling argument to justify the proposed research. Some key components of this section are shown in Table 6.1. It should succinctly summarize what has been done by the investigators and others in the specific and related areas of research, it should highlight what deficiencies exist and what additional information is needed, and it should state how the proposed research will address those needs. It is important to stress the unique characteristics of the proposed research, which may involve new methods, unique patients, a new intervention, an innovative study design, or other new approaches that distinguish the proposed research and warrant its conduct. This should all logically flow to a concise statement of the hypothesis addressed by the proposed research and be concluded by a statement of the significance of the anticipated results, whether they confirm or fail to confirm the hypothesis.

The importance of this section cannot be overstated as it provides the first impression of the investigators to reviewers, funding agencies, and others who may have to approve or support the proposed research. It offers these others a glimpse of the investigators thought processes, their analytic and synthetic abilities, the thoroughness of their methods, and their objectivity. Finally, it should be written in a style that is suitable to both scientific and nonscientific lay persons who may be members of reviewing and approving bodies.

Table 6.1 Components of the background and rationale section of the clinical trial protocol

• General description of the disease being treated/managed and why improved treatment/intervention/management is needed
• Description of current treatment/management of the disease/condition and any problems with available therapy/management
• Description of known properties of the proposed treatment/management intervention that justify its use
• Brief summary of relevant preclinical and clinical experience with the proposed treatment/management intervention
• Rationale for the current study and its role in the overall research program
• Statement of the hypothesis and objectives of the proposed research
• Brief description of the significance of the study

Statement of Hypothesis

The hypothesis (described in detail in Chap. 3) must be asserted early in the protocol. Therefore, we offer a few key points here on how it should be stated in the protocol.

The introductory section should logically lead to a statement of the hypothesis of the proposed research. This section is the key to the entire protocol as it describes the purpose of the trial and guides the rest of the protocol which, subsequently, is developed to provide the details about the methodology to be used in assessing the stated hypothesis. In other words, the hypothesis addresses the primary question by providing a tentative answer. The rest of the protocol describes how the hypothesis will be tested to provide a more definitive answer.

The section stating the hypothesis or hypotheses (there may be more than one in a given study) typically begins with a broad description of the overall goal of the research within the context of the investigators' overall research program. For example, the investigators may have an interest in seeking new treatments for a given disease, and the broad purpose of the proposed study is to test a new drug for treating that disease. The broad purpose in this case is an attempt to answer a new question. In some situations, the broad purpose might be to confirm previous preliminary work in the field in a larger or different patient population. The overall purpose might also be preliminary in nature as a "proof of concept" study to assess whether a hypothesized pathogenetic mechanism plays an important enough role in a disease such that it might be a therapeutic target.

In addition to stating the broad programmatic goal of the proposed research, the statement of the hypothesis also presents a more specific broad objective of the research followed by some more detailed specific aims of the research. For example, a broad objective might be to test the hypothesis that a new drug improves symptoms in patients with the disease of interest to the overall research program. The specific aims might be to determine whether certain of those symptoms improve by a specified amount over a specified period of time without producing major side effects. The specific aims typically include major outcomes (primary endpoint [s]) that essentially drive the study design and other outcomes of lesser importance (secondary endpoints) that provide supportive information, as will be discussed in greater detail below.

The statement of hypothesis should be succinctly phrased and should provide a basis for the overall study design being employed to test it, i.e., to determine whether the hypothesis is supported by the study results. As noted in Chap. 3, the operational restatement of the hypothesis should, at minimum, clearly identify the patient population, intervention (if any), primary endpoint, key methods, duration, and anticipated outcomes.

Significance of the Research

The Introduction should conclude with some discussion, even if largely speculative, about the significance of the proposed research and its possible outcomes. If the hypothesis is confirmed, what does that mean in terms of the initial objectives? Is it conclusive or does it indicate a direction for future research? Results which are not confirmatory may lead to outright rejection of the hypothesis or may imply a need for modification of the research approach. Finally, some findings of the study may generate new hypotheses to be addressed by future research.

Table 6.2 Components of the study design summary

- Statement of study type (e.g., controlled clinical trial)
- Overview of study design
  - Parallel-group, crossover
  - Level of blinding (e.g., open-label, single-blind, double-blind)
  - Method of treatment assignment (e.g., randomization, stratification)
- Statement of treatment/intervention to be used
  - Investigative drug or device
  - Dosage of drugs or usage of devices
  - Type of control (e.g., placebo, active drug, no treatment)
- Description of study population
  - Planned sample size
  - Source of patients
  - Number of centers
  - Note any unique patient characteristics (age, race, sex) required
- Description of the disease or condition being studied and any characteristics of that disease/condition that might affect patient eligibility or study outcomes
  - Duration
  - Etiology
  - Severity
  - Treatment
- Sequence and duration of study visits
- Description of study endpoints

Overview of Study Design Summary

It is common practice and helpful to include an overall summary or synopsis of the study design before embarking on the detailed discussion of the various protocol components that will ensue. This summary is especially useful to certain reviewers, e.g., research administrators, funding agency officials, or institutional review board (IRB) members, who may not be scientists or may not require the level of detail of the full protocol in order to perform their specific review or critique functions. Thus, this section is typically very brief and to the point, as details of everything addressed here will be provided in the sections that follow. Table 6.2 shows the key components of this summary.

The summary should include a statement of the nature of the study design (e.g., whether it is controlled or uncontrolled, parallel or crossover, blinded or unblinded, and the number and nature of treatment arms). A brief description of any randomization methods should be provided (the details of which should be given in the Statistical Considerations section). It also should indicate the number of centers involved (single or multicenter), total number of patients to be enrolled, and the geographical area included, e.g., United States, North America, Europe, China, or a region of a country. The study population should be characterized, especially any unique demographic characteristics, e.g., women only, African-Americans only, or a certain age group. In addition to patient demographics, a brief description of their underlying disease condition being studied should be mentioned along with any important information about the current status, duration, severity, and treatment of the condition that might affect patient eligibility as well as outcomes. The active intervention being tested, along with any control interventions, should be briefly described. In addition, the frequency and duration of the intervention should be stated along with the total study duration, which may be longer than the intervention period. Finally, the primary study endpoint should be described along with a statement about how it will be assessed, when it will be assessed, and how often it will be assessed. Key secondary endpoints may be simply listed.

Endpoints

It is desirable to present the study endpoints early in the protocol, as these tend to drive the rest of the study design which is developed to measure an effect on those same endpoints. Thus, the sample size, methodology, duration of study, and analytical methods are all influenced by the choice of endpoints.

The endpoints are defined as primary and secondary. The *primary endpoint* is usually a single one, though it may include two endpoints, or may consist of a single composite endpoint made of two or more components. It is important to strictly limit the number of primary endpoints, as attempts to address multiple primary endpoints almost invariably lead to methodological inconsistencies and difficulties, resulting in a trial that fails to achieve any meaningful result in terms of primary endpoints. The primary endpoint(s) should be specifically defined, along with an explanation of how and when it will be measured. The *secondary endpoints* may be more numerous than the primary ones. They may represent additional measures of efficacy or safety but also may be included for other reasons such as exploration of mechanisms, particular safety concerns, and development of data for future research. The secondary endpoints also should be specifically defined, and the timing and methodology of their measurements should be briefly stated.

Factors considered in the selection of endpoints (especially the primary endpoints), such as relevance, practicality, acceptability, validation, and experience should be discussed. Clearly, it is necessary to establish that the endpoint chosen is relevant to the patients and conditions being studied; that is, it addresses real and significant needs such as improving symptoms, survival, diagnosis, or other outcomes. In addition, the endpoints should be practical, not only by addressing real needs but by utilizing readily applied methods of objective measurement. Furthermore, the methods used must be acceptable to both investigators and patients in terms of ease of application, safety, comfort, and cost. Optimally, they should be standard methods that are appropriate for the group under study to avoid the necessity of validating them, which usually must be done in separate preliminary studies [3]. Validation involves establishing (via the literature or the investigator's own work) that the proposed methods perform as intended in both the patients and conditions being studied. The investigators must indicate that they have sufficient experience with the successful use of the proposed methods. Finally, it is critical that there be a consensus regarding study endpoints among all investigators, study administrators, and committees before the study starts in order to avoid disputes when the final results become available [4]. Table 6.3 lists guidelines for describing the key components

Table 6.3 Primary study endpoints

• State the primary study endpoint(s)
• Briefly mention the appropriateness and relevance of the endpoint
• Describe the methods, timing, and frequency for assessing the endpoint
• As needed, describe and special personnel performing the assessment (e.g., an unblinded assessor in a double-blind study)
• Additional details about collecting endpoint data may need to include: – Details about the use of subjects diaries – Any instructions on timing/conditions of assessment – Details about unusual collection, storage, or analysis of laboratory samples
• Provide information about the standardization and validation of the methods to be used for endpoint measurement
• Describe the investigator's experience with the methods to be used
• As needed, describe any training that might be required in using the methods for endpoint measurements

of primary study endpoints; secondary endpoints should follow this same sequence, though with less detail.

It should be noted that endpoints, as discussed above, refer primarily to clinical trials. Other kinds of studies, such as nonprospective observational studies that evaluate associations or distributional characteristics (e.g., prevalences) rather than intervention effects may not employ endpoints as described above for their study objectives. Observational studies are discussed in greater detail in Chap. 4.

Study Population

This section is a detailed description of the patients/subjects to be included in the study and should provide a broad description of the study population, the source of patients, and a comprehensive listing of the inclusion (eligibility) and exclusion criteria for study participation.

Although the terms "patients" and/or "subjects" often are used interchangeably or may be established according to convention of the sponsoring group, we prefer to use the term "patients" for those individuals with a medical diagnosis or condition that is the target of the proposed research. We reserve the term "subjects" for normal healthy individuals that typically are included in some studies as the control population but who also may represent the primary population, e.g., in studies of the clinical pharmacological properties of a new drug before it is given to patients.

General Description of the Study Population

The study population should be described in terms of its general demographics, as well as the characteristics of the disease or condition being studied that the patients should have, along with the number of such patients that will be recruited and enrolled. The *demographic characteristics* typically describe the sex and age group of patients and, if appropriate, their race. If any of these characteristics are particularly restrictive, the reason for that restriction should also be given. For example, if one is studying only Asian females in their 20s, the reason for focusing on that population should be presented. In many instances, this may have been addressed in the introductory sections and need not be gone into in great detail in this section. The selection of these demographic characteristics (especially age) should not be taken lightly, as they may have important effects on adverse events and study outcomes [5]. In fact, it has been suggested that these kinds of patient characteristics may impact study results more than other features of the study design itself [6]. These characteristics will be expanded upon in greater detail as needed in the list of inclusion/exclusion criteria, as discussed below. The *medical condition* these patients must have in order to participate in the study also should be described in terms of its diagnostic criteria, duration, etiology (if appropriate), treatment, present status, and severity. If normal subjects are included, then operational criteria for defining the normal subject also must be presented. Subjects may be required to be completely normal, with no significant past or current medical conditions, especially if these subjects constitute the primary study population. If normal subjects are included as a control group, they may only be required to be "relatively" normal, i.e., they should not have the same disease as the other patients in the study. These disease characteristics will be expanded upon in greater detail in the list of inclusion/exclusion criteria. This section also should include a description of the *number of patients* to be studied. Whereas a sample size estimate typically is included in the statistical analysis section (see below), that estimate usually refers to the number of patients needed to complete the study. Since, typically, some patients fail to complete a trial for several different reasons, it is necessary to try to estimate the total number of patients that will be recruited in order to achieve the number needed to complete the trial. Depending on the disease, study population, and treatment, patients may drop out of the trial for many reasons, including death and side effects of the treatment. In addition to these reasons, which will vary, some patients withdraw consent, move, or just never return for follow-up. The investigator must make every attempt to estimate the number of expected "dropouts" and decide what to do about them, i.e., to replace them or not in the study. It is critical to estimate the number of patients that need to be recruited not only in order to achieve the desired number of study "completers" but also to properly estimate resource needs, e.g., study medications, case report forms, and laboratory supplies.

Patient Sources

The techniques to be used for recruiting patients for the trial should be discussed in detail in this section. One should describe the number and location of investigative sites that will provide patients and/or participate in the trial. Not all sites may actually have study investigators; some may serve only as sources that will identify and refer patients to an investigator's site. Methods to be used for finding patients should be described. These may include various ways of publicizing the study, ranging from notices within the local institution to advertising in various media. These techniques and the individuals responsible for implementing them should be described. It also is necessary to describe how patients, once identified, will be further screened and by whom. A detailed description of the screening process to determine eligibility should be included, listing the specific initial parameters that will be used preliminarily to identify potential eligible patients. It is common practice to identify patients who meet initial screening criteria by history, then follow them for a brief interval to determine whether they subsequently meet all study eligibility criteria. For example, in a study of treatment of hypertension, patients initially may be screened on the basis of having a history of hypertension or of having a single reading of elevated blood pressure. Typically, such patients would be followed for a limited period to see if they, in fact, do currently have hypertension.

The location of screening procedures should be specified. This could involve screening of clinic records, emergency room logs, diagnostic laboratory reports, etc., depending on the population being sought. For example, in a study of patients with documented coronary artery disease, one might screen the cardiac catheterization and intensive care unit logs. The protocol should describe who will do this, when it will be done, and how it will be done. Unlike some sections of the protocol (e.g., endpoint definitions, patient inclusion/exclusion criteria, and analytic methods to be used), the screening procedures are not "carved in stone" and may be modified as needed.

For a more detailed description of recruiting techniques and the many issues that may become involved, the reader should consult standard references and the medical literature [1, 7–11].

Inclusion/Exclusion Criteria

A list of all inclusion and exclusion criteria to be used in determining eligibility of patients for the trial must include a detailed description of all the requirements a patient or subject must meet to be eligible for enrollment in the trial, along with a detailed description of all variables that would render the patient ineligible for enrollment. Each patient enrolled must satisfy all of the inclusion criteria and none of the exclusion criteria, without exception, in order to be enrolled in the trial.

It is important that the list be very detailed, leaving no ambiguities for the study personnel who must use the list to screen for potential patients. Thus, specific criteria, along with any relevant methods needed to apply them, should be provided for each item on the inclusion/exclusion list. For example, eligibility for inclusion in a trial of antihypertensive treatment might require that the patient have a systolic blood pressure above 140 mmHg or a diastolic pressure above 90 mmHg, as determined by the average of 3 readings taken 5 min apart with the patient seated and using a standard sphygmomanometer. In addition, if the study is to include untreated patients, the exclusion criteria might state that "A patient may not be included if he/she has received any antihypertensive drugs within the past 6 months, specifically any diuretics, beta-blockers, calcium blockers, ACE-inhibitors, angiotensin-receptor blockers, or alpha-blockers. For other agents with possible antihypertensive activity, the investigator must obtain approval of the study chairperson before enrolling the patient." It is extremely important that this list be as comprehensive and detailed as possible since it will serve as a checklist for many of the personnel involved in the study, including those doing the screening, designing the case report forms, developing the database, analyzing the results, and auditing the study's conduct.

Since the inclusion/exclusion criteria are critical to defining the study population (whose characteristics, in turn, may greatly impact the study results), it is mandatory that these criteria be carefully thought through and decided upon prospectively. It is highly undesirable to change these in any way after the study has started as such post hoc changes may introduce bias, thereby impacting the results and their interpretation, and raise doubts about the validity of the study in adequately testing the original hypothesis. Occasionally, circumstances can arise that may mandate a change in patient eligibility criteria, but these are rare and usually involve ethical issues. For an example, an effective new treatment may become available for some or all of the patients in the trial, making it potentially unacceptable to leave them on a placebo or on an unproven treatment. It generally is unacceptable to change eligibility criteria simply because the investigators have found it extremely difficult to recruit patients meeting the current criteria. In such instances, it may be wiser to terminate the study and start a new one with different eligibility criteria. Obviously, such decisions have important consequences and should never be taken lightly.

Table 6.4 shows some items to be considered when constructing an inclusion/exclusion criteria list. The first requirement is written informed patient consent. Without this, it would not be permissible to proceed to the subsequent criteria which require obtaining confidential medical historical information from the patient. The criteria list follows a structured progression from the general demographic characteristics to those that are more related to a specific disease, and concludes with criteria that relate to characteristics that might confound the conduct or outcomes of the study or that might impair the patient's ability to complete the study. The exclusion criteria often mirror the inclusion criteria by stating the converse of the corresponding inclusion criteria, thereby providing a means of "double checking" the patient's eligibility. For a more detailed discussion of how to construct an inclusion/exclusion list, the reader should consult standard references [1].

Table 6.4 Patient eligibility considerations

Category	Inclusion criteria	Exclusion criteria
Patient characteristics	• Provision of written informed consent • Demographics (age, sex, race) • Body weight • Pregnancy or childbearing potential • Behaviors (alcohol, smoking, activity, diet) • Mental status	• Failure to provide written informed consent • Hypersensitivity/intolerance to study interventions • Medical history (current or preexisting conditions and treatments) • Allergies/food intolerance • Occupational risk/hazard • Breast feeding
Characteristics of disease being studied	• Diagnostic criteria • Duration • Etiology • Status/severity • Treatment (required, permitted)	• Nonpermitted treatment • Status/severity that might bias results • Confounding concomitant conditions/complications
Screening examinations	• Within limits specified • Meets all run-in requirements (compliance, stability)	• Outside of limits specified • Fails to meet run-in criteria
Other factors	• Cooperative attitude • Occupation • Availability for all study requirements for full duration	• Inability to perform study requirements/procedures • Lack of availability • Increased risk of lack of cooperation • Current/recent participation in another clinical trial

Implementation of the Intervention, Study Visits, and Observations

Once the study endpoints and population have been defined, one must provide the detailed methods by which the actual study data will be generated. This section provides all interested parties with a precise description of how the patients will be entered into the study, how they will be started and followed while on the study intervention, how and when required observations will be made, and when and how the patient's participation in the study will be terminated.

Study Initiation

After eligible patients have been defined, screened, identified, and consented, they are ready to be enrolled in the study and begin their active participation. Depending on the specific study design and intervention, patients may be started immediately in the active phase of the study or may be observed during a preliminary phase (run-in period), before entering the active phase of the study.

Run-In Periods

It is common to have patients enter a run-in period between the time that they qualify for a clinical trial and the time that they begin active involvement, i.e., are started on the actual study intervention. There are several reasons for using a run-in period. Common reasons include establishing final patient eligibility, demonstrating stability, and assessing compliance. Not all inclusion/exclusion criteria may be completely available for assessment at the time of screening, especially if there is a requirement for recent laboratory or diagnostic information. A run-in period just before starting a new drug or a special procedure may be used to allow for obtaining any assessments that must be current (e.g., an echocardiogram to document presence of abnormal cardiac function) to confirm that the patient actually has the medical condition required for study participation. A run-in period also may be used to demonstrate that a patient has the required status of the condition being studied. For example, it may be required that a patient have stable symptoms while taking all standard treatment for the condition in order to minimize difficulty in interpreting changes in the patient's condition after starting active treatment. If the patient was not stable or if other treatments were started after the study intervention, it would be extremely difficult to assess the cause of a change in the patient's condition. Another common reason for using a run-in is to assess the tolerability of the study intervention. A patient may have difficulty complying with an intervention if it produces significant side effects or is difficult to administer. Furthermore, patient compliance may be influenced by other patient conditions or behaviors, e.g., substance abuse or alcoholism. A run-in period may be useful to assess the patient's likelihood of complying with and completing all study requirements.

Treatment during run-in periods may vary. If the purpose is only to acquire final inclusion/exclusion information, no treatment may be needed. Obviously, if the purpose is to assess stability and/or compliance with an intervention such as a study drug, it would be necessary that it be given according to the same regimen that would be used in the active phase of the study. This phase usually involves either active study intervention in all patients if its purpose is primarily to assess tolerability or placebo in all patients to assess patient compliance for reasons other than tolerability of the intervention. Clearly, the patient is kept blinded to treatment if the active phase is to be double-blinded.

Finally, the duration of the run-in periods should be as short as possible, typically not more than 2–3 weeks. In general, less time is needed to obtain laboratory tests, and more time would be needed to assess tolerability or compliance. The problem with excessively long run-in periods is that patients may change during this time. In cases where a run-in period has had to be extended, it is common practice to terminate that patient from the study at that point and restart him/her as a "new patient" in the screening phase. Another potential risk and criticism of run-in periods is that they may introduce bias by selecting the better responders to the active study intervention [12].

Start of Study Treatment/Intervention

Once all inclusion criteria are satisfied and no exclusion criteria are met, whether at the end of screening or after a run-in period, the patient is ready to initiate study-mandated activities. At this time, the patient will be assigned his/her study treatment or intervention. If the study is not controlled, the patient will be started on the study intervention. If the study is controlled, the patient is randomized to his/her study treatment. The method of randomization, e.g., consulting a list, opening an envelope, or contacting a central randomization center should be briefly described here. If the intervention being evaluated in the trial includes pharmacological therapy, the study drug may also be dispensed at this time or arrangements may be made for procuring it. The patient should be given any applicable instructions at this time and scheduled for the next clinic visit. Typically, the details of the randomization technique, and the administration and management of the intervention, respectively, are provided in the statistical and administrative sections of the protocol.

Schedule of Visits and Observations

The protocol must provide a schedule of patient visits with details about when these will be conducted and what information will be collected at each visit. This section is used and closely adhered to by study personnel, much as a recipe is followed by a cook. Study visits typically consist of a baseline or study initiation visit, follow-up interim visits, a final on-treatment study visit, and a post-study follow-up visit. It is important to specify the timing of these visits, with a window of plus or minus a small number of days, if possible, to allow the patient some flexibility in scheduling appointments. Typically, the time is set relative to randomization or baseline, i.e., at some time ± a time window following the date of randomization or the baseline visit. The observations recorded at each visit often are variable, with fewer items observed at interim visits.

Baseline Visit

The baseline visit is performed at or very close to the time when the patients are randomized to study treatment/intervention, whether or not that treatment/intervention has actually been instituted. This is a critical visit as all observations recorded at this time will be the basis for comparison with all observations made while on study treatment. Thus, a complete medical history and physical examination usually are performed, along with laboratory tests. All concomitant medications are recorded with details about dose and duration of administration. In addition to this general medical examination, there is usually information collected that is specific to the status of the medical condition being studied, e.g., its duration, severity, history of complications, current symptoms and status, and current treatment. Any special tests, assessments, or procedures relating to study endpoints are carried out at this visit or are scheduled to be obtained very soon after this visit, if not yet already done. One cannot overemphasize the importance of all baseline determinations. They must be thorough and comprehensive, as any medical and/or laboratory findings that appear later must be ascribed in some way to study participation if they were not present at baseline. In trials evaluating experimental medications, the baseline visit is concluded by dispensing any study drugs or other required materials to the patient, scheduling the next visit, and arranging for any procedures or tests needed for the next visit.

Interim Visits

Following the baseline visit, the patient is seen at intervals specified in the protocol to occur at some set time, e.g., every 3 months ± 1 week from the date of the baseline visit. These interim visits primarily are intended to monitor the patient's progress and his/her tolerability of the study intervention. A brief medical history and physical examination are carried out, with the emphasis on looking for any adverse events or findings. Information on one or more study endpoints may be collected, but not necessarily the primary endpoint, especially if that involves a special procedure, e.g., cardiac catheterization, which might be done only at the end of the study or once during an interim visit. In trials evaluating medications, patient compliance usually is assessed, typically by having the patient bring any unused study medications with him/her and calculating the percentage of pills taken relative to those prescribed. The interim visit also is concluded by dispensing any study drugs or other required materials to the patient, scheduling the next visit, and arranging for any procedures or tests needed for the next visit.

Of course, patients may develop complications and may need to be seen between scheduled visits. All clinical trials must include provisions for patients to be seen by physicians who may be associated with the study in order to deal with clinical necessities whether or not a visit is specifically related to a protocol-based assessment. The reasons for, and findings obtained during, any unscheduled visits must be recorded as study data on appropriate forms.

Final Visit

The final visit is the last one during which the patient is still receiving the study intervention. Its observations include essentially the same as those obtained at the baseline visit and are just as critical since they represent the study results and outcomes that will be compared to those from the baseline visit. In addition, the same kind of information collected at the interim visits is obtained to cover the interval since that preceding interim visit.

Whereas a final visit is obtained routinely in all patients at the end of the study, it may be necessary to perform a "final visit" if a patient terminates his/her study participation prematurely, as might happen for intolerable side effects or other

Table 6.5 Template schedule of study events in protocol no. XXXX

Evaluation	Screening (Day xx)	Baseline Day 0	Treatment period Day #	Day #	Day #	Day #	Follow-up Day #
Informed consent	X						
Inclusion/exclusion criteria	X	X					
Demographics	X						
Medical history	X						
Full physical examination	X	X				X	
Partial physical examination			X	X	X		X
Laboratory tests	X	X				X	
Special tests/procedures		X			X	X	
Randomization		X					
Vital signs and weight	X	X	X	X	X	X	X
Study intervention administration			X	X	X	X	
Adverse event assessment	X	X	X	X	X	X	X
Concomitant medication assessment	X	X	X	X	X	X	
Terminate study drug						X	

reasons. In such cases, every attempt must be made to have the patient return and perform all the procedures and observations required at a regularly scheduled final visit. Without this, that patient's entire dataset may be useless and exclude the patient from the study analysis. In most instances, "final visit" data obtained even prematurely may still be analyzable and allow the patient to be included in the results.

At the end of the final visit, study drug/intervention is terminated, and the patient is scheduled for a study follow-up visit.

Post-study Follow-Up Visit

Often by regulatory requirement, but more in the interests of good clinical practice, patients should be seen at least once after completing their study participation to ensure that they are not experiencing any sequelae that might be attributed to their study involvement. Such visits usually are scheduled at 1 week to 1 month after the final "on treatment" study visit, depending on the possible duration of effects of the study intervention. (As used here, the term "on treatment" means the patient is still receiving a study-mandated intervention, regardless of whether he/she is receiving active therapy or an inactive control substance [or other control condition].) In some instances, especially by regulatory requirements, it may be mandatory to attribute any side effects or complications occurring during this period to the study intervention. These post-study visits also are of value in helping to document patient status and to protect all study personnel and institutions in the event of any future allegations stemming from the patient's study involvement. It is strongly suggested that a flow chart of all scheduled visits and related procedures be included, a template of which is shown in Table 6.5.

Data Management

A clinical trial, along with its data generation and acquisition, is driven by the thoroughness and objectivity of the research protocol. The research data to be generated, collected, processed, and stored in the clinical database must support the objectives of the study, as specified in the protocol. This, in turn, relies on designing data management processes that correctly capture the required research data. All data generated by the trial must be captured and managed to ultimately yield the results of the trial. Data management has been enhanced dramatically in recent years as a result of technological advancements including computerization of databases, bioinformatics, and Internet applications to facilitate acquisition and processing of data [13–15]. As a consequence, modern data management processes involve specialized personnel and methods which are discussed in detail in Chap. 7. For all these processes to be properly carried out, it is necessary that a detailed, comprehensive, and unambiguous protocol be developed, as the protocol drives the data management processes which tend to follow the protocol in a chronological fashion. Obviously, the tools used for data collection will be developed in accordance with protocol specifications. Ideally, data management processes should be developed in advance of data collection because post hoc changes potentially introduce a risk of bias, threatening the validity and credibility of the results, as noted above.

The data management plan closely follows the structure and sequence of the protocol. A well-written data management section will provide detailed descriptions of each data item to be collected, how it will be collected, and when it will be collected. The data management group must work very closely with the team that is preparing the actual protocol to help ensure that all the data described are readily obtainable, complete, unambiguous, objective, and easily programmable and quantifiable. Furthermore, it must be ascertained that all of the data generation methods are generally accepted and that the research team is adequately experienced in using these methods so as to help ensure reliability and validity of the data obtained.

Whereas trials generally try to limit the amount of information collected to that which is necessary to obtain valid results, it is common to collect additional information, especially at baseline, because this is the last time one can make observations before the effects of the trial interventions come into play. Just being in a clinical trial may affect patient outcomes because of the level and frequency of care provided (see also Chap. 5). It is critical that every attempt be made to capture all the required data at the times specified by the protocol, as incomplete, inaccurate, and/or missing data can undermine the reliability and credibility of results. The completeness, accuracy, and timeliness of data collection are key indicators of the quality of conduct of the study; as such, they are commonly audited after study completion to help ascertain the validity and reliability of the study conclusions.

Safety Monitoring Procedures

A complete protocol should describe all procedures that will be in place to ensure and assess the safety of study participants. Whereas much of this information already is included in different parts of the protocol, e.g., on the schedule of visits and procedures, it is recommended that a specific section be devoted to summarizing all safety monitoring procedures. It should summarize how often patients will be seen, that an interim history and physical examination will be performed, and that laboratory tests will be obtained. It is important to point out any special visits, examinations, tests, or procedures that will be conducted specifically to look for known side effects of the treatment. For example, liver function tests would be obtained in a trial of a new drug suspected of possibly producing liver toxicity, or the eyes would be examined often in a trial of an intervention that could potentially be associated with cataract formation.

In addition to describing what will be done and how often, it is important to specify who is responsible for carrying out these procedures and what will be done with the information in case something is found, i.e., instructing the investigators whom to contact, how to establish contact, and the timeframe for making contact. It is important that all study personnel know what constitutes an adverse event or serious adverse event. These are not simply clinical impressions but are specifically defined by regulations. These regulations also establish what information about the adverse event must be collected (start date, duration, severity, drug dose, concomitant drugs, action taken, outcomes, etc.) and who must be notified within the specified time frame (other investigators, IRBs, study administrators, regulatory agencies, etc.). Instruction also should be provided to the investigators regarding possible discontinuation of the study drug, premature termination of the patient's study participation, unblinding of any study medication, etc.

It is critical that all study personnel understand that an adverse event is any undesirable sign, symptom, or medical condition that occurs after starting study participation regardless of its relationship to the study intervention, i.e., even if a cause other than the study intervention is present. Any condition that was present before starting study participation must be considered an adverse event if it worsened. Furthermore, the seriousness of an adverse event is not synonymous with its severity or potential outcomes. An adverse event is considered serious if it is (1) serious or life-threatening, (2) requires or prolongs hospitalization, (3) is significantly or permanently disabling or incapacitating, (4) constitutes a congenital anomaly or birth defect, or (5) requires medical/surgical intervention to prevent any one of the preceding. There is no mention of severity or potential seriousness. Thus, a severe symptom or abnormal laboratory finding that does not meet one of these criteria is not considered a serious adverse event.

Above all, it is critical that adverse events be looked for, recognized, recorded, and reported as quickly as possible to the appropriate study governing personnel to allow any necessary actions to be taken to safeguard all other study participants.

Ethical Considerations (See Also Chap. 12)

The protocol must state that all patients will provide *informed consent* prior to being enrolled in the study. The consent form must be written in language the patient can fully understand and must contain certain elements. These include a description of the study; what is expected of the patient; what risks are involved with any tests, procedures, and treatments; what alternative treatments' are available; and assurance that the patient will be given the best available treatment for his/her condition whether or not he/she chooses to participate initially or to terminate prematurely. The patient should also be informed that his/her study records may be reviewed by the sponsor, auditors, or other regulatory authorities and that his/her study information may be used in publications. In any of these instances, the patient must be assured that his/her identity will be kept strictly confidential. The process of obtaining informed consent offers an excellent opportunity to establish good communications and rapport between the patient and the investigators and, as such, may impact the study outcome [21–23]. It is important to recognize that consent for study participation contains important elements that distinguish it from consent to a procedure, be it a routine clinical procedure or one required as part of the study; thus, consent to participate in a research study should be obtained separately from other permissions obtained in caring for a patient [24]. The informed consent form itself is considered a part of the protocol. The protocol also should contain a statement that IRB approval will be obtained and that the investigators and all study personnel will obtain all periodic re-approvals and comply with all other requirements of that review board.

In addition, the protocol often includes a description of the *investigators' responsibilities* regarding patient safety. This description typically points out the research policies, regulations, and requirements of governmental, international, institutional, and sponsoring bodies. The investigators are required to comply with all of these. In addition, the investigators agree to accept full responsibility for protecting the rights, safety, and welfare of patients under their care during the study. The principles of good clinical practice mandate that the investigators provide the best available care, themselves or by appropriate referral, for any medically related problems that arise during the study, regardless of their relationship to the study itself.

Statistical Considerations

All protocols should contain a section that describes trial-specific statistical evaluation plans. For randomized controlled clinical trials, such considerations typically include (but are not limited to): the specific nature of the study design and related issues, the specifics of the randomization procedure and rationale employed, justification of sample size and associated power (see also Chap. 11), the statistical analysis planned for assessing primary and secondary outcome measures, and a statement of the null hypothesis for primary efficacy comparison. When appropriate (e.g., a randomized controlled trial evaluating high-risk patients), this section also may articulate statistically-based "stopping rules" for premature termination of the study (e.g., early evidence of efficacy in the absence of safety problems).

Protocol Implementation and Study Conduct

Recent observations suggest that the conduct of certain types of clinical trials have decreased, raising concerns about adequacy of planning and implementation. For example, "late phase" clinical trials represented about 20% of all clinical trials in 1994 whereas in 2008, they accounted for only 4.4% of all clinical trials [16]. Possible reasons that may contribute to this apparent decline include inadequate organization and infrastructure, lack of coordinated research team effort, and insufficient training [16–18]. No matter how well a protocol is written, it is of little value if it cannot be implemented and carried out to completion.

Study Organization, Structure, and Administration

In addition to describing how the study will be done, protocols typically address issues which help safeguard the well-being of patients during their study participation, while ensuring the integrity and proper conduct of the study. Many of the topics discussed in this section are addressed at great length in other publications and reference materials which the reader should consult [1, 9]. We will focus here on some of these topics, especially those that are typically required for inclusion in a protocol by sponsoring institutions, funding agencies, and regulatory authorities.

Studies typically encounter unforeseen problems and questions during their conduct. In addition, some potential issues can be foreseen prior to study initiation; these need to be prospectively addressed so that solutions can be decided quickly according to plan should they, indeed, arise during the course of the study. Examples of such issues include endpoint criteria, rules for early termination of the study, need for protocol changes, etc. It is important for any study, and is mandatory for multicenter studies, that the protocol identify those individuals responsible for making decisions about the study's conduct. Thus, the protocol should specify the individuals and committees who are responsible for study leadership and charged with making the kinds of decisions mentioned above.

Multicenter studies should have a chairperson who is empowered to make and/or delegate day-to-day decisions regarding such things as deciding if a patient satisfies all inclusion/exclusion criteria or if a patient or center has violated protocol requirements, etc. In addition, there may be a steering or executive committee to address broader issues, e.g., protocol changes, and to address recommendations of any subcommittees. The subcommittees may typically include an independent data safety and monitoring board (DSMB) that periodically reviews study data to assess the need for possible premature termination of the study if a clear benefit or risk appears that makes it unethical to continue the study. Another subcommittee might analyze study endpoint outcomes, e.g., cause of death or reason for hospital admission. It is mandatory that subcommittees and committees prospectively define the rules and criteria to be used in arriving at any decisions they make and that information required to satisfy these rules be included as a part of the protocol. Subcommittees and other committees generally make recommendations to the steering or executive committee who has responsibility for making final decisions based on those recommendations.

In summary, the leadership of the study is responsible for the general satisfactory conduct of the study in all of its aspects. This includes resource recruitment and allocation, providing any training required, ensuring timeliness of patient recruitment, overseeing data management, and reporting of the results.

Resource Allocation and Management

Key resources include funds, manpower, and supplies. Funding may be available prior to study initiation in some settings with predetermined budgets, e.g., industry. In other settings, funding must be applied for, and its procurement often depends heavily on the quality of the research proposal and/or protocol. Once funds are secured, the study leadership must oversee their allocation, accountability, and continuing availability, as well as identify the individuals who will be responsible for these matters.

The success of the study also will depend on the availability of sufficient and qualified personnel to carry out all the required functions. For certain functions, especially those that might only be required from time to time to address specific issues that might arise, it may be preferable to use consultants. For example, if patient recruitment lags, the advice of persons specialized in recruitment techniques might be sought. It is critical that all personnel be qualified to carry out whatever responsibilities they are assigned and that the study leadership provides the proper training needed to ensure their qualifications.

Availability of all supplies needed to carry out the study is critical and may be a rate-limiting factor in starting and completing the study in a timely fashion. Obviously, the study cannot start without materials for gathering and reporting data, e. g., case report forms (see also Chap. 7). Similarly, study drugs and/or devices must be available and ready for use, i.e., properly coded and allocated for a randomized trial. Any supplies for laboratory tests and study procedures also must be available. Not only is it important that all supplies be available to start the study, but it also is necessary to assure that they will continue to be available throughout the study until its conclusion. A key responsibility of study leadership is to oversee the individuals responsible for ensuring timely availability of supplies. In addition, study leaders must be readily available to these same individuals to try to resolve any supply problems that might arise.

The protocol should contain information about *study materials* the patient will need, including study drugs, laboratory kits, questionnaires, diaries, etc. Information should be provided on who is responsible for procuring and dispensing these materials, how and where they will be procured, how they will be supplied (kits, bottles, etc.), how they will be labeled to correctly identify content and the study patient, and instructions for their use. There also should be a description of how the supplies will be stored. Finally, there must be an accurate inventory of all materials, with dates of receipt, dispensing, names of recipients, etc. There also must be a procedure for returning study material and recording their receipt. All of these records are mandatory for accountability of supplies and are subject to strict regulations, especially when any controlled substances are involved. This section is critical to the study sponsor who generally provides the materials and must be able to show that adequate instructions for their correct handling were provided to investigators.

Recruitment of Study Participants

The recruitment of eligible patients/subjects into the study in a timely fashion is one of the key rate-limiting processes that has a major impact on study results. Failure to recruit patients in a timely manner may have serious consequences by precipitating retrospective protocol changes, such as relaxing eligibility/exclusion requirements or modifying procedures and observations. Any such changes can significantly affect the study and potentially undermine its original intent and capacity to properly test the study hypothesis, thus yielding results that may not be valid and conclusive relative to the original intent. Failure to recruit patients quickly enough in sufficient numbers can lead to early termination of the study itself as well as discontinuation of its funding, thereby jeopardizing the power of the trial to achieve its projected sample size needed to achieve statistically conclusive results.

Techniques for recruiting study subjects vary considerably and represent a specialized topic in and of itself [1, 19, 20] that is beyond the scope of this chapter. The study leadership must identify the individuals responsible for recruitment and provide them with adequate resources and training for whatever recruitment techniques are employed. The specific techniques to be used should be spelled out in detail in the protocol. Numerous recruitment techniques are available and include screening subjects from (1) the local research site (office, clinic, hospital, etc.), (2) collaborating local sites, and (3) collaborating regional, national, and/or international sites. Within each of these sites, local areas of interest must be identified, e.g., office, laboratory, and emergency room. Screening-type trials seeking large or broad populations of subjects may establish recruitment centers in churches, schools, supermarkets, shopping centers, commercial establishments, etc., to identify appropriate patients. In addition, advertising through various media should be utilized to reach potentially eligible participants. Other sources are colleagues, bulletin board notices, direct mailings, and telephone screening [1]. The final decision regarding recruiting methods will depend on the overall number and kinds of patients/subjects needed. Importantly, the duration of active recruiting efforts commonly is specified in a protocol. These timelines should be closely monitored and adjusted as needed by the study leadership.

Study Monitoring

Implementation of the protocol should be carefully monitored. The persons assigned this task should be identified and adequately trained in the monitoring procedures to be used. These individuals should identify the personnel responsible for overseeing study conduct at the various centers and should ensure that all personnel at the center are well aware of and able to properly carry out all the investigators' responsibilities. It is important to describe the procedures that these individuals will follow to ensure (1) adherence to the protocol, (2) provision of complete and accurate data, (3) response to queries, and (4) compliance with auditing. Instructions on record keeping and record retention should also be provided.

Monitoring techniques vary and may include simple periodic telephone or e-mail contact with mailing or electronic submission of study documents between investigator sites and the monitors. Monitors may visit sites on a periodic basis to retrieve and deliver study materials as well as directly observe the site's performance. For a more detailed description of monitoring methods and procedures, the reader should consult standards references on the subject [1].

Data Acquisition and Processing

The principles of data acquisition and management are described in detail in Chap. 7. From the study conduct perspective, it is important that adequate numbers of qualified personnel are available for data processing and management. Furthermore, these individuals must have expertise or be trained in the required methods to be used for acquiring and processing data. Similarly, study leadership must ensure that all appropriate materials, especially equipment, hardware and software, are available to properly process the data.

End of Study Procedures

Once all study visits have been completed in all subjects, the study itself can be terminated. Procedures for terminating the study may include a final monitoring visit to retrieve all outstanding study materials such as case report forms and study supplies. Data processing procedures, e.g., quality control and source document verification, should be initiated and completed. Record retention procedures should be implemented.

The final results should be tabulated, analyzed, and presented in a final study report to be submitted as required to funding agencies, IRBs, regulatory agencies, etc. Most importantly, it is strongly recommended that all final results be published. Only in this manner can the study be critically analyzed by all those with a stake in its outcome as well as be replicated if deemed desirable.

Overview of the Interventional Clinical Trial

Most of what is discussed above has derived from, and has been best defined by, interventional clinical trials which represent the culmination of clinical research and merit special consideration because of their impact on clinical research methodology. Interventional clinical trials are designed and conducted for the primary purpose of testing a treatment or management strategy in patients with a specific disease. Such trials typically are sponsored by large research organizations, such as the United States National Institutes of Health (NIH), or by private organizations such as pharmaceutical companies or medical device manufacturers.

An interventional clinical trial is a formal experiment designed to elucidate and evaluate the relative efficacy and safety of different treatments or management strategies for patients with a specific medical condition [25]. Healthy volunteers often are used in the early phases of assessment of a new therapy primarily to assure sufficient safety of an intervention before applying it to patients with the disease targeted by the intervention. Such studies typically involve establishing the proper dosing and/or administration of the intervention along with demonstrating that the intervention is tolerated well enough to permit further studies in patients. However, healthy human volunteers provide only indirect evidence of effects on patients. Therefore, ultimately, clinical trials of putative interventions must be conducted among individuals with disease. The results obtained from this limited sample then are used to make inferences about how treatment can be applied in the diseased population in the future [25]. Most commonly, a clinical trial takes the form of a prospective study comparing the effect of an intervention, usually a new drug or device, with a comparator or control (i.e., a placebo or a treatment already available) [26]. The fundamental design of the clinical trial can be widely applied to many different disciplines or areas of clinical research. (For a comprehensive discussion of contemporary clinical trial methodology, the reader is referred to the seminal writings of Spilker [1]). Clinical trials can be employed to evaluate many forms of therapy, including surgical interventions and radiation therapy. In addition, clinical trials can be used to test other nontherapeutic approaches to patient care, such as diagnostic tests or procedures [27]. Thus, the NIH classifies clinical trials into five categories according to their purpose, i.e., treatment trials, prevention trials, diagnostic trials, screening trials, and health-related quality of life trials. These categories reflect the way in which clinical trials fit within the entirety of the clinical research spectrum, as they can be instrumental in assisting clinical efforts to improve not only the treatment of a particular disease (as is most often the case) but also its prevention and detection [27].

The clinical trial is the most widespread application of experimental study design in humans [26]. Indeed, it is the adherence of the trial to the principles of scientific experimentation, perhaps more so than a reliance on therapeutic comparison, that most aptly validates the results of the trial. Along this vein, a number of general characteristics of the scientific method play a substantial role in the modern conduct of clinical trials including, most notably, the control of extraneous factors that might influence outcome variability, selection bias, or interpretation of results [28]. For example, an important feature of the randomized controlled trial, which is widely accepted as the primary standard of evidence when interventions are evaluated, is the requirement to randomly allocate patients to alternative interventions, strengthening the internal validity of the study (see also Chap. 5).

In any clinical trial, regardless of which interventions or tests are administered, investigators must carefully follow the progress of recruited subjects, collecting data for a prespecified time interval according to the requirements of the study protocol; subsequently, statistical analyses are performed that might yield valuable conclusions relevant to predefined research objectives. Some studies might involve more tests or medical visits than are clinically necessary, while others interfere only minimally with normal patient care practices. In general, the details of the procedure, including the specific conceptual plans for observation, data capture, follow-up, and analysis depend on what type of clinical trial is being conducted. Due to their broadening scope of applicability since the mid-1900s, clinical trials currently play a paramount role in examining the impact of interventions among human subjects. What has further cemented the clinical trial as a valuable tool for the clinical investigator has been the recognition by health-care professionals that, if insights into disease prevention and improvement to patient care are to be gained, experimental methodology should be followed as rigorously in a clinical setting as it is in basic science[28]. Proper preparation of the research protocol, therefore, is essential to the successful and ethical application of the clinical trial to modern clinical research.

Conclusions

The study protocol is the most important and critical document available to the investigator and is central to the conduct of any study. It provides the necessary guidance and serves as the main reference for all study personnel, while also providing for the welfare and safety of all study participants. It must be detailed and comprehensive and must be prospectively defined. Whereas it is not possible to foresee all things that might occur during the course of the study, it behooves the investigators to plan for all foreseeable developments in the protocol. Virtually, anything that must be done post hoc has the potential to introduce bias and undermine the credibility and validity of the study. The degree to which the investigators can achieve these requirements will serve as testimony to their thoughtfulness, attention to detail, and overall quality of work. A high-quality protocol should allow others who follow it rigorously to obtain the same results. Most importantly, a high-quality protocol will likely lead to a valid and credible conclusion, whether it confirms or refutes the hypothesis, thereby reducing the likelihood of needing a costly repeat study because of a faulty protocol.

Take-Home Points

- A protocol is the most critical document in a research study.
- It plays a central role in the conduct of a study by describing how a hypothesis will be tested.
- It provides the necessary guidance and serves as the main reference for all study personnel, while also providing for the welfare and safety of all study participants; it must be prospective, detailed, and comprehensive.
- A protocol is organized in chronological divisions; the background and rationale provide the first impression of the investigators; study endpoints, especially the primary ones, drive the rest of the study design.
- The study population schedule of visits/procedures, and methods for ensuring patient safety, along with other human subjects issues, must be described in detail.
- A high-quality protocol will enhance the likelihood of drawing valid conclusions, whether they confirm or refute the hypothesis, thereby reducing the likelihood of needing a costly repeat study.

References

1. Spilker B. Guide to clinical trials. New York: Raven; 1991.
2. Treweek S, McCormack K, Abalos E, Campbell M, Ramsay C, Zwarenstein M, PRACTIHC Collaboration. The trial protocol tool: the PRACTIHC software tool that supported the writing of protocols for pragmatic randomized controlled trials. J Clin Epidemiol. 2006;59:1127–33.
3. Sellier P, Chatellier G, D'Agrosa-Boiteux MC, Douard H, Dubois C, Goepfert PC, Monpère C, Saint Pierre A, Investigators of the PERISCOP study. Use of non-invasive cardiac investigations to predict clinical endpoints after coronary bypass graft surgery in coronary artery disease patients: results from the prognosis and evaluation of risk in the coronary operated patient (PERISCOP) study. Eur Heart J. 2003; 24:916–26.
4. Mahaffey KW, Harrington RA, Akkerhuis M, Kleiman NS, Berdan LG, Crenshaw BS, Tardiff BE, Granger CB, DeJong I, Bhapkar M, Widimsky P, Corbalon R, Lee KL, Deckers JW, Simoons ML, Topol EJ, Califf RM, For the PURSUIT Investigators. Disagreements between central clinical events committee and site investigator assessments of myocardial infarction endpoints in an international clinical trial: review of the PURSUIT study. Curr Control Trials Cardiovasc Med. 2001;2:187–94.
5. Marang van de Mheen PJ, Hollander EJ, Kievit J. Effects of study methodology on adverse outcome occurrence and mortality. Int J Qual Health Care. 2007;19:399–406.
6. Borgsteede SD, Deliens L, Francke AL, Stalman WA, Willems DL, van Eijk JT, van der Wal G. Defining the patient population: one of the problems for palliative care research. Palliat Med. 2006;20:63–8.
7. Chin Feman SP, Nguyen LT, Quilty MT, Kerr CE, Nam BH, Conboy LA, Singer JP, Park M, Lembo AJ, Kaptchuk TJ, Davis RB. Effectiveness of recruitment in clinical trials: an analysis of methods used in a trial for irritable bowel syndrome patients. Contemp Clin Trials. 2008;29:241–51.
8. Sisk JE, Horowitz CR, Wang JJ, McLaughlin MA, Hebert PL, Tuzzio L. The success of recruiting minorities, women, and elderly into a randomized controlled effectiveness trial. Mt Sinai J Med. 2008;75:37–43.
9. Armitage J, Souhami R, Friedman L, Hilbrich L, Holland J, Muhlbaier LH, Shannon J, Van Nie A. The impact of privacy and confidentiality laws on the conduct of clinical trials. Clin Trials. 2008;5:70–4.
10. Anisimov VV, Fedorov VV. Modelling, prediction and adaptive adjustment of recruitment in multicentre trials. Stat Med. 2007;26:4958–75.
11. Abbas I, Rovira J, Casanovas J. Clinical trial optimization: Monte Carlo simulation Markov model for planning clinical trials recruitment. Contemp Clin Trials. 2007;28:220–31.
12. Franciosa JA. Commentary on the use of run-in periods in clinical trials. Am J Cardiol. 1999;83:942–4.
13. Romano P. Automation of in-silico data analysis processes through workflow management systems. Brief Bioinform. 2008;9:57–68.
14. Lacroix Z. Biological data integration: wrapping data and tools. IEEE Trans Inf Technol Biomed. 2002;6:123–8.
15. Shah AR, Singhal M, Klicker KR, Stephan EG, Wiley HS, Waters KM. Enabling high-throughput data management for systems biology: the Bioinformatics Resource Manager. Bioinformatics. 2007;23:906–9.
16. Nussenblatt RB, Meinert CL. The status of clinical trials: cause for concern. J Transl Med. 2010;8:65–8.
17. Smith A, Palmer S, Johnson DW, Navaneethan S, Valentini M, Strippoli GF. How to conduct a randomized trial. Nephrology. 2010;15:740–6.
18. Paschoale HS, Barbosa FR, Nita ME, Carrilho FJ, Ono-Nita SK. Clinical trials profile: professionals and sites. Contemp Clin Trials. 2010;31:438–42.
19. Bader JD, Robinson DS, Gilbert GH, Ritter AV, Makhija SK, Funkhouser KA, Amaechi BT, Shugars DA, Laws R. X-ACT collaborative research group. Four "lessons learned" while implementing a multi-site caries prevention trial. J Public Health Dent. 2010;70:171–5.
20. Treweek S, Pitkethly M, Cook J, Kjeldstrøm M, Taskila T, Johansen M, Sullivan F, Wilson S, Jackson C, Jones R, Mitchell E. Strategies to improve recruitment to randomised controlled trials. Cochrane Database Syst Rev. 2010;4:MR000013.
21. Helgesson G, Ludvigsson J, Gustafsson Stolt U. How to handle informed consent in longitudinal studies when participants have a limited understanding of the study. J Med Ethics. 2005;31:670–3.
22. Jones JW, McCullough LB, Richman BW. Informed consent: it's not just signing a form. Thorac Surg Clin. 2005;15:451–60.
23. Albrecht TL, Franks MM, Ruckdeschel JC. Communication and informed consent. Curr Opin Oncol. 2005;17:336–9.
24. del Carmen MG, Joffe S. Informed consent for medical treatment and research: a review. Oncologist. 2005;10:636–41.
25. Pocock SJ. Clinical trials: a practical approach. New York: Wiley; 1983.
26. Portney LG, Watkins MP. Foundations of clinical research: applications to practice. 2nd ed. New Jersey: Prentice-Hall; 2000.
27. Basic questions and answers about clinical trials. Rockville (MD): Food and Drug Administration (US). Last Updated: 07/16/2009. http://www.fda.gov/forconsumers/byaudience/forpatientadvocates/hivandaidsactivities/ucm121345.htm Accessed 11 Aug 2011.
28. Piantadosi S. Clinical trials: a methodologic perspective. New York: Wiley; 1997.

Data Collection and Management in Clinical Research

7

Mario Guralnik

Introduction

As noted elsewhere in this volume, all successful clinical trials begin with a good study question or questions, optimally framed as one or more hypotheses, and an appropriate research design that clearly defines appropriate study endpoints as well as other key variables. As in most serious endeavors, the old adage "Failing to plan is planning to fail" applies when conducting clinical research, where poorly conceived study objectives and incompletely defined endpoints can almost guarantee that a study's conclusions will be faulty. In such cases, the best the researcher may hope for are anecdotal observations of questionable validity; at worst, they could mislead the community of patients, clinicians, and/or health policy decision makers for whom the research was conducted.

Once these elements have been rigorously defined, the next most important step is the designation of the data to be collected among the subjects to be included in the trial and the manner of data collection. Optimally, these will be detailed in procedural manuals, which outline the plans and processes for data flow, entry, and quality control and represent the essential documents for managing the conduct of the research. Not surprisingly, most data are collected to address the research study objectives. However, trial administration and compliance data also are often collected to provide evidence of the quality of the conduct of the study.

Having developed the proper study design and data definitions, the researcher next is faced with the challenge of selecting the systems to be used to collect and manage the trial data. Well-designed data management processes, collection tools, and systems will help ensure the validity and integrity of the data to be analyzed. Only data whose sources can be trusted as accurate, complete, and protected from tampering can be used to substantiate conclusions about a trial's outcomes. Also, clinical research inherently raises issues of patient privacy and data security; thus, data management processes and systems used in clinical trials must address both of these areas as well. Overall, defects and inefficiencies in methods and procedures of data identification, collection, and management translate into defects in documented evidence and waste in the conduct of the trial itself [1]. These problems may be compounded when studies are large, are long-term, or utilize multiple centers [2]. Therefore, well-designed trials and data management

M. Guralnik, PhD (✉)
Synergy Research Inc, 3943 Irvine Blvd #627,
Irvine, CA 92602, USA
e-mail: Mario@guralnik.com

P.G. Supino and J.S. Borer (eds.), *Principles of Research Methodology: A Guide for Clinical Investigators*,
DOI 10.1007/978-1-4614-3360-6_7,

methods are essential to the integrity of the findings from clinical trials and containing the costs of conducting them.

The methods by which data are collected must be addressed during the research design step. Attention must be paid to identifying existing or creating new research documents or devices into which trial observations can be recorded. Selecting the documents/devices that provide the most reliable and valid data is a critical component of the research design process. Historically, the cornerstone of data collection has been the structured paper case report form (CRF) into which the required data are transcribed from the research documents. However, inherent inefficiencies are present in paper-based data collection due to its time and resource-intensive nature and the error-prone aspects of data transcription and database entry. Not surprisingly, in the last decade, studies once steadfastly done on paper now routinely use electronic data capture (EDC) in an attempt to overcome these inefficiencies. Specifically, these EDC systems reduce redundancy, trap errors in real time (allowing their prompt resolution), and promote the uniform collection of data which can be analyzed and shared in a more consistent and timely manner. Procedural manuals typically outline processes for data generation, flow, entry, and quality control. They are essential for managing the conduct of the research. Verifying, validating, and correcting data entered into a clinical research database are critical steps for quality control. Several data cleaning processes are available for this purpose.

This chapter will consider the tools and processes that support the development of accurate clinical research data and efficient trial management. These tools and processes are designed to satisfy the requirements of funding agencies, Institutional Research Boards (IRBs), and other regulatory bodies with regard to protecting human subjects, provide timely access to safety and efficacy data, and maintain patient confidentiality. Topics to be covered include the various types of data used in clinical research, basic source and research documents, data capture methods, and procedures for monitoring and securely storing data.

Data Types

The term "data" in clinical research refers to observations that are structured in such a way as to be "amenable to inspection and/or analysis" [3]. In other words, they represent the evidence for conclusions drawn in a trial. All data collected in biomedical research studies are either numerical or nonnumerical. Nonnumerical data typically are based on written text but also could include data from sources ranging from digital photography to voice dictation. Any individual study may collect either or both of these data types. The approaches required to analyze, summarize, and interpret each type vary, so the differences between the various approaches must be considered when designing a study and collecting the data [4].

Quantitative Data

The data collected in randomized clinical trials (RCTs), where the effectiveness and safety of new clinical treatments are evaluated, primarily are quantitative (numerical) in nature. Such data may be discrete or count-based (e.g., number of white blood cells or hospitalizations) or continuous measurements (e.g., dimensions, temperature, flow) and are collected using such methods as objective (laboratory) testing or patient response questionnaires and surveys that ask the respondent how much or how many. Quantitative data may be displayed graphically or summarized and otherwise analyzed through the use of descriptive and/or inferential statistics. Descriptive statistics, including distributional characteristics of a sample (e.g., frequencies or percentages), measures of central tendency (e.g., means, medians, or modes), and measures of variability (e.g., ranges or standard deviations), provide a way by which the voluminous numerical data collected can be reduced to a manageable and more easily interpretable set of numbers. Inferential statistics provide levels of probability by which the research hypotheses can be tested and conclusions drawn (see Chap. 11 for an in-depth discussion of these methods).

Qualitative Data

Exploratory trials, in which one of the purposes is to generate information for use in the planning and design of RCTs, rely heavily on nominal and other forms of nonnumeric data produced using such methods as patient free-text opinion surveys, diaries, and translations of verbal communications (e.g., interviews). The summarization and analysis of nonnumeric data typically involve the use of descriptive statistics (as is the case for quantitative study data), but additional work is required before the descriptive statistics can be calculated. Specifically, the nonnumeric data first must be translated into numeric codes based on a coding scheme preferably specified in the protocol or, at least, prior to the collection of the data. The coding scheme, however, is by its very nature a subjective process which has the potential for investigator bias resulting from selective collection and recording of the data (or from interpretation based on personal perspectives). The potential bias can be minimized by having at least two researchers independently collect and record the data based on the same information and coding scheme.

Reliability and Validity

Reliability and validity are concepts that reflect the rigor of the research and the trustworthiness of the research findings [5]. Reliability describes the extent to which a particular test, procedure, or data collection method (e.g., a questionnaire) will produce similar results under different circumstances. Highly reliable data are in evidence when the research tool or method used in the collection of the data provides similar information when used by different individuals (interrater reliability) or at different times (reproducibility). Validity is a subtler concept which describes the extent to which what we believe we are measuring accurately represents what we intended to measure. Internal validity indicates the accuracy of causal inferences drawn from a study's findings. External validity indicates the extent to which a study's findings can be applied to other similar groups of people or situations. Additional information about validity and reliability can be found in Chaps. 5 and 8.

Principles of Data Identification and Collection

As previously described, the research data to be collected in any clinical trial and stored in the clinical database must support the objectives of the study and be specified in the protocol. This, in turn, relies on designing data collection instruments and computer databases that correctly capture the defined research data. To support trial administration and to document compliance with regulations and Good Clinical Practice (GCP), source documents also are expected to capture subject participation data, though such data are not necessarily included in the research database [4].

The research data represent the information that is analyzed to answer the questions being stated in the study objectives. In most protocols, addressing primary and potentially secondary objectives requires collection of both efficacy and safety endpoints. To appropriately design the data collection documents and collection methods, it is important to consider the value or weight that each study objective contributes to the overall outcome of the study. Emphasis must be placed on accurate and complete collection of the specific data points necessary to investigate the study's primary objectives, while the collection of extensive data in support of secondary objectives should never be allowed to detract from satisfying the study's primary objectives.

When considering the collection of administrative source data to help with the management of a trial, the amount of such data required depends to a large degree on the complexity of the trial structure. For example, in a small, single-institution trial, much less information typically is needed than in a large multicenter trial [4]. The specific types of data to be collected will depend on the details of the trial and could include information about transport of study materials, monitors assigned to each site, dates of monitor visits, or drug supply levels at each site [4]. Regardless of the amount and the type of administrative data collected, it is not uncommon for trial management information to be manually and/or electronically stored separately from the clinical trial research results.

Other administrative data include personal patient information. The *Study Coordinating Center* must be able to link a patient to a specific institution and maintain a roster of contact details for that institution (e.g., patient name, address, telephone and fax numbers, and names, titles, and e-mail addresses for key trial personnel at that institution) [4]. However, due to privacy considerations, the patient identification information must be stored separately from the trial database which contains uniquely assigned patient and possibly randomization numbers, which can also be used to link data from multiple sources to the same patient (e.g., laboratory data, demographic information, and medical history).

Most studies also will need some documentation of compliance with regulatory requirements. The level of detail for such compliance data depends on the type and purpose of the trial. Studies to be submitted to regulatory agencies in support of *New Drug or Product License Applications* typically require the most complete set of compliance source data. Types of documentation can include ethics committee approvals for the protocol, original copies of patient consent forms, and personnel qualifications and training at participating sites [4].

Bottom line, in most clinical trials, a large volume of data is collected. According to a recent review of data monitoring in clinical trials [6], the more data that are collected, the more cumbersome and complicated data management becomes. Therefore, one goal in trial design should be to minimize the volume of noncritical data required so as to increase the integrity and quality of the study's results. This requires a realistic appraisal of the ability of investigators and other study personnel to manage the amount of data collected with a minimum of confusion and error.

Data Sources

During the research design step, attention must be paid to identifying existing or creating new research source documents or electronic devices into which trial observations can be recorded. Selecting the source documents/devices that provide the most reliable and valid data to investigate the research study objectives is a critical component of the research design process. Data may be extracted from *research-independent sources*, e.g., health insurance databases or electronic health records (EHRs), or *research-dependent sources*, e.g., lab reports generated from the performance of procedures conducted according to a trial protocol's schedule. Both types of sources may provide data for a research study and are described, in greater detail, below.

Source Documentation and the Concept of "Original Ink"

Source documents for research can be defined as all information contained in original records and certified copies of results, observations, and other aspects required for the reconstruction and evaluation of a study and its conduct [7]. Source documentation in a clinical trial includes medical or physiological, social, and psychological indicators of health that can be used to determine the effectiveness of a clinical intervention. These can involve copies of any or all of the following original confidential medical records: pharmacy dispensing records, physician's notes, clinic and office charts, nurse's notes, clinical laboratory reports, diagnostic imaging reports, patient diaries and questionnaires, hospital admission records, hospital discharge records, emergency room reports, autopsy reports, electronic diagnostic or research test results, vital sign records, electronically captured original study data, photographs, diagrams, and sketches. Source documents also can be created or provided by a trial sponsor by a third party (e.g., a contract research organization

[CRO] or a site management organization [SMO]) or by the investigator or site staff, and may include study *case report forms* (CRFs) *or electronic case report forms* (eCRFs) *if* used as the first point of data capture. A source document could even be a cafeteria napkin containing laboratory results or other observations, although a more formal data collection source document would be much preferred.

Use of the "original ink" concept can help to differentiate a source document from subsequent documentation. Original ink is a term that may be used to define the first-ever written documentation of an event or observation pertaining to the study subject. Thus, documents containing original ink are considered source documents for research. The US Food and Drug Administration (FDA) as well as other regulatory agencies also recognize a CRF as source documentation when it has captured the original ink of an event or observation in a clinical trial. In contrast, transcriptions or reproductions are considered "subsequent documentation" based on the source "original ink" document. With today's use of advanced computer technology, ranging from digital photography to voice dictation, we must consider other forms of original ink or, more appropriately termed, original electronic chronicles. These include voice, electronic, magnetic, photo-optical, and other source documentation and records. For further information on the FDA's position on source documentation, the reader is referred to Guidance for Industry: Electronic Source Documentation in Clinical Investigations (2010) [8].

Confusing these issues can lead to misrepresentation of clinical trial data. For example, after site staff has collected a subject's history directly on sponsor-designated CRFs, the study monitor might remind the investigator's staff that pre-printed sponsor source documents exist and that they are designed to assist the site in capturing all necessary data elements. The site staff might then proceed to transcribe data from the CRF onto the sponsor's source documents. To further confuse the matter, subsequent monitoring or query resolution activities by the sponsor would then rely on the transcribed sponsor's source documents to be the accurate and overriding data points for resolution. Simply stated, erroneous data could be considered the factual representation of an event or observation. A simple but effective tool for avoiding such situations is to define in advance on a site-by-site, as well as a form-by-form, basis what is and what is not "source documentation." When clarifying the definition of source documentation, an important point to keep in mind is that the study staff may habitually record original ink data in certain places. For example, a patient's temperature and pulse may be routinely taken at the bedside by the study coordinator and recorded on a copy of the CRF. If the patient's blood pressure is then taken from the physician's notes and recorded on the copy, then that copy becomes the source documentation for the first two measurements, but not for the third. Interviewing the staff prior to source document verification is an effective time-saving tool. When done early in the study initiation process, this method can very effectively clarify potential discrepancies.

Research-Independent Data Sources

A wealth of medical information is generated every day for nonresearch purposes. A significant source of such data, accessible for research purposes, are the patient medical records maintained by hospitals, clinics, and doctor's offices. Even the simplest medical records could contain important information for research purposes, such as sociodemographic data, clinical data, administrative data, economic data, and behavioral data. Additional potential research-independent primary data sources are (a) claims data (such as those from managed care databases), (b) encounter data (such as those from a staff/group model of health maintenance organizations), (c) expert opinions, (d) results of published literature, (e) patient registries, and (f) national survey databases. Since these data sources contain historical as well as current data that are updated on an ongoing basis, these sources provide data that are potentially useful in both retrospective studies (designed to investigate past events) and prospective studies (designed to investigate events occurring after patients have been enrolled in a study).

Research-Dependent Data Sources

Controlled evaluation of investigational products or interventions requires prospective data collection which typically involves identifying one or more patient groups, collecting baseline data, delivering one or more products or interventions, collecting follow-up data, and comparing the changes from baseline among the different patient groups. Although there may be some research-independent sources collected in these controlled evaluations (e.g., demographic, characteristics, medical history), most of the baseline data and, obviously, the follow-up data must be collected from research-dependent sources. Well-designed investigations of this nature specify, prior to the initiation of the study, the data to be collected and the collection methods to be used.

Data Collection Methods

The study design and the study data to be collected dictate the methods by which the data are to be collected. Laboratory data (e.g., hematology, urinalysis, serology) and vital signs (e.g., height, weight, blood pressure) may be required in a clinical trial to evaluate efficacy and, often, to evaluate patient safety. These data typically would be collected using standard methods for these data types and recorded in the patient's medical records, often designed specifically for the research study. Other data collected to address the research question(s) may require clinical information (e.g., events experienced by the patient, nonstudy medications used by the patient), tracking information (e.g., timing and amount of study medications received, alcohol consumption, sexual activity), or subjective information (e.g., personal opinions of medical condition or ease of treatment). These data must be obtained directly from the patient, most often through the use of a questionnaire or survey.

Questionnaires and surveys consist of a predetermined set of questions administered verbally, as a part of a structured interview, or nonverbally on paper or an electronic device. The responses to the questions may be discrete bits of data or may be grouped as measures of study outcomes (e.g., psychological scales). If the questionnaire is intended to measure study outcomes, establishing its reliability and validity and minimizing bias are essential. Administering a published questionnaire for which reliability and validity have been previously determined is recommended when possible. However, the use of some published questionnaires requires permission of their authors and may have a cost associated with their use. When the use of published questionnaires is not feasible, new questionnaires will need to be developed. Such questionnaires should be pretested systematically (i.e., "piloted") with a small subgroup of the patient population in order to identify and correct ambiguities or biases in the way the questions are stated. Training interviewers who verbally administer a questionnaire will also increase the quality of the data generated both from published or newly developed data collection instruments. (See Chap. 8 for a detailed description of various item formats used in questionnaires and general rules to consider when constructing questionnaire items.)

Data Capture

Paper-Based Methods

Efficient analysis, summarization, and reporting of biomedical research data require that data be available in an electronic database, such as a spreadsheet or one of several available databases, some of which have been designed specifically for clinical research data. The manner in which the data are entered into these databases has been evolving. Historically, most data in biomedical research, particularly in RCTs, were entered from a set of paper CRFs specifically designed for the study. Figure 7.1 shows an example of a typical paper CRF used to collect data obtained from physical examination.

INSTITUTION CODE	PARTICIPANT ID	VISIT TYPE	VISIT DATE (MM/DD/YYYY)
______	______	______	__ __/__ __/__ __ __ __

Examination Date (MM/DD/YYYY): __/__/__ ☐ Not Done		
Height: __ __ __. __ __ ☐ cm ☐ in ☐ Not Obtained	Weight: __ __ __. __ __ ☐ kg ☐ lb ☐ Not Obtained	Temperature: __ __ __. __ __ ☐ °C ☐ °F ☐ Not Obtained
Pulse Rate: ☐ Not Obtained	Respiration Rate: ☐ Not Obtained	Blood Pressure: __ __ __/__ __ __ ☐ Not Obtained Systolic (mm Hg)Diastolic (mm Hg)
Performance Status: ☐ 0 ☐ 1 ☐ 2 ☐ 3 ☐ 4		

Check here if NO body systems were examined: ☐

Body System/Site	Normal	Abnormal	Not Examined	Comments (Required if Abnormal; provide condition/diagnosis)
Appearance	☐	☐	☐	
Skin	☐	☐	☐	
H/E/E/N/T	☐	☐	☐	
Thyroid	☐	☐	☐	
Chest	☐	☐	☐	
Lungs	☐	☐	☐	
Breasts	☐	☐	☐	
Heart	☐	☐	☐	
Abdomen	☐	☐	☐	
Musculoskeletal	☐	☐	☐	
Genitalia	☐	☐	☐	
Pelvis	☐	☐	☐	
Rectal	☐	☐	☐	
Prostate	☐	☐	☐	
Vascular	☐	☐	☐	
Neurological	☐	☐	☐	
Lymph Nodes	☐	☐	☐	

Fig. 7.1 Example of a paper CRF used to collect research data from a physical examination. Downloaded from the National Cancer Institute at the National Institutes of Health, Division of Cancer Prevention. http://dcp.cancer.gov/Files/clinical-trials/FINAL_DCP_CRF_Templates_Version_3.doc (Accessed 10 Nov 2011)

Electronic Systems

Despite their long-term use, paper-based systems for data collection and management have been found to be inefficient and error prone because of multiple iterations of data transcription, entry, and validation [9]. Thus, due to recent technological advances, paper-based CRFs are being replaced by eCRFs into which the data are entered directly into trial databases from source documents. Features of eCRFs are presented in Table 7.1, but they may vary depending on the computer software upon which they are based.

Table 7.1 Features that may be available for electronic CRFs depending on the clinical trial data management software used (Reproduced with permission from Brandt et al. [2])

Feature	Function
Primary electronic data entry	Data entered into CRF by interviewer or subject (rather than into a paper form first)
Context-sensitive help	Help is given in the context of the problem (immediately)
Default values set	Based upon predefined criteria, or previously entered date, values of fields may be set
Skip patterns	Disabling of questions that become inapplicable based on response to a previous question
Computed (derived) values	Certain questions may be based on values of other questions (such as body mass index (BMI) that is derived from height and weight). Computed values may also control skip patterns on a CRF. If BMI exceeds a present threshold, questions related to high BMI may be enabled
Interactive validation	Immediate checking of the values entered into the CRF based upon predefined criteria such as ranges, other values in the CRF or study, etc.

Principles of Case Report Form Design

Regardless of whether a CRF or eCRF is used, meaningful collection of high-quality data begins with a CRF that is based on the trial protocol [8]. Hence, consistency with source documents is an essential feature of a well-designed CRF. However, an analysis of source document verification performed by the sponsors of clinical trials has identified areas of inconsistency in 70% of cases [10]. Several items were either covered in the CRF but not in the source documents (including those pertaining to patient history and informed consent) or were described in the source documents but not in the CRF (including those regarding patient history, complications, adverse events, and concomitant drugs or other therapies). Sources of such discrepancies need to be resolved before a trial begins. Although CRFs play a pivotal role in the successful conduct of a trial, the design of these forms often is neglected in the haste to launch a trial. [11]. The content, format, coding, and data-entry requirement principles of good CRF design, described more than 20 years ago by Bernd [11], remain applicable today (Table 7.2).

To avoid the excessive costs and delays often associated with printing CRFs, sponsors that use paper-based data capturing have found alternatives

Table 7.2 Content, format, and data-entry principles of good case report form design

CRF content principles

- Collect data that support questions (as defined in the protocol) that are to be answered by the statistical analysis.
- Define terminology and scales.
- Avoid questions that address ancillary issues.
- Ask each question only once.

CRF format principles

- Ask questions directly and unambiguously, using conventional and professional terminology.
- For long-term studies, provide a separate CRF for each visit and group of visits.
- Arrange the questions in a logical sequence (i.e., the order in which a physician would ordinarily collect the data).
- Specify how precise answers should be (i.e., whether values should be rounded off or carried to one or more decimal places).
- When possible, collect direct numerical measurements rather than broad categorical judgments.
- Use design techniques that simplify reading and completing the form:
  - Balance white space with text.
  - When possible, use check-off blocks instead of asking for a code, value, or term.
  - Block sections of the form to make them easy to locate and complete.
  - Use variations in size and boldness to show the hierarchy of headings.
  - Highlight areas of the form where entries are needed.

CRF coding and data-entry requirements

- Use consistent reference codes (e.g., if code [1] represents "no" for one question, it should not represent "yes" for another question).

to the traditional outsourcing of this task. Desktop-publishing systems and precollated no-carbon-required paper (NCR) allow printing, collating, and binding of CRFs, with multicolored two- or three-part sets [11]. Over the course of a longitudinal study, CRFs often are improved or refined, including the addition of new entries and modification or deletion of entries on previous versions [2]. Some newly requested data (such as information about the patient's history) may be obtainable later, whereas time-dependent observations (such as measurements taken at a certain clinic visit) will not. Data for new or modified questions that cannot be obtained must be treated as "missing." Conversely, when a question is deleted, data for patients evaluated under the older CRF version must be archived or purged or both [2]. Regardless of the types of changes made, the FDA requires that the sponsor preserve all electronic versions for agency review and copying [12].

Electronic systems are designed to support data entry where data are entered directly from source documents with most data validations executed real time as the data are entered and errors promptly resolved typically by study site staff. As will be noted below, EDC systems also support the monitoring, cleaning, storage, retrieval, and analysis of research data [2], as well as promote the uniform collection of data, which can then be more easily analyzed and shared across a variety of platforms and databases [13].

EDC systems, however, are not without their own constraints. To be useful in multicenter trials, EDC systems must allow electronic submission of data from different sites to a central data center, be easy to implement and use, and minimize disruption at the clinical sites [9]. Timing is essential to the successful implementation of an EDC system. Considerable information technology (IT) support is needed to build the eCRFs, and considerable time must be dedicated to educating the trial site staff on the proper use of the new systems. To be successful and reap the benefits of EDC systems, this effort should be undertaken prior to the initiation of any research study [14].

Although EDC systems are most often used by formally organized research centers with data management staff, many clinical investigators in private practice or in academia conduct studies without the support of qualified biomedical informatics consultants and sophisticated EDC systems [15]. Nevertheless, EDC systems are available that can be implemented without specialized software for investigators with small budgets or limited access to data management staff.

Data collection has naturally evolved alongside with computer and information technology. Major milestones in this evolution include personal computers, relational databases, user-friendly interfaces for software once reserved for engineering and systems design staff, and broadened connectivity options such as computer to computer, internet networking, wireless to Ethernet, and cellular data connectivity. These advances along with the availability now of mobile computing and electronics devices, like the iPad, have a potentially huge impact on how we gather data, as well as where data capture is heading.

The iPad is a major step forward for clinical data management. These truly remarkable devices, resting in the hands of all members of the research team, would allow quick access to tools for capturing data, real time or otherwise. They also offer two-way connectivity along with the portability and functionality of the hardware, thereby lending them the exact adaptability needed for clinical medicine and research roles.

Newer generation iPads allow data to migrate from text-based field entry, or PDF form data entry, through to server-based relational databases. Using methods from e-mail as a carrier to internet-connected applications, the data stream can be instantaneous, allowing for immediate two-way data efforts, relaying back from sponsor to investigator. Third-party communications further enhance the iPad platform. All of this has begun to evolve because the iPad platform has simplified the process of data capture and transfer via its accessible hardware and novel data management applications.

Electronic Training Manuals

Procedural and training manuals—core documents of any clinical study—outline plans and processes for study coordination, creation of CRFs, data entry, quality control, data audits, data-entry verification, and site/data restrictions [2, 16]. The recent technological advances have not only made possible efficiencies in data collection and data processing but also made possible electronic manuals created with HTML-based content which offer several advantages over paper-based core documents. Special software can be used to edit multiple discrete documents, organize them hierarchically, and provide hyperlinking between related topics. When a manual is produced in this way, many authors can work simultaneously on different topics that are subsequently integrated with a version-control system as the content evolves. The version-control software can also manage changes and updates to protocol documents. Other advantages of this system over simple text documents include the capability for single-source authoring with generation of multiple output formats (e.g., JavaHelp), distribution of the complete manual through a dedicated web site of the complete manual (with hyperlinks to support online browsing) and support for highly efficient, full-text searching, with results ranked by relevance [2].

Data Error Identification and Resolution

Verifying, validating, and correcting data entered into a clinical research database are critical steps for quality control. Several data cleaning processes are available, including the following: double computer data entry which captures entry inconsistencies (though it cannot detect errors made by the person supplying the data without additional exploratory data analysis), random data-entry audits (which are based on a predetermined level of criticality for each data category), and electronic data validation (which identifies entry errors by their deviation from allowable and expected responses and interactively prompts for corrected data). Compared with paper-based systems, EDC systems can more efficiently clean data by reducing the number of data discrepancies and requests for clarifications, as well as lower the cost of each data query resolution by lessening the amount of manual input required.

Data-Entry "Cleaning"

"Cleaning," the process of verifying, validating, and correcting data entered onto the CRF or into the database, is essential to verifying quality control in a clinical trial. Double data entry, the most common way to verify data entered onto CRFs [17], begins with reentry of data from the CRF into the study database at a later point than the original entry; often, this step is performed by a person other than the operator who made the first entry. Next, the two versions are automatically compared, and any discrepancies are corrected [17]. Despite the widespread use of this method, the quality of data so corrected has been debated for many years [18]. Commenting that "…the concept of typing a final report twice to check for typographical errors is almost laughable," one group questioned "why double data entry but not double everything else?" Because double data entry rests on the assumption that original records are correct and all errors are introduced during data entry, this system can never trap errors made by the person completing the form without exploratory data analysis (EDA) [19]. EDA, which challenges the plausibility of the written data on the CRF, should therefore be performed either as data entry is ongoing or as the first stage in an analysis when double data entry is used.

Random data-entry audits are another way to check the quality of data on a CRF. This method is based on a predetermined level of criticality (assigned by the data management/ investigator team) for each data category, with respect to the adverse consequences of entering erroneous data.

For each category, a proportion of the CRFs is sampled by a random-sample-generating program, and entered data are compared with the source documents for discrepancies. For very important categories (i.e., data that are central to the study objective and must be correct), as many as 100% of CRFs may be sampled [2, 6]. Noncritical data, which should be correct but would not affect the study outcome if incorrect, would require a lower proportion of CRFs to be checked [6]. After sampling, the number of discrepancies is reported and corrective action taken. The proportion of audited CRFs for any category may be modified for a given site in light of site-specific discrepancy rates [2].

Electronic data validation identifies entry errors by their deviation from allowable and expected values or answers. These include laboratory measurements, answers that contradict answers to other questions entered elsewhere on the CRF, spelling errors, and missing values [2]. Because of their concrete nature, these errors can easily be identified.

Data Queries

To support the full process of study monitoring and auditing, the data management system should have querying tools in place [2]. After the data entry/verification process discovers an entry that requires clarification and determines that the data were accurately entered into the database, the data coordinator sends the participating institution a paper or electronic query. Examples of entries that warrant queries include missing data values, values out of range, values that fail logic checks, or data that appear to be inconsistent [20]. The query should include protocol and patient identifiers, specific descriptions of the form/data item in question and the clarification needed, and instructions on how and when to send a response. In turn, the coordinating center should have a mechanism for recording the issue and response to each query [20].

EDC systems have a proven superiority to paper-based systems with respect to the querying process. The use of eCRFs in combination with manual ad hoc queries by study monitors has been able to reduce data discrepancies and the consequent need for clarifications by more than 50%. The enhanced ability to clean and analyze data has resulted in the generation of more accurate data [21]. Moreover, compared with a paper-based system, EDC systems with built-in error checking for data quality have been shown to reduce the total number of queries and decrease the cost of each query resolution from $60 to $10 [14].

Document Retention, Security, and Storage

Retention

All clinical investigators should ensure that relevant forms such as CRFs are always accessible in an organized fashion. Informed-consent forms, CRFs, laboratory forms, medical records, and correspondence should be retained by the investigator until the end of the study and, thereafter, by the sponsor for at least 2 years after clinical development of the investigational product has been formally discontinued or 6 years after the trial has ended. Even after the completion of the study, side effects or benefits of the intervention may be present and the relevant forms may need to be retrieved. Factors to be considered are the availability of storage space and the possibility of off-site storage if there is insufficient storage space [22].

Security and Privileging

Both during and after completion of a study, investigators and their staff must prevent unauthorized access, preserve patient confidentiality, and prevent retrospective tampering/falsification of data. Under the FDA's Title 21 Code of Federal Regulations [23], access must be restricted to authorized personnel, the system must prevent malicious changes to research data through selective data locking, and an audit trail must exist [2].

Consideration should be given for software that provides:

- ***Privileging***: Study-specific role-based privileges should be assigned, with roles requiring adequate training and documentation of such training prior to system use. In the case of multisite studies, it is especially important to be able to assure investigators from each site that other sites can be restricted from altering their data or, in some cases, even seeing their data while the study is in progress. Also, different users should have different data access and editing privileges. Software should allow site restriction of data and the assignment of both role-based and functional privileges. The software should allow the level of restriction to be changed as appropriate.
- ***Storing of De-identified Data***: For studies where breach of patient confidentiality could have serious repercussions, the software should support storing of de-identified data. It is important to note that the Health Insurance Portability and Accountability Act (HIPAA) does not prohibit the storing of patient-identifiable information: it requires only that it be secure, be made accessible strictly on a need-to-know basis, and that accesses to such information be audited. The drawback of not storing patient-identifiable information in every study is that many of a system's useful workflow-automation features, such as generation of reminders to be mailed to patients periodically, cannot function seamlessly and personalization of reminders requires manual processes. Also, in prospective clinical studies for life-threatening conditions such as cancer, where decisions such as dose escalation are based on values of patient parameters, the storage and selective echoing of protected health information (PHI) provides an added safeguard to ensure that data are being entered, or the appropriate intervention is being performed, for the correct patient.
- ***Generation of De-identified Data***: The software should be able to de-identify the data when required in order to share data and should utilize information about user role-based privileges as well. For example, an investigator may have privileges to view patient identifying information, but other personnel, such as biostatisticians performing analyses, may view only de-identified data.
- ***Data Locking***: The software should allow a study coordinator to lock all the data in the system by study, subject, or CRF level when required. All investigators, particularly those involved in any type of human subjects research, must be sure to take adequate steps to preserve the confidentiality of the data they collect. Investigators must specify who will have access to the data, how and at what point in the research personal information will be separated from other data, and how the data will be retained at the conclusion of the study.

The following guidelines for preserving patient confidentiality should be followed [24, 25]:

- In general, all information collected as part of a study is confidential: data must be stored in a secure manner and must not be shared inappropriately.
- Information should not to be disclosed without the subject's consent.
- The protocol must clearly state who is entitled to see records with identifiers, both within and outside the project.
- Wherever possible, potentially eligible subjects should be contacted either by the person to whom they originally gave the information or by another person with whom they have a trust relationship.
- Information provided to prospective subjects should include descriptions of the kind of data that will be collected, the identity of the persons who will have access to the data, the safeguards that will be used to protect the data from inappropriate disclosure, and the risks that could result from disclosure of the data.
- Academic and research organizations should establish patient privacy guidelines for non-employee researchers.

Other Responsibilities and Issues

GCP guidelines mandated through the Code of Federal Regulations require that institutions (or when appropriate, an IRB) maintain records of all research proposals reviewed (including any scientific evaluations that accompany the proposals), approved sample consent documents, progress reports submitted by investigators, and reports of injuries to subjects [25]. Institutions also must maintain adequate records on the shipment of the drug product to the trial site and its receipt there, the inventory at the site, use of the product by study participants, and the return to the sponsor of unused product and its disposition [26–28]. Because drug-accountability records must be accurate and clear, especially for an audit of the study site [29], electronically based inventory management systems have been devised. In addition to describing current inventory [20], some of these systems have "look ahead" capabilities to assess and fulfill future inventory needs [30].

Oversight of Data Management: Role of Institutional Review Boards

As will be noted in Chap. 12, IRBs have a wide range of responsibilities in the design, conduct, and oversight of clinical trials, and it is important that clinical researchers be familiar with them. IRB functions that are particularly germane to those managing data include oversight of protection of the privacy and confidentiality of human subjects (identifiers and other data), monitoring of collected data to optimize subjects' safety, and continuing review of findings during the duration of the research project [31].

Confidentiality and Privacy of Research Data

Information obtained by researchers about their subjects must not be improperly divulged. It is essential that researchers be able to offer subjects assurance of confidentiality and privacy and make explicit provisions for preventing breaches. For most clinical research studies, assuring confidentiality typically requires adherence to the following routine practices: substituting codes for patient identifiers, removing face sheets (containing such items as names and addresses) from survey instruments that contain data, properly disposing of computer sheets and other documents, limiting access to data, and storing research records in locked cabinets. Although most researchers are familiar with the routine precautions that should be taken to maintain the confidentiality of data, more elaborate precautions may be needed in studies involving sensitive matters such as sexual behavior or criminal activities to give subjects the confidence they need to participate and answer questions. When information linked to individuals will be recorded as part of the research design, IRBs require that data managers ensure that adequate precautions are in place to safeguard the confidentiality of the information; thus, numerous specialized security methods have been developed for this purpose and IRBs typically have at least one member (or consultant) who is familiar with the strengths and weaknesses of the different systems available. Researchers should also be aware that federal officials have the right to inspect research records, including consent forms and individual medical records, to ensure compliance with the rules and standards of their programs. In the USA, FDA rules require that information regarding this authority be included in the consent forms for all research regulated by that agency.

Monitoring and Observation

One of the areas typically reviewed by the IRB is the researcher's plan for collection, storage, and analysis of data. Regular monitoring of research findings is important because preliminary data may signal the need to change the research design or the information that is presented to subjects or even to terminate the study early if deemed necessary. Thus, for an IRB to approve proposed research, the protocol must, as appropriate, include plans for monitoring the data collected to ensure the safety of subjects. Investigators sometimes misinterpret this requirement as a call for annual reports to the IRB. Instead, US Federal regulations require that, when appropriate, researchers provide the IRB with a description of their plans for analyzing the data during the collection process. Concurrent collection and analysis enables the researcher to identify flaws in the study design early in the project. The level of monitoring in the research plan should be related to the degree of risk posed by the research. Furthermore, when the research will be performed at foreign sites, the IRB at a US institution may require different monitoring and/or more frequent reporting than that required by the foreign institution. Under normal circumstances, however, the IRB itself does not undertake data monitoring. Rather, other independent persons (e.g., members of a data safety monitoring board [DSMB]) typically are responsible for monitoring trials and for decisions about modification or discontinuation of trials. It is the IRB's responsibility, though, to ensure that these functions are carried out by an appropriate group. The review group should be required to report its findings to the IRB on an appropriate schedule.

Continuing Review

At the time of its initial review, the IRB determines how often it should reevaluate the research project and will set a date for its next review. Some IRBs set up a complaint procedure that allows subjects to indicate whether they believe that they were treated unfairly or that they were placed at greater risk than was agreed upon at the beginning of the study. A report form available to all researchers and staff may be helpful for informing the IRB of unforeseen problems or accidents. US Federal policy requires that investigators inform subjects of any important new information that might affect their willingness to continue participating in the trial. Typically, the IRB will make a determination as to whether any new findings, new knowledge, or adverse effects should be communicated to subjects, and it should receive copies of any such information conveyed to subjects. Any necessary changes to the consent document(s) and any variations in the manner of data collection must be reviewed and approved by the IRB. The IRB has the authority to observe, or have a third party observe, the consent process and the research itself. The researcher is required to keep the IRB informed of unexpected findings involving risks and to report any occurrence of serious harm to subjects. Reports of preliminary data analysis may be helpful both to the researcher and the IRB in monitoring the need to continue the study. An open and cooperative effort between the researcher and the IRB protects all concerned parties.

Summary and Conclusions

Clearly defined study endpoints combined with well-designed source documents, CRFs, and systems for capturing, monitoring, cleaning, and securely storing data are essential to the integrity of findings from clinical biomedical research trials. Because IRBs have a wide range of responsibilities in the design, conduct, and oversight of clinical trials, it is also essential that clinical investigators be familiar with their requirements.

The inexorable shift from paper-based to EDC systems in large trials promotes the efficient and uniform collection of data that can be analyzed and shared across a variety of platforms and databases. EDC systems can build quality control into the data collection process from its inception—a more productive approach than building checks onto the end [19]. Although modern software tools unquestionably improve the potential for data collection and management, "…systems alone are worthless without pro-active study coordinators and investigators who create and enforce policies and procedures to ensure quality" [2]. Therefore, a trial's data collection system and its findings are only as sound as the commitment by individuals who formulate and carry out document design, study procedures, training, and data management plans.

Take-Home Points

- Well-designed trials and data management methods are essential to the integrity of the findings from clinical trials, and the completeness, accuracy, and timeliness of data collection are key indicators of the quality of conduct of the study.
- The research data provide the information to be analyzed in addressing the study objectives, and addressing the primary objectives is the critical driver of the study.
- Since the data management plan closely follows the structure and sequence of the protocol, the data management group and protocol development team must work closely together.
- Accurate, thorough, detailed, and complete collection of data is critical, especially at baseline as this is the last time observations can be recorded before the effects of the trial interventions come into play.
- The shift from paper-based to electronic systems promotes efficient and uniform collection of data and can build quality control into the data collection process.

References

1. Liu EW. Clinical research the six sigma way. JALA. 2006;11:42–9.
2. Brandt CA, Argraves S, Money R, Ananth S, Trocky NM, Nadkarni PM. Informatics tools to improve clinical research study implementation. Contemp Clin Trials. 2006;27:112–22.
3. Piantadosi S. Clinical trials. A methodologic perspective. 2nd ed. Hoboken: Wiley; 2005.
4. McFadden E. Data definition, forms, and database design. In: Management of data in clinical trials. 2nd ed. New York: Wiley; 2007.
5. Roberts P. Reliability and validity in research. Nurs Stand. 2006;20:41–5.
6. Williams GW. The other side of clinical trial monitoring; assuring data quality and procedural adherence. Clin Trials. 2006;3:530–7.
7. Crerand WJ, Lamb J, Rulon V, Karal B, Mardekian J. Building data quality into clinical trials. J AHIMA. 2002;73:44–56.
8. Guidance for industry: electronic source documentation in clinical investigations. Rockville: Food and Drug Administration (US). 2010. Office of Communication, Outreach and Development, HFM-40. Accessed 28 Oct 2011.
9. Kush R, Alschuler L, Ruggeri R, Cassells S, Gupta N, Bain L, Claise K, Shah M, Nahm M. Implementing Single Source: the STARBRITE proof-of-concept study. J Am Med Inform Assoc. 2007;14:662–73.
10. Takayanagi R, Watanabe K, Nakahara A, Nakamura H, Yamada Y, Suzuki H, Arakawa Y, Omata M, Iga T. Items of concern associated with source document verification of clinical trials for new drugs. Yakugaku Zasshi. 2004;124:89–92.
11. Bernd CL. Clinical case report forms design—a key to clinical trial success. Drug Inf J. 1984;18:3–8.
12. US Food and Drug Administration. Code of Federal Regulations:21CFR11.10. Title 21—food and drugs. Chapter I, subchapter A—general. Part 11—electronic records; electronic signatures. Subpart B—electronic records. Sec. 11.10—controls for closed systems. http://www.accessdata.fda.gov/scripts/cdrh/cfdocs/cfCFR/CFRSearch.cfm?fr=11.10. Accessed 25 Feb 2008.
13. Meadows BJ. Eliciting remote data entry system requirements for the collection of cancer clinical trial data. Comput Inform Nurs. 2003;21:234–40.
14. Welker JA. Implementation of electronic data capture systems: barriers and solutions. Contemp Clin Trials. 2007;28:329–36.
15. Kashner TM, Hinson R, Holland GJ, Mickey DD, Hoffman K, Lind L, Johnson LD, Chang BK, Golden RM, Henley SS. A data accounting system for clinical investigators. J Am Med Inform Assoc. 2007;14:394–6.
16. Argraves S, Brandt CA, Money R, Nadkarni P. Informatics tools to improve clinical research. In: Proceedings of the American Medical Informatics Association Symposium, 22–26 Oct 2005; Washington, DC.
17. Kawado M, Hinotsu S, Matsuyama Y, Yamaguchi T, Hashimoto S, Ohashi Y. A comparison of error detection rates between the reading aloud method and the double data entry method. Control Clin Trials. 2003;24:560–9.
18. King DW, Lashley R. A quantifiable alternative to double data entry. Control Clin Trials. 2000;21:94–102.
19. Day S, Fayers P, Harvey D. Double data entry: what value, what price? Control Clin Trials. 1998;19:15–24.

20. McFadden E. Software tools for trials management. In: Management of data in clinical trials. 2nd ed. New York: Wiley; 2007.
21. Trocky NM, Fontinha M. Quality management tools: facilitating clinical research data integrity by utilizing specialized reports with electronic case report forms. In: Proceedings of the American Medical Informatics Association Symposium, 22–26 Oct 2005; Washington, DC.
22. Saw SM, Lim SG. Clinical drug trials: practical problems of phase III. Ann Acad Med Singapore. 2000;29: 598–605.
23. http://www.datagovernance.com/adl_FDA_21_CFR_USA.html.
24. Department of Health and Human Services. IRB Guidebook Chapter IV: Consideration of research design, 2007. http://www.hhs.gov/ohrp/irb/irb_chapter4.htm. Accessed 25 Apr 2008.
25. US Food and Drug Administration. Code of Federal Regulations: 21CFR56.115. Title 21—Food and drugs. Chapter I, subchapter A—general. Part 56—institutional review boards. Subpart D—records and reports. Sec. 56.115—IRB records. http://www.accessdata.fda.gov/scripts/cdrh/cfdocs/cfcfr/CFRSearch.cfm?fr=56.115. Accessed 24 Feb 2008.
26. US Food and Drug Administration. Code of Federal Regulations: 21CFR312.59. Title 21—Food and drugs. Chapter I, subchapter D—drugs for human use. Part 312—investigational new drug application. Subpart D—responsibilities of sponsors and investigators. Sec. 312.59 —disposition of unused supply of investigational drug. http://www.accessdata.fda.gov/scripts/cdrh/cfdocs/cfcfr/CFRSearch.cfm?fr=312.59. Accessed 24 Feb 2008.
27. US Food and Drug Administration. Code of Federal Regulations: 21CFR312.61 Investigational New Drug Application. Title 21—Food and drugs. Chapter I, subchapter D—drugs for human use. Part 312—investigational new drug application. Subpart D—responsibilities of sponsors and investigators. Sec. 312.61—control of the investigational drug. http://www.accessdata.fda.gov/scripts/cdrh/cfdocs/cfcfr/CFRSearch.cfm?fr=312.61. Accessed 24 Feb 2008.
28. US Food and Drug Administration. Code of Federal Regulations: 21CFR312.62. Title 21—Food and drugs. Chapter I, subchapter D—drugs for human use. Part 312—investigational new drug application. Subpart D—responsibilities of sponsors and investigators. Sec. 312.62—investigator recordkeeping and record retention. http://www.accessdata.fda.gov/scripts/cdrh/cfdocs/cfcfr/CFRSearch.cfm?fr=312.62. Accessed 24 Feb 2008.
29. Siden R, Tankanow RM, Tamer HR. Understanding and preparing for clinical drug trial audits. Am J Health Syst Pharm 2002;59:2301,2306,2308.
30. DDOTS, Inc. IDEA Web-based software for investigational drug inventory management. http://www.ddots.com/idea_product_overview.cfm. Accessed 24 Feb 2008.
31. Department of Health and Human Services. IRB Guidebook Chapter III: Basic IRB Review. 2007. http://www.hhs.gov/ohrp/irb/irb_chapter3.htm. Accessed 25 Apr 2008.

Constructing and Evaluating Self-Report Measures

8

Peter L. Flom, Phyllis G. Supino, and N. Philip Ross

A self-report measure, as the name implies, is a measure where the respondent supplies information about him or herself. Such information may include self-reports of behaviors, physical states or emotional states, attitudes, beliefs, personality constructs, and self-judged ability among others. A self-report may be obtained via questionnaire, interview, or related methods. Questionnaires typically are written documents that are administered without the involvement of an interviewer, whereas interviews usually (but not always) are administered orally [1]; both are sometimes termed "surveys."

Self-reports are important in medical research because while some variables can be evaluated through physiological measures, chart review, physical exam, direct observation of the respondent, or by reports by others, other variables only can be assessed from information directly furnished by the patient or other subject. Indeed, the subject often can provide valuable information about social, demographic, economic, psychological, and other factors related to the risk of disease or to adverse outcomes of disease. The choice between self-report, observational, and biophysiological measures will depend on the data that are available and the nature of the research questions and hypotheses. It is important to note that while the range of biophysiological measures is constantly increasing, and while these measures may permit objective evaluation of clinically relevant attributes, they are not perfectly reliable (i.e., free from measurement error). Even more importantly, they may fail to capture the specific quality that the investigator wishes to evaluate. For example, if an investigator is interested in blood pressure, this may be evaluated biophysiologically. However, if the aim of the investigation is to examine the effects of mood on blood pressure, mood can be evaluated only by self-report as there are no biophysiological measures of mood (though there may be biophysiological correlates, and even causes and consequences of biophysical factors). Observational data also may provide useful information, but their use has its own perils as individuals do not always accurately observe the actions of others. For these reasons, information directly reported by patients and other subjects commonly is collected by clinicians, clinical investigators, and other health-care professionals, and can be used as a tool for patient management or for research. Topics commonly examined by self-report include physical or mental symptoms, level of

P.L. Flom, PhD (✉)
Peter Flom Consulting, LLC,
515 West End Ave, New York, NY 10024, USA
e-mail: Peterflomconsulting@mindspring.com

P.G. Supino, EdD
Department of Medicine, College of Medicine,
SUNY Downstate Medical Center,
450 Clarkson Avenue, Box 1199,
Brooklyn, NY 11203, USA
e-mail: phyllissupino@aol.com

N.P. Ross, BS, MS, PhD Statistics
SUNY Downstate Medical Center,
9006 Kirkdale Road, Bethesda, MD 29817, USA
e-mail: ross@statlogic.net

P.G. Supino and J.S. Borer (eds.), *Principles of Research Methodology: A Guide for Clinical Investigators*,
DOI 10.1007/978-1-4614-3360-6_8,

pain or stress, activities of daily living, health-related quality of life, availability of social support, use and perceived effectiveness of strategies used to cope with ill-health, satisfaction with the doctor-patient interaction, and adherence to medication schedules (though the latter might, at least in theory, also be evaluated through objective testing).

Although self-report instruments are relatively easy to use, their construction and validation can be difficult. This chapter will cover fundamental aspects of, and distinctions among, questionnaires, interviews, and other methods of self-report and will indicate the circumstances under which a new self-report measure may be needed. It also will describe methods of generating and structuring responses; discuss approaches to asking about sensitive information; describe the rationale for, and processes involved in, pilot testing, evaluating, and revising a measure; review related ethical and legal aspects; and provide a general guide to the entire process.

What Is a Questionnaire?

A questionnaire is a type of self-report instrument that is designed to elicit specific information from a population of interest. Questionnaires may be standardized but often are designed (or adapted) specifically for a particular study. Depending on the objective of the study and resources, the questionnaire, like other self-report measures, may be administered to all subjects in the available sample or to a defined subsample. As noted below, the most common method of administration is direct mailing to subjects, though other methods exist. Deciding upon the sampling strategy is a complex process. It can range from a simple random sample to a very complex hierarchical design involving multiple strata and sampling procedures, as reviewed in Chap. 10. For additional information on this subject, the reader is referred to Kish (1995) [2], Groves et al. (2004) [3], and Cochran (1977) [4].

The questionnaire usually is in the form of a written document, though sometimes it may be administered by audio or with pictorial methods. Questionnaires, like tests, can produce a total score or subscores, but also can yield different types of information that can be separately analyzed. Questionnaires are almost always a necessity when direct contact with the subject is not possible. Under these circumstances, questionnaires typically are administered by mail to the respondent who, in turn, completes and returns them to the sender. In other circumstances, questionnaires may be read to the respondent over the telephone or in-person as part of a structured interview, or they may be administered via the Internet in a variety of ways. A questionnaire can cover virtually any topic, although here we will emphasize those that capture information related to medical issues or health-related topics including, but not limited to, diseases, symptoms, and a patient's experiences with doctors and other health professionals. Some well-known questionnaires used in medical research are the *Brief Symptom Inventory* (a 53-item questionnaire covering nine dimensions of psychological health [5]); the *SF-36* (a 36-item patient-centered questionnaire about general physical and mental health-related quality of life [6]); the 26-item *World Health Organization Quality of Life Questionnaire* (*WHOQOL*) [7] assessing general, physical, emotional, social, and environmental health quality; the *Minnesota Living with Heart Failure Questionnaire* (*MLHFQ*) (comprising 21 questions that measure the patient's perceived limitations due to heart failure [8]); and the *Morisky Scale* (a series of six questions about medication adherence [9]).

Interviews and Related Methods

There are a large variety of interview and related methods that also can be used to collect self-report data. These can be categorized along several dimensions: level of structure of the interview, number of respondents involved (one vs. two or more), and use of subject narrative (historical or anecdotal methods). In addition, these types of measures are usually qualitative (i.e., focus groups, in-depth/unstructured interviews, ethnographic interviews) as opposed to quantitative (e.g., structured interviews and questionnaires) in nature. This chapter provides an overview of some of these qualitative methods, but the construction of these methods and the analysis of the data generated from qualitative methods are quite complicated and outside the scope of this chapter. For further information on qualitative methods and data analysis, see Strauss and Corbin (1998) [10].

Level of Structure

Unstructured interviews (also known as "in-depth" interviews [11]), contain very little organization; the developers of unstructured interviews may have only a general idea of what sort of information they need or they may wish to allow the respondents to develop their responses with minimal interference. Unstructured interviews often resemble conversations, proceeding from a very general question to more specific ones (the latter dependent upon responses to the general question). They are advantageous because they produce data that reflect an exact accounting of what the respondent has said and can elicit important information that the interviewer had not considered before the interview. However, they suffer from a number of limitations. An important one is reproducibility, that is, the same interview, conducted twice with the same subject, can yield quite different results due to variations in the circumstances of the interview (including, but not limited to, the influence of unintended responses by the interviewer) [1]. Other disadvantages include the potential for digressions by the respondent that can cause this type of interview to be excessively time-consuming, complexities of coding and categorization of responses, and difficulty generalizing responses to the reference population (as unstructured surveys typically are performed on relatively small numbers of subjects). An example of an unstructured interview can be found in the work of Cohen et al. who studied patients' perceptions of the psychological impact of isolation in the setting of bone marrow transfusions, which began with the question "What was it like to have bone marrow transplantation?" [11]. Another type of unstructured interview, often found in the anthropological literature, is termed "ethnographic." With ethnographic methods, there is even less structure than with traditional unstructured interviews, as the process begins with the interviewer simply listening. Perhaps the best known example of a medical ethnographic study can be found in the book *The Spirit Catches You and You Fall Down* [12], which describes the horrific experiences of a young Hmong immigrant child and her American doctors, caused by the collision of their vastly differing cultural views about illness and medical care.

Sometimes investigators may prepare a topic guide or a list of questions of interest, but the respondents are free to respond in any way they choose. Interviews of this nature are termed "semistructured" and can be useful when there is concern about imposition of bias or constraint of potential responses. Typically, in a semistructured interview, follow-up questions are simple probes, such as "tell me more," but occasionally they may be more complex. Because the questions contained in the interview are not fully articulated before the interview, interviewers using these methods must be thoroughly trained [13]. Semistructured interviews have been used in a number of biomedical and health education studies. For example, this methodology has been used to ascertain cancer patients' views about disclosing information to their families [14] and to evaluate the consumption and perceived usefulness of nutritional supplements among adolescents [15].

As the name implies, a structured interview delineates the questions in advance, usually with the aid of a written questionnaire or other instrument [11]. This approach provides more uniformity than is possible with a semistructured or unstructured questionnaire, but it lacks some of their advantages. Probably the best-known examples of highly structured interviews are polls, where the respondents' choices are strictly limited. Although polls are most familiar in political contexts, they also can be used in medical research aimed at, for example, eliciting information about patient preferences regarding types of care or provider characteristics. A greater degree of structure generally is appropriate when specific hypotheses are involved and when the field of study is well developed. A lesser degree of structure is more appropriate earlier in the development of a field of knowledge or when the particular research is highly exploratory.

Number of Respondents

While the traditional interview typically entails a one-on-one interaction between interviewer and an interviewee (respondent), the "joint interview" involves two (or sometimes several) individuals who know each other, commonly a couple or a family [16]. Joint interviews differ from focus group methods (described below) where those being interviewed may be strangers. They have value in survey research because different individuals may have very different perspectives that may be illuminated by the interaction between or among them. These different perspectives, in turn, may provide the researcher with greater insight into the problem at hand; however, to accomplish this objective, the interviewer must be able to prevent one respondent from dominating the discussion. Joint interviews have been used to study family reactions to youth suicide [17] and to study reliability of reports of pediatric adherence to HIV medication by interviewing both patients and their caregivers [18]. Note that the term "joint interview" sometimes is used when there are two interviewers, rather than two subjects. This approach can be used as a vehicle for interviewer training and for determination of inter-rater reliability, but it also can be used to provide better answers to health-care questions, as when a psychiatrist and an internist jointly interview a patient to obtain information from varying perspectives [19].

In a "focus group," typically four or more individuals (usually a fairly homogenous group) collectively discuss an issue, guided by a moderator. Focus groups are useful for exploring a particular issue in depth. However, to provide useful information, members of the focus group must be properly selected. In addition, moderators must be matched well to the subjects, they must know the subject matter very well, they must be able to elicit information from those who do not offer it spontaneously [20], and (as in the case of the joint interview) they must have sufficient skill to ensure that one member of the group does not dominate the discussion. Focus groups have been used in medical research to uncover attitudes about a particular illness or difficulty. For example, Quatromoni and colleagues used focus groups to explore the attitudes toward, and knowledge about, diabetes among Caribbean-American women [21], whereas Hicks et al. used focus groups to explore ethical problems faced by medical students [22].

Narrative Methods

- ***Life Histories, Oral Histories, and Critical Incidents***: "Life histories" are narrative self-disclosures about personal life experiences, typically recounted orally or in writing in chronological sequence [1]. They commonly are used as an ethnographic tool for identifying and elucidating cultural patterns, but the technique also can be of value for eliciting the experience of patterns and meanings of health care in populations of interest. "Oral histories" are similar to life histories, but they focus on personal recollections of thematic events rather than on individual life stories. The "critical incident" technique, pioneered by Flanagan [23] in the mid-1950s, is widely used in many areas of health sciences and health sciences education. More focused than life or oral history methods, the critical incident technique requires respondents to identify and judge past behaviors and related factors that have contributed to their success or failure in accomplishing some outcome of interest. The critical incident method has been used to explore such wide-ranging topics as adverse reactions to sedation among children [24], attitudes of third-year medical students toward becoming physicians [25], and reasons why physicians changed their areas of clinical practice [26].
- ***Diaries***: A diary is not technically an interview, as no one is asking questions. Nonetheless, because diaries have some similarities with interview methods, sometimes they are classified with them. A diary is a written

record kept by the respondent, usually over a fairly lengthy period of time. Diaries may have any degree of structure or content; for example, in a study of diet, a diary might include only what the respondent ate each day. On the other hand, in a study of reactions to medication, the diary might include any reactions that a patient may have experienced after taking the medication. If subjects are not literate, diaries may need to be orally recorded. Diaries have been used in clinical research to describe somnolence syndrome in patients after undergoing cranial radiotherapy [27], to measure morbidity of children experienced at home [28], and for improving heart failure recognition after intervention [29]; the methodology has been particularly useful for monitoring symptoms in individual patients in the setting of "N of 1" randomized clinical trials [30] (see Chap. 5).

- ***Think-Aloud Methods***: With "think-aloud" methods, respondents are asked to dictate their thoughts into a recorder while they are trying to solve a problem or make a decision. These methods produce inventories of decisions as they occur in context [1]. One fundamental aspect of think-aloud methods that differentiates them from other approaches is that they are concurrent with the process involved—that is, information is gathered while active reasoning is taking place. Think-aloud methods have been used to examine nurses' reasoning and decision-making processes [31] and have been shown to produce useful information in hospital settings [32]. For further information about this approach, the reader is referred to the seminal writings of Ericsson and Simon (1993) [33].

Making the Choice: Questionnaires Versus Interviews

This choice is, in some ways, a false one. Similar questions may be asked in interviews and questionnaires, and as noted above, interviews may be guided by written questionnaires. Either approach may be relatively structured or unstructured. There are even questionnaires that may be completed by couples or groups. Nevertheless, these methods differ in certain important respects. As noted, questionnaires *tend* to be more structured; some forms of interview, such as those conducted with focus groups, cannot be conducted as a questionnaire and require a trained moderator. In addition, some individuals (e.g., young children, stroke patients, nonnative speakers) may be more comfortable with spoken than with written English and may have a diminished ability to read, which would limit their ability to complete a paper and pencil questionnaire. These factors notwithstanding, some types of questions, particularly those that are relatively complex, are better suited to questionnaires, particularly when "skip patterns" are clear. (The skip pattern refers to the idea that some questions will be passed over appropriately depending on answers to earlier questions or when the questions do not apply to the respondent.) For example, in a questionnaire about general health, women might answer questions on topics such as menstruation and pregnancy, whereas men would not answer these questions. In addition, because it takes less time to read a question than to speak it, questionnaires can contain more items, yet be completed within the same amount of time as an interview covering fewer items. Finally, self-completed questionnaires may be viewed as less intrusive than face-to-face interviews. Thus, the choice is a complex process, and a variety of factors must be weighed.

When Is a New Self-Report Measure Needed?

Creating a new self-report measure entails considerable time and effort for item construction and for pilot testing, refinement, and validation. Before undertaking such a project, it makes sense to be sure it is necessary to do so. As noted above, answers to some questions can be obtained through biophysiological methods or through direct observation and some cannot. Should the investigator decide that answers to a research question can be obtained only through use of a self-report measure, he or she should first determine whether a suitable measure already exists. (The Internet site http://www.med.yale.edu/library/reference/publications/tests.html provides directories of tests and measures in medicine, psychology, and other fields; other good sources are *Tests in Print* [34], the *Mental Measurements Yearbook* [35], and the *Directory of Unpublished Experimental Mental Measures* [36].) Should an existing measure be selected (even if widely used and psychometrically sound in other populations), the investigator should ensure that it has been successfully employed and, optimally, validated in the population under study. If an appropriate preexisting measure cannot be identified, it may be possible to identify two (or more) measures that together may serve the needs of the study, though the investigator should be aware that combining multiple measures (or rewording items) can impact the psychometric properties of their constituent parts.

Sources of Items

The first source of items for a self-report measure is the existing literature, which, as noted, includes existing tests and measures. In some cases, there may be a strong conceptual basis for a set of questions in which case the theoretical or discursive literature may be helpful for item generation. An additional source of items is observation and interview. One profitable long-term research strategy is to begin with relatively qualitative methods (such as unstructured interviews or observation), administered among relatively small samples, and use the findings obtained with these methods to develop more structured forms that can be administered to significantly larger samples. On the other hand, unexpected responses to a highly structured method may provide the impetus to developing less structured surveys that can further explore those areas.

Structuring Questions: Key Points

- ***The Respondent's Reading Level***: When developing a questionnaire, the potential respondents' reading level and related characteristics must be kept in mind. How educated will they be? In which languages will they be fluent? If subjects are excluded who are not fluent in the language used in the questionnaire, how will lack of fluency bias the sample? Answers to all of these questions will vary by sample and by location. If, for example, an investigator is surveying a group of professionals (e.g., doctors or nurses) in the United States [USA], England, or in another country in which the native language is English, it probably is safe to assume that the respondents will have a reasonable command of English as well as a high level of education. On the other hand, if patients are being surveyed from among a heterogeneous population where geographic variations in language exist, it must be assumed that the patients' language proficiency in the country's primary language (and their use of alternative languages) will vary by location and that at least some may have little formal education. These assumptions can be examined by administering various tests of reading level. If reading level is low, alternative formats can be used including auditory or pictorial methods. For example, pain scales exist that use faces representing different levels of pain [37]. These can be particularly useful with young children or with illiterate respondents. (Issues regarding need for and methods of translating questionnaires are discussed below.)
- ***Clarity***: Not only must questions be readable by the target population, they also must be clearly framed to render the survey process as simple as possible for the respondent. It is very common to assume that a question that is clear to the investigator will be clear to others. However, this often is not the case. The best route to assess clarity is thorough pilot testing. Questions that are unclear may be skipped by the respondent or, worse, may be answered in unexpected ways. Unlike readability, lack of clarity affects respondents at all levels of education and language proficiency, although it may be more problematic at lower levels. Ironically, sometimes it can be more

problematic at higher levels of proficiency, as readers may overinterpret the questions. Lack of clarity can arise from the use of vague or uncommon words whose meaning is imprecise and not evident in context. However, even common words such as "assist," "require," and "sufficient" may be misunderstood [38]. The respondents' perception of clarity will depend greatly on the population being surveyed. For example, if the population comprises medical professionals, it may be clearer to use a less common word because, often, the less common word is more precise. For example, the choice between "abdomen" and "stomach" might depend on whether the survey is of medical professionals (for whom the former term is more precise) or the general population (for whom it may be obscure). Vague words often are found in the response options associated with the questions. For example, when asking about the frequency with which a subject does something, words like "regularly" and "occasionally" are vague—it would be better to specify a frequency (e.g., "three times a week"). Other common vague words are "sometimes," "often," "most of the time," and "rarely." Clarity also can be negatively impacted by *ambiguity*. Could a word, a sentence, or a question mean more than one thing within a given context? For example, if respondents are asked about how much money they made in the last year, is the question soliciting information about "before-tax" or "after-tax" income? Does the question imply individual income, household income, or family income? If the latter, does the term include individuals not living with the family who contribute financially or individuals living with the household who are not family members? Should unearned income, illegal income, odd jobs, capital gains, etc., be included? Complex questions such as these may be better asked as several questions [39]. Ambiguity also can arise when pronouns are used in unclear ways [40]. Consider, for example, being asked to agree or disagree with the statement: "Doctors and nurses must educate patients. Otherwise, they will be at risk." Is it the doctors, the nurses, or the patients who will be at risk? To ensure clarity, it may be helpful to operationally define terms within the survey process [39]. However, if definitions of terms are provided, they should be provided to all respondents, not only to those who ask for them. Fowler [39] provides a particularly good example of an unclear question of this nature, in which respondents were asked how often they visited doctors. Those who asked for clarification were told that "doctors" included psychiatrists, ophthalmologists, and anyone else with a medical degree, whereas those who did not seek clarification may have excluded psychiatrists and ophthalmologists, or may have included individuals without medical degrees (e.g., psychologists, nurses, individuals trained in alternative medicine who did not have MD or similar degrees), rendering interpretation of these data very difficult.

- ***Avoiding Leading Questions***: A leading question is one that guides a respondent's answers and represents a significant source of bias in any questionnaire or interview. This can be deliberate or accidental and can occur in a single question or in a series of questions. For example, "Do you smoke, even though you know it causes cancer and many other health problems?" is a leading question framed within a single question. Similarly, if the respondent is first asked questions about the many dangers of smoking, and these questions are followed with one that asks the respondents if they smoke, different answers may be obtained than if the question about the respondent's smoking history had been posed without the initial background questions. More subtle leading questions include those that start with negative wording (e.g., "Don't you agree that ….?" rather than "Do you agree or disagree that ….?") [38].
- ***Avoiding Double-Barreled Questions***: A double-barreled (or multibarreled) question is one that combines multiple questions. For example, a subject may be asked to respond to the statement "I exercise regularly and get plenty of sleep." If the respondent answers

affirmatively, it will not be clear whether he or she exercises, sleeps adequately, or does both. A negative response is similarly uninterpretable [38]. A more subtle double barrel is a question that incorporates a particular reason, for example, "I support civil rights because discrimination is a crime against God." Such a question may lead to confusion among individuals who support civil rights for other reasons [40].

- ***Question Order***: There are several universal criteria that must be met for proper ordering of questions. Below is a guide:
  - Group similar questions so that respondents can remain focused on one area.
  - When testing ability, arrange items from easy to difficult to build confidence.
  - Arrange items from interesting to dull so that respondents do not stop answering questions.
  - As noted below (see section "Asking About Sensitive Information"), if the survey includes questions that are potentially sensitive, these are best asked after relatively neutral questions to increase respondent comfort level.
  - Arrange items from general to specific to avoid biasing the answers. For example, if querying patients about their general and specific experiences in a hospital, the general question should be asked first; otherwise, respondents may answer the general question as the sum of the specific questions, ignoring factors that were not included in the specific questions (even if those factors were important to the respondents).
  - Ideally, all questions should apply to each respondent. When this is not possible, "skip questions" or conditional logic should be used to guide respondents through the survey so that they are not required to answer irrelevant items or sections. Alternatively, a "not applicable" category can be included as a response option to avoid confusion. "Not applicable" is not equivalent to "no opinion"; rather, it indicates that the question does not apply to the respondent (e.g., questions about complications during pregnancy apply neither to men nor to women who have never been pregnant).
  - *Translation issues*: If large numbers of potential respondents are not fluent or in the primary language spoken by the population to which results are to be extrapolated (e.g., English in the USA), excluding those individuals may introduce sampling bias. However, including them, but asking questions only in English, may bias their responses. Under these circumstances, the survey may need to be translated. Preparatory to this process, it will be necessary to ascertain the primary languages spoken by members of the sample. Then, for each language spoken by large numbers of the sample, questions and answer choices will need to be carefully translated. (If self-reported data are to be collected via an interview rather than by questionnaire, it will be necessary to recruit interviewers who are fluent in these various languages.) After translation, the material will need to be "back-translated" to identify potential linguistic problems. However, even these steps may not suffice. Not all words and phrases have exact equivalents in other languages, and some concepts vary strongly from culture to culture. Chang and colleagues [41] investigated premenstrual syndrome in Chinese-American women. Using a questionnaire that had been translated and back-translated, they asked bilingual women to respond to both the Chinese and English versions. While intraclass correlations indicated moderate to high levels of equivalence for total scores and scales, some questions showed very little consistency between languages.
  - *Asking the same question in more than one way*: Rephrasing a question also can help to minimize ambiguity and avoid honest or dishonest errors. As an example, studies have found that respondents tend to provide more precise and accurate information when they are asked for birth dates compared to when they are asked to state their ages [42]. This phenomenon may be due to intentional mistruth or to poor recall. Thus, commonly, those collecting self-report data often will ask for both the respondent's

birthday and his or her age. However, it is important to be selective, as asking all questions in multiple ways not only will make for a very long survey, it will invariably irritate the respondents. Therefore, it is best to include intentionally redundant items only for key areas and under conditions where ambiguity is difficult to avoid.

Structuring Potential Responses

There are two broad types of questions that can be included in a self-report measure: *open-ended* (also known as "open") questions and *closed-ended* (also known as "closed") questions. These differ according to who (the developer of the survey or the respondent) is responsible for defining possible answers to the questions.

- ***Open-Ended Questions***: Open-ended questions are those for which the respondent supplies the answer. These are subcategorized into (1) *numeric* open-ended questions that may ask for responses expressed as quantities (e.g., "How much out-of-pocket money did you spend on medications during the past week?" "How much weight did you gain during the last year?" "How old were you when you had your first heart attack?") versus (2) *free text* questions (sometimes called "verbatims"). The latter, often seen at the end of surveys, ask about experiences or satisfaction with services (e.g., "Do you have any other comments you'd like to share?"). Open-ended questions are the question-level equivalent of unstructured surveys and share some of the same problems (in particular, they may be difficult to code). The chief advantage of open-ended questions is that they do not constrain the range of possible responses. Indeed, they permit respondents to freely respond to the question, allowing them to describe their feelings about, attitudes toward, and understanding of the topic at hand. As such, they potentially can generate more information about the topic than other formats. Open-ended responses also tend to reduce the response error associated with answers supplied by others (i.e., the survey developer). But this approach has its perils. If a survey includes a question such as "When did you move to New York?" then, given an open-ended format, respondents may name a year, a date, or may refer to a time in their lives (e.g., "right after I got married") or to the history of the area (e.g., "just before the big blackout"). For a question such this, it is better to ask for a specific type of response (e.g., either "How old were you when you moved to New York?" or "In what year did you move to New York?") because, under these circumstances, it is unlikely that any response given would be unduly constrained.
- ***Closed-Ended Questions***: Closed-ended questions are those in which the respondent is asked to choose from a preexisting set of response options that have been generated by the individuals developing the survey. Closed-ended questions, therefore, limit the answers that the respondent can provide. Their primary advantages are that they are easier to code and analyze, provide more specific and uniform information for a given question, and generally take less time to answer than open-ended questions. Closed-ended questions can be subclassified into those calling for *dichotomous responses* versus *polychotomous* (*multiple choice*) responses. Dichotomous responses are those that have only two possible values—most commonly, "yes" or "no." Examples of questions that may generate such responses are legion ("Did the patient die?" "Do you have a physician?" "Have you ever had surgery?"). When items are framed as statements rather than as questions, typical dichotomous responses include "true"/"false" or "agree"/"disagree" response options. Items calling for dichotomous responses sometimes are combined into scales that can yield an aggregate score. One well-known example is *Thurstone scaling*. Thurstone scaling refers not to a method of soliciting responses to single unrelated items, but to a method of constructing and scaling several related items. The essential idea is to construct several dichotomous statements about a respondent's attitudes, each of which may be answered "Agree" or "Disagree". This method of scaling can be used to classify respondents with different levels of an attribute [40].

For example, if the area of inquiry entailed nurses' attitudes about doctors' orders, the following series of items might be presented:

(a) A nurse must always follow every order that a doctor gives, even if he/she thinks it is wrong.
□ Agree □ Disagree
(b) A nurse should almost always follow a doctor's orders, but may raise questions on rare occasions.
□ Agree □ Disagree
(c) A nurse should generally follow a doctor's orders, but should also voice his/her opinions about those orders.
□ Agree □ Disagree
(d) Nurses should be equal partners in all decisions about patient care and should regard doctors' orders as advice.
□ Agree □ Disagree

In contrast to questions soliciting dichotomous responses, multiple choice questions include three or more response options. These, in turn, can be differentiated into questions calling for *nominal*-level responses and those that call for *ordinal* responses.

As noted in Chap. 3, nominal variables are simply names—they have no order. There are two primary types of questions that call for nominal responses. The first includes items for which the respondent can provide only one answer, as the available response options are mutually exclusive. Examples include questions about demographic characteristics (e.g., religion, gender), other characteristics such as hair color and blood type, and so on. The second type includes questions where the respondent can select more than one response (i.e., "choose all that apply" questions). The latter may provide very useful information but pose data entry and analytic challenges that need to be considered when designing the survey instrument. To counter these, special techniques are needed. For example, if one is interested in learning about why patients have gone to the hospital, it is advisable to divide the main question into two subquestions: the first asking the respondent whether he or she has been to the hospital and (if answered in the affirmative) a follow-up question asking about reasons for the hospitalization, with responses entered into separate columns of a spreadsheet.

Ordinal responses are those that have a meaningful sequence, but no fixed distances between the levels of the sequence. Questions about subjective responses are often ordinal. For example, responses to a question such as "How much pain are you in?" could range from "none," to "a little," to "some," to "a lot," to "excruciating." They are considered to be ordinal rather than interval because while they arguably proceed from least to most pain, it is not at all clear whether the difference between, for example, "none" and "a little" is larger, smaller, or the same as the difference between, for example, "a lot" and "excruciating." As noted, ordinal response scales typically include a number of possible answers. Usually, an odd number of responses (typically five or seven) is chosen to allow the respondent a "neutral" or midrange option, though there is no consensus about how many choices to include. There are a variety of different ordinal response scales. The most common are given below:

- ***Traditional Ordinal Rating Scales***: These rating scales ask the respondent to evaluate an attribute such as performance by checking or circling one of several ordered choices. Rating scales often are used to measure the direction and intensity of attitude toward the target attribute. An example of a traditional rating scale is given below:

  □ Excellent □ Good □ Fair
  □ Poor □ Very Poor

- ***Likert Scales*** represent another traditional type of rating scale that asks the respondent to indicate his or her level of *agreement* with a given statement, with the center of the scale typically representing a neutral point [40]. Likert scales are most frequently used for items that measure opinion and take the general form shown below:

  □ Strongly Disagree □ Disagree □ Neither Agree Nor Disagree

  □ Agree □ Strongly Agree

- ***Semantic Differential Scales***: Semantic differential scales measure the respondent's reactions to stimulus words and concepts using rating scales with contrasting adjectives at each end [43]. For example, one might ask a question where the polar extremes are "good" and "bad," with gradations between these extremes provided as response options.

Good — — — — — — — Bad
−3 −2 −1 0 1 2 3

- ***The Behaviorally Anchored Rating Scale (BARS)*** is a complex approach to performance appraisal that combines the elements of traditional rating scales with critical incident methods. It was developed to counter concerns about subjectivity associated with traditional rating scales and, thus, to facilitate relatively more accurate ratings of target behaviors or performance versus other approaches. A BARS is constructed by compiling examples of ineffective and effective behaviors (usually based on the consensus of experts), converting these behaviors into performance dimensions, and identifying multiple "incidents" per dimension to form a numerical scale in which each item is associated with a particular type of behavior [44]. Respondents may rate their degree of agreement with each item by checking or circling the appropriate level of the accompanying rating scale. Shown below is a 7-point BARS that could be used to evaluate an academic faculty member's research productivity in terms of number and types of publications produced during a given period (a dimension of interest to faculty leaders). Note each scale value (1 = "extremely poor performance," 2 = "very poor performance," 3 = "somewhat poor performance," 4 = "neither good nor poor performance," 5 = "somewhat good performance," 6 = "very good performance," 7 = "outstanding performance") is anchored in specific behaviors related to the dimension of interest. Unlike traditional rating scales, which are presented horizontally, BARS typically is arrayed vertically, comprising between 5 and 9 scale points (values); when the number of scale values are uneven, the midpoint of the scale typically represents a neutral response (as is the case in many rating scales).

During the past year, Dr. Heartly has:

Outstanding performance	7	Independently published (as sole or first author) two or more research manuscripts in top-tier journals, with others in draft
Very good performance	6	First authored one research manuscript in a well-regarded peer-reviewed journal, with minimal input from senior faculty
Somewhat good performance	5	Coauthored one or more published research manuscripts in a peer-reviewed journal, with support from senior faculty members
Neither good nor poor performance	4	Presented a first-authored abstract at a scientific meeting but has not completed the manuscript
Somewhat poor performance	3	Actively coauthored a research abstract, but provided very limited assistance in manuscript development
Very poor performance	2	Provided minimal contribution as coauthor on a research abstract but no participation in manuscript development
Extremely poor performance	1	Made no progress in developing scientific manuscripts or abstracts, due to competing priorities or interests

- ***Visual Analog Scales***: Visual analog scales (VAS) are similar to Likert scales or semantic differential scales, except, rather than checking a box or circling a predefined response option, the respondents indicate their responses by making a mark (denoted here by the x) along a line anchored by terms describing opposite values of an attribute, as shown in the hypothetical example below:

Good ________x________ Bad

VAS have the dual advantages of being very sensitive, and, in cases where the measure is repeated over time, the respondent will not be able to intentionally duplicate his or her previous response. However, different individuals may encode physical space differently. Thus, a mark halfway between "good" and "bad" may not mean the same thing to all respondents. VAS have been used commonly for the clinical measurement of chronic and acute postoperative pain. In one study, designed to formally assess its psychometric performance in the latter setting, DeLoach and coworkers [45] administered the VAS to 60 patients in the immediate postoperative period, using the scale anchors "no pain" and "worst imaginable pain." The authors found good correlations between the VAS and a traditional numeric measure though individual VAS estimates tended to be relatively imprecise.

- ***Rank Order Scales***: With this form of measure, respondents are asked to rank alternatives in order, rather than rate them on a scale. For example, if members of a medical school class all had the same professors in one semester, they could be asked to grade them in relation to one another, as shown below:

  Please rank each of your professors from best to worst, where 1 = "best" and 5 = "worst":

  Adams _____ Bassett _____ Cochran _____
  Davis _____ Edwards _____

Advantages and Disadvantages of Categorizing Responses

Many times, responses that are fundamentally continuous in nature are transformed into categorical responses by the design of the questionnaire. Instead of asking "How old are you?" a respondent can be asked "Are you: (a) under 18, (b) 19–24, (c) 25–34, (d) 35–44, (e) 45–54, (f) 55–64 or (g) over 65?" This approach, however, has several important drawbacks. First, categorical responses cannot be reconverted into continuous responses. Second, it can limit comparisons with other questionnaires that utilize different breaks between categories. Third, breaks must be meaningful, with variations occurring only between those that have been included. Sometimes the survey developer may choose breaks that are inappropriate. For example, if, after data collection, it is determined that most respondents are over age 65, it is not possible to reverse course and redo the survey adding additional breaks for 65–74 and 75–84. Nonetheless, there can be advantages to categorical scaling. The primary advantage is that some respondents may be more willing or able to answer some questions in categorical form than in numerical form. This is particularly true of income questions, where respondents may not know their precise income, but they will know it approximately. (Ironically, self-reported age follows an opposite pattern as individuals appear to be better able and more willing to give their birthdates than their ages.)

Asking About Sensitive Information

What is sensitive information? The answer to this question depends on the respondent, because what is sensitive to one person is not to another. In general, questions about stigmatized or illegal behaviors, or unusual beliefs and opinions will be judged to be more sensitive by those who engage in those behaviors or hold those beliefs than by those who do not [39]. Highly personal questions (e.g., income, weight, some health conditions) or questions about traumatic events (e.g., rape or child abuse, or other forms of abuse) also may be viewed as sensitive. When asking about sensitive information, "warm up" questions often are used to set the respondent at ease, thereby increasing the likelihood that the sensitive questions will be answered. It also may be useful to include a "cool-down" or "cool-off" phase that can reduce the possible stress induced by the sensitive questions. Typical warm-up questions include those about nonsensitive demographics (e.g., county of residence, birth order); cool-down questions often are quite trivial (e.g., pet ownership, taste in music, food preferences, and similar items).

Sensitive questions can be uncomfortable to the respondent and may raise ethical concerns. When included within a research protocol, the investigator may need to demonstrate to his or her institutional review board (IRB) the need for such questions and provide assurances that the respondent will not be compelled to answer them. When asking highly sensitive questions, interviewer training is essential, and interviewers may need to be aware of referral services that can be offered if the respondent reveals high-risk behavior, for example, being involved in an abusive relationship, being suicidal, or using illicit drugs. In addition, becoming aware of certain types of behavior via self-report may impose ethical responsibilities on certain classes of professionals. For example, clinical psychologists have a duty to report certain behaviors. Clinical researchers typically are obligated to report nonadherence to (or adverse outcomes associated with) treatment. More generally, anyone who is a member of a group that has licensure will need to investigate his or her own specific requirements for such disclosure.

Modes of Administration

Self-reported information can be obtained via a variety of methods. These include face-to-face interviews, mailed questionnaires, e-mail and web-based surveys, telephone surveys, computer-assisted response systems, and randomized response methods.

Face-to-Face Interviews

The chief advantages of face-to-face administration are that response rates are optimized and that it provides an opportunity for the interviewer to clarify confusing items. Disadvantages include expense (both time and money), the possibility that interviewer behaviors may influence (bias) responses, and the fact that some individuals may be reluctant to answer some questions in the presence of an interviewer due to embarrassment (especially sensitive items) or concerns about revealing illegal behavior.

Mail (Postal) Surveys

Administering a questionnaire by mail is relatively inexpensive and helps to avoid interviewer bias. However, unless care is taken, response rates are likely to be suboptimal (i.e., <85%) [46], and respondents may not be a random sample of any particular population, precluding generalizability of conclusions. These limitations apply even to mail surveys that have been published in medical journals, where average response rates have been shown to be approximately 60% [47].

E-mail and Web-Based Surveys

E-mail and web-based surveys are less costly to administer than traditional postal mail surveys, but have several limitations. Anonymity can be difficult to ensure, response rates may be low, and responses may not be random (often, there is no way of knowing exactly who is answering the questions). Response rates with Internet surveys have been found to differ from those obtained by postal methods, depending on the group surveyed. Younger individuals tend to respond more frequently than older individuals to e-mail, whereas older individuals more to traditional mail [48]; in one study, medical doctors have been found to respond more frequently to traditional mail than to Internet-based methods [49].

Telephone Surveys

Telephone surveys are less costly than face-to-face interviews, but the telephone-based approach may lead to significant nonresponse. Assuming that the subject can be reached, the lack of personal contact between the interviewer and respondent may increase the likelihood that the latter will decline the interview. In addition, in the current era, many potential respondents lack landline telephones, and some have multiple telephones creating difficulties in achieving a random sample. A recent study using telephone survey methodology found response rates of only 39% [50].

Computer-Assisted Interviews (CAI)

The availability of computers over the last several decades has created new methods of administering and responding to surveys. Among the most common are the Computer-Assisted Personal

Interview (CAPI), the Computer-Assisted Telephone Interview (CATI), and the Audio Computer-Assisted Self-Interview (ACASI). With CAPI, the interviewer typically uses a computer screen to read questions to respondents in the setting of a face-to-face interview. With CATI, the interviewer follows a script provided by a software application to ask questions by telephone. Depending on the system used, the respondent may have the options of interacting with a "live" interviewer or listening to a recorded interview and may answer questions by voice or touch phone mechanisms. CATI also provides the advantages of automating initial calls and call-backs and keeping notes on the status of the interviews. With ACASI, the respondent uses a headphone connected to a computer to listen to preprogrammed questions and enters his or her responses directly into the computer via a keyboard or keypad. If respondents have limited computer literacy, these systems can be engineered to employ a touch screen mechanism whereby the respondent simply pushes a patch of a certain color. Because absence of an interviewer protects privacy (broadly defined as control of access of oneself to others), some respondents may feel more comfortable answering sensitive questions in this format. Indeed, studies have shown that respondents are more likely to admit use of illicit drugs and to report sensitive or stigmatized sexual behaviors with ACASI than when interacting with an interviewer in person or by telephone [51, 52]. CAI methods have distinct advantages over traditional "paper-and-pencil" surveys. They improve turnaround time, avoid problems associated with skip patterns and branching in complex surveys, and facilitate entry validation and internal consistency checks. They also minimize (or entirely eliminate) the requirement for secondary data entry and cleaning, further improving data quality by avoiding additional keystroke errors [53]. The primary limitation of CAI is their relatively high initial setup costs. In medicine, computer-assisted methods have been shown to be of value for obtaining information from stroke victims [54] or others with limited ability to use a pen. They also have been used to improve patient care in the setting of HIV infection [55].

Randomized Response

Randomized response is a useful method of assessing the rate of stigmatized behaviors. In brief, respondents flip a coin (in private) or use some other randomizing device to determine whether they are about to answer an innocuous question (e.g., "Is today Monday?") or a sensitive one (e.g. "Have you ever used heroin?"). They report their answers ("yes"/"no") without the investigator being aware which question the respondent was asked, thus protecting the latter's privacy. At the conclusion of the assessment, a statistical algorithm is used to calculate out overall prevalence of the target behavior. Variations on randomized response methods also exist for ordinal and interval level variables. Randomized response methodology has been widely used for highly stigmatized behaviors such as illegal drug use [56] and homosexual sex [57] and has been found to yield more accurate data than direct surveys [58].

Methods for Boosting Response Rates

There is a large literature comprising methods for increasing response rates to surveys, some of which involve paying or providing other incentives to respondents for their participation. Their appropriateness is largely dependent on the population with which the investigator is working as well as the nature and magnitude of the inducement. For example, if participants are members of a low-income, nonprofessional group, offering modest compensation for time and effort would be ethically appropriate and could encourage participation in a survey, whereas offering large sums of money or valuable goods for such participation would be viewed as coercive. Among more advantaged respondents, offering an inducement could backfire (if the respondent viewed the inducement as insulting). For such subjects, a reasonable alternative is to offer money to a charity of the respondent's choice. Other effective methods, frequently adopted in other domains such as marketing but applicable to medical research, include making the survey interesting, including questions that are relevant to the respondent and keeping the survey short and simple (KISS). Strategies specific to mail surveys include the use of personalized questionnaires and/or cover letters that orient the respondent to the purpose and importance of the study and invite their participation. Additional strategies include the use of colored ink, first class mail and recorded delivery, stamped return envelopes (or permitting use of facsimile), contacting participants before sending surveys, maintaining follow-up contact with participants, and providing nonrespondents with replacement questionnaires when the initial questionnaires were not readily accessible [59]. In one study, the combined use of replacement questionnaires and chocolate (the inducement) was found to significantly increase response rates versus either method alone [60]. Strategies specific to telephone surveys include allowing the respondent to return the call using a toll-free number and sending alerts prior to initiation of the survey. (For more possibilities, the reader is referred to the website www.guidestarco.com/Increasing-survey-response-rates.htm.)

Evaluating Psychometric Properties of a Self-Report Measure

Before a self-report measure can be used with confidence, it must be rigorously evaluated to determine whether it is psychometrically sound; that is, that it measures the construct of interest (e.g., quality of life, satisfaction, emotional state of health) accurately in the population of interest. Such an assessment not only is essential for all newly developed instruments, it also is important for instruments that have been validated for other populations. By accuracy, we mean that the quantitative or qualitative assessment provided by the instrument should provide as true a measure of the underlying construct as possible. Unfortunately, all measurement is accompanied by the possibility of error which is either systematic or random as no data collection technique is perfect. Whenever we measure a patient characteristic, be it by objective testing or by more subjective methods, the measurement instrument provides only an estimate of the quantity of interest. By an estimate, we mean that the recorded value is not a direct measure of the underlying quantity of interest or the "true" value. For example, if we are measuring the blood pressure of an individual, the observed value for the systolic pressure may be 124 mmHg. However, the true value cannot be observed and is equal to the 124 plus or minus some value reflecting measurement error as well as other sources of error.

Two fundamental components of *accuracy*, both inversely related to the error of an observation, are *validity* and *reliability*. Physicians and others using self-report measures for research should have a fundamental understanding of these concepts if they are to form judgments about the quality of outcomes based on these measures or develop their own measures. In the setting of tests and measures, validity relates to how well the instrument measures what it purports to measure and reliability relates to how consistently the instrument measures whatever it is that it measures. These qualities exist on a continuum rather than as absolutes, that is, inferences drawn from an instrument are neither "valid" nor "invalid" nor are they "reliable" or "unreliable"; rather, they are valid to a certain degree and reliable to a certain degree for a given population and setting (i.e., are "sample dependent"). Together, validity and reliability reflect the ability of the instrument to provide an accurate quantitative estimate of the characteristic of interest to the researcher.

Validity

Validity has been defined as the degree to which conclusions drawn from the results of any assessment are "well-grounded or justifiable, being at once relevant and meaningful" [61]. When the term validity is applied to measurement, it refers to the extent to which the instrument measures the actual parameter of interest [62]. Thus, a well-built scale should, on average, produce readings that permit a meaningful conclusion about a person's actual weight; a well-constructed measure of clinical depression should yield data that are useful for drawing meaningful conclusions about the presence and severity of depressive symptoms; and a properly designed measure of health-related quality of life should provide responses that are value for drawing meaningful conclusions about health status or health utility from the perspective of the patient. In each of these cases, the quality of the instrument is judged according to the soundness of the conclusions that can be drawn from the responses that it provides. Therefore, though the term "valid" is commonly used as a descriptor for various tests and measures, validity, as Cook and Brown have noted, represents a property of the inference rather than the instrument itself [63]. Because these inferences are influenced by the circumstances under which the instrument is administered, there is no such entity as a generically valid instrument. Indeed, all instruments should be validated for each interpretation, including the specific populations and contexts in which it will be used. For example, a test that measured knowledge of basic addition and subtraction might be used to draw valid inferences about mathematics proficiency among first-grade students but would not be useful for drawing similar inferences about college mathematics majors. Similarly, a scale that has been validated for one disorder (e.g., depression) would need to be re-evaluated to establish its validity in the setting of another (e.g., anxiety). Moreover, an instrument that has been shown to permit valid inferences under research conditions or in highly selected patients may need further evaluation before use in a general clinical population [63].

Validation of a measurement instrument is a complex process, in part, because validity encompasses various dimensions. The most common of these are summarized below:

- ***Face Validity***: Face validity (validity "at face value"), also known as "representation validity," is concerned with how a measurement instrument or procedure appears to be relevant to a construct, as judged by a potential respondent. It is the simplest type of validity to gauge and, typically, is assessed early in the validation process. Does the assessment seem like a reasonable way to gain the information the investigator is attempting to obtain? Does it look as though it will measure what it is supposed to measure? Does it seem well designed? [64] For example, the *Beck Depression Inventory*, which is widely used in clinical medicine, asks questions about depression; more specifically, it asks about such attributes as sadness, suicide, and loss of pleasure [65]. It has face validity because these (and other) items are what most people think of as depression.
- ***Content Validity***: Content validity reflects how well the items comprising a measure cover (sample) the subject of interest or "domain." When a domain is well defined, content validity is relatively easy to ascertain. If the domain is less well defined, ascertainment of content validity may require having experts in the field review the measure [40]. The content validity of a test of knowledge of women's health was called into question by comparing the domains it covered with those covered by a set of curriculum guides [66], and the content validity of the SF-36 health questionnaire was affirmed by comparing it with the longer instrument from which its items were drawn [67].
- ***Construct Validity***: Construct validity is the degree to which a measure is related to other measures or attributes, as dictated by theory. It reflects the extent to which the construct under study (e.g., depression), even if it cannot directly be assessed, has been properly labeled (operationalized) by the items comprising the measure. In other words, does the instrument measure what it was designed to measure? Thus, construct validity is a key part of validity—no instrument has any value unless it satisfies this criterion. Inferences about construct validity can be evaluated by a variety of methods. A common approach to construct validation entails assessment of the *convergent* and *divergent* (or *discriminant*) validities of a measure. Convergent validity indicates that the measure correlates highly with other measures of similar constructs, whereas

divergent validity indicates that it correlates poorly with measures of other constructs. For example, we would expect a measure of depression to correlate more highly with measures of anxiety than with measures of most physical characteristics. Similarly, we would expect measures of post-traumatic stress disorder to correlate more highly with measures of similar stressors than with measures of age. A related approach is *known groups* analysis, which evaluates the extent to which scores on a measure discriminate between individuals known to possess an attribute versus those who do not. Known groups validity analysis has been used to provide support for the construct validity of the *Pediatric Evaluation of Disability Inventory* by demonstrating different scores among individuals with different levels of disability [68]; the method also was used to support the construct validity of the *Multidimensional Fatigue Inventory* by demonstrating scores consistent with greater fatigue among patients presenting with chronic fatigue-like symptoms or chronically unwell patients versus healthy controls [69]. An alternative approach involves the use of factor (exploratory or confirmatory) analysis or principal components analysis to identify clusters of related items on a scale. Collectively, these methods are useful for (a) determining how many "latent variables" or dimensions underlie a set of items (thereby helping to elucidate or confirm the structure of the instrument), (b) condensing a relatively larger number of items into a smaller number of variables to facilitate statistical analysis, and (c) clarifying the meaning of these variables [39]. As examples, principal components analysis was used to define two distinct higher-order clusters reflecting mental and physical health from among the eight scales comprising the *Medical Outcomes Study Short Form (SF) 36* [70]; exploratory factor analysis was used to identify three subdimensions of climate (clarity, challenge, support) in a work-group climate assessment tool for improving the performance of public health organizations [71], and confirmatory factor analysis was used to substantiate the single-factor structure of a mental well-being scale [72].

- ***Criterion Validity***: Criterion validity (also known as criterion-related or instrumental validity) refers to how well the results obtained by an instrument correlate with or predict some real world behavior or other attribute. It estimates the accuracy of the measure by comparing it with some preexisting indicator that has been demonstrated to measure the same construct (i.e., a "gold standard"). There are two primary forms of criterion validity: concurrent and predictive. *Concurrent validity* is evaluated by comparing two measures in parallel and determining whether they are concordant. For example, the concurrent validity of a test of fitness could be defined by determining the extent to which it correlates with maximum oxygen uptake measured at (or approximately at) the same time [73]. *Predictive validity* implies that the measure forecasts an expected result. As examples, a self-report measure of functioning in the elderly was found to predict mortality [74]; a measure of readiness to change was used to predict change in drinking behavior in excessive drinkers [75]; and a measure of adherence to medication instructions was affirmed by predicting blood pressure 5 years later [9].
- ***Responsiveness to Change***: A primary goal of clinical management and target of clinical investigation is assessment of change over time in a patient's status in response to treatment. As Portney and Watkins have noted, the use of change scores as a basis for assessing treatment outcomes is pervasive throughout clinical research [76]. While some methodologists contend that the sensitivity of an instrument to change (i.e., its "responsiveness") is distinct from validity [77], others argue that responsiveness is, indeed, an important component of validity [76, 78]. An instrument is considered to be responsive if it can accurately detect change when (and only when) it has occurred [79]. In other words, it should produce the scores that change in proportion to the change in the patient's status, but remain stable when the patient is unchanged [76].

Two forms of responsiveness are recognized: "internal" and "external" [80]. Internal responsiveness represents the instrument's capacity to detect change from before to after exposure to an intervention of acknowledged efficacy [81]. Typically, it is evaluated in the setting of repeated measures designs that incorporate assessments before and after the intervention in the same individual. These designs can involve a single group of subjects followed over time (i.e., a "treated" cohort, where intra-subject change is expected) or include two groups (including an untreated control where change is unexpected). External responsiveness refers to the degree to which changes in a measurement correlate with changes in other putatively related changes in health status [81]. Both forms of responsiveness are influenced by reliability and scale characteristics. Scales that are unreliable will produce too much noise to allow for determination of meaningful change over time. Scales with too few response categories may fail to detect all but very large changes. Scales producing "ceiling" effects (due to restriction at the upper level of the range of possible values) may leave little room for improvement on subsequent testing just as those producing "floor" effects (where data cannot take on lower values) will be insensitive to clinical decline even when there is a worsening of status or functioning. When instruments with varying scaling characteristics (type, length, directionality, etc.) are compared to determine their relative responsiveness, unit-free statistical approaches including standardized scores and comparisons (e.g., effect sizes or standardized response means) must be used. (For an excellent discussion of these techniques and their interpretation, the reader is referred to Liang et al. [82] and Angst et al. [83]).

As noted throughout this volume, the validity of any study can be threatened by bias, which broadly is defined as known or unknown systematic error in the design, sampling, measurement, or other critical aspects in the conduct of an investigation that can produce distortions of findings. Unlike a random error, described below, a systematic error consistently affects the measurement of the variable in the same way each time that the measurement is done. It provides an incorrect measure of the variable, and the error will be the same for every subject.

There are several types of bias that specifically affect responses obtained in self-report measures; some of the most common are listed below. (For a fuller list, the reader is referred to Aiken and Mardegan [44] and Choi and Pak [38].) Although adequate quantitative data are not available for purposes of comparison, there is general agreement that the extent and impact of these biases vary greatly from discipline to discipline and from one population to another.

- ***Social Desirability Bias***: Social desirability bias (sometimes termed "faking good" bias) refers to the tendency of respondents to answer questions in ways that make them look good, rather than honestly [40]. This positive response bias may be of two types—some respondents may deliberately tell falsehoods in order to appear acceptable to those conducting the survey, whereas others may have internalized the dishonest response. (The latter occurs more commonly than generally recognized [84].) The social desirability bias can compromise most forms of self-report, but its potential impact should be anticipated when asking about stigmatized behaviors or attitudes (e.g., when questions involve issues of criminality, violence, or sexual orientation), or when the respondent has reason to believe that a socially nondesirable response could cause him or her to lose something of critical value (e.g., a belief by a patient that nonadherence to a health-care provider's instructions could negatively impact future interactions with that provider). Although it may not be possible to eradicate this form of bias, the extent of its potential influence can be examined by embedding, in the self-report measure, an item or two that ask the respondent to answer a question such as "I have never intentionally told a lie" or "I always know the difference between right and wrong" or through formal testing. A common test of social desirability is the *Marlowe-Crowne* scale [85]; a shorter version of this scale has been created by Strahan and Gerbasi [86].

- ***Agreement Bias***: Agreement bias (also known as *acquiescence bias*) is the tendency to say "yes" or "I agree" to every item regardless of content. It is subtly different from social desirability bias as agreement bias includes admission to possessing socially undesirable traits. For example, respondents manifesting agreement bias might respond affirmatively to the question, "Have you ever used illicit drugs?" whereas those exhibiting social desirability bias would likely provide the opposite response. The phenomenon is thought to have multiple causes. First, it has been argued that most respondents desire to be polite and respectful and, thus, not wish to disagree with the questioner [87, 88]. Second, respondents may feel that they have lower standing than the questioner and agree with questions based on this perceived status differential [89]. Third, respondents may select an agreeable (but not necessarily truthful) answer to complete the survey as rapidly as possible [90]. Whatever the cause, agreement bias can be detected (and sometimes resolved) by including a balance of positively and negatively worded items [91], though care must be taken to minimize confusion to the respondents.
- ***"Faking Bad" Bias***: In contrast to social desirability (or "faking good") bias, the "faking bad" bias occurs where failure (in the usual sense) is a goal. In the context of self-reported information, faking bad is a negative response bias that is caused by the respondent's desire to appear worse (e.g., manifest symptom amplification) than he or she really is either to avoid duty or responsibility (i.e., malinger) or to qualify for goods or services [38]. If faking bad bias is suspected, methods exist to detect it. (For a comprehensive discussion of one such method [the *Fake Bad Scale*], the reader is referred to Nelson et al. [92].)
- ***Halo Effect***: The halo effect is a systematic bias that occurs when respondents fail to rate individual attributes of a person, object, event, or service in isolation but instead let overall impressions guide their ratings. It is suspected whenever respondents assign similar ratings to each dimension measured in a survey (e.g., rate all aspects of performance as "excellent" or all components of a course or program as "very good"). The phenomenon, empirically confirmed by Thorndike in 1920 [93], is thought to result from a cognitive bias, whereby one particular trait, especially a positive characteristic, influences or extends to perception of other traits. A commonly cited example is judging an attractive person as more intelligent. Its logical opposite is sometimes termed the "devil," "horns," or "reverse-halo" effect whereby individuals judged to have a single undesirable trait (e.g., unattractiveness) are subsequently judged to have other undesirable traits (e.g., lack of intelligence) based on the evaluator's tendency to allow a single weakness to influence the totality of impressions [94]. In the setting of a survey, a respondent's prejudices, recollections of previous observations, and even answers to previous questions also may influence responses. Thus, the halo (and reverse-halo) effects collectively represent an important bias that must be recognized and, if possible, minimized to improve the accuracy of individual ratings. Several approaches have been recommended including proper introduction of the purpose of the survey (to emphasize the importance of the respondents' ratings), increasing the number of attributes to be rated (bearing in mind that an excessive number of questions may cause the respondent to abandon the survey), and/or physically arranging scales so that their favorable and unfavorable ends alternate.

Reliability

Reliability is related to the question "how consistent or reproducible are the scores that an instrument produces?" Like validity, reliability technically is considered to be a property of the measurement rather than of the instrument itself because the same instrument administered in different settings and to different subjects under varying conditions can yield widely varying reliability estimates [63]. Reliability is considered to be a necessary, but insufficient, element of validity [95, 96]. This is because valid conclusions cannot be drawn from an instrument that yields inconsistent observations [63]. At the same time, reliability does not imply validity because an instrument can produce consistent errors.

The concept of reliability can be illustrated using the metaphor of a bathroom scale. For example, if you are like many people, you probably will step on your bathroom scale in the morning, check your weight, step off, and step back on the scale to recheck the reading. You have learned through experience that the measurement displayed by a bathroom scale the first time you weigh yourself is not always the same as the second time you try, but usually it is very close. A good scale might vary by half a pound or so, but if measured weight differs significantly (e.g., more than 5 lb) at 7:00 a.m., 7:01 a.m., and 7:02 a.m., the readings that the scale produces would have very limited reliability. Similarly, if an instrument is designed to measure a patient's self-confidence, then it should yield approximately the same result each time it is administered to the same subject.

Whereas validity is diminished by systematic error, reliability is reduced by random (chance) error. There are many sources of random error in research measurement. The most common are those caused by factors related to the subject, researcher, environment, and instrumentation. For example, a subject who is tired, sick, hungry, angry, irritable, or confused may produce measurements that are different than they would be if the subject were not so afflicted. Indeed, any changing physical, emotional, or psychological state of the subject, including the subject's awareness of the researcher's presence, can introduce error into the measurement process. The researcher can introduce random error in measurement simply by his or her physical appearance, demeanor, or other personal attributes or by becoming fatigued, impatient, bored, ill, or distracted. Many factors that cause random error in measurement can arise from perturbations of the research setting (e.g., unintended variations in temperature, lighting, noise, or interruptions). Finally, many factors causing random error have their source in the instrument. For example, unclear questions or directions, inadequate item sampling, suboptimal format, or even the order in which the questions are posed are potential sources of random error. Random error (like systematic error) must be considered in interpreting the results of studies; the greater the error, the less we can rely on the results of the measurement process for decision-making. In designing or selecting among instruments, we are constantly striving to create or identify those that not only measure the attribute of interest but which measure that attribute reliably.

Like validity, reliability can be classified according to several dimensions. These include the stability of the measurement over time, the congruence of a measurement when defined by different assessors (or determined by different methods), the consistency (homogeneity) of items within a measure or scale, and the correspondence of parallel measures. These dimensions, typically expressed as reliability coefficients, are evaluated using various methodological approaches, as described below:

- ***Test-Retest Reliability*** (***Temporal Stability***): Test-retest reliability is the most commonly recognized form of reliability. It is evaluated by administering the same item, scale, or instrument to a sample of individuals twice over a relatively short period (the period depending on the intrinsic stability of the variable under study) and comparing the results using *Pearson's product moment correlation* for interval data or *Spearman's rank order correlation* for ordinal data. Typically, test-retest correlation coefficients ranging 0.70–0.80 generally are considered to be satisfactory to good (though criteria for acceptability vary according to discipline). This measure of reliability is most appropriate for assessing relatively enduring characteristics such as personality traits, aptitude, and chronic health status in stable populations where subjects are willing to undergo multiple administration of the same measure. It is less appropriate for estimating temporal consistency of attitudes, mood, and knowledge that can be influenced by experience(s) or for health states that have been altered by intercurrent events between measurements.

- ***Interobserver (Inter-rater) Reliability***: Inter-rater reliability reflects the agreement between or among two or more assessors who independently rate the same item, scale, or instrument administered within a sample of individuals at a single point in time. *Cohen's Kappa* (*k*) is a commonly used statistic for estimating agreement between two raters for binary data (e.g., heart failure present vs. absent); a related statistic ("Weighted Kappa") may be used for ordinally ranked data such as those obtained via Likert-type scales. If the raters are in complete agreement, then $k=1$. If there is no agreement beyond that which would be expected by chance, then $k=0$ (values <0 signify that agreement is even less than that which would be attributable to chance). Although there is no universal consensus, in the range of values indicating better than chance agreement, statistics 0.01–0.20 have been interpreted as "slight agreement," 0.21–0.40 as "fair agreement," 0.40–60 as "moderate agreement," 0.61–0.80 as "substantial agreement," and ≥.81 as "almost perfect agreement" [97]. When data are at the interval level, inter-rater reliability can be established via computation of the Pearson's correlation coefficient (r) when sample size is relatively large and by the interclass correlation coefficient (ICC) when sample size is smaller (i.e., <15) [98], and is interpreted in the same manner as Kappa.
- ***Internal Consistency***: Internal consistency is an approach to reliability assessment that estimates the homogeneity of items in a scale that are intended to measure the same construct. The essential idea is that the various items on a scale all should correlate highly and positively; that is, when one item is answered in a particular way, other related items ought to be answered similarly. This approach is preferable to test-retest methods for instruments that are highly sensitive to change and which, when evaluated as repeated measures, can falsely create the impression of relatively low reliability [99]. Internal consistency reliability customarily is evaluated by a variety of approaches, each of which assesses equivalence of responses within a related group of items during a single administration of the instrument to the same subjects. The most common are given below:
  - ***Split-Half Reliability*** is one of the oldest methods for evaluating internal consistency. It is calculated by dividing a scale into two parts, computing a correlation coefficient between those parts, and adjusting the correlation using the *Spearman-Brown prophecy formula* to correct for foreshortened test length (as shorter scales tend to yield lower reliability estimates). As a rule of thumb, coefficients between .70 and .80 indicate adequate reliability, and .90 or greater indicates high reliability. If the two "half" measures are highly correlated, this provides evidence that they are measuring the same attribute. Two common methods for performing this analysis are to choose the first N items and the last N items, or to choose odd numbered items and even numbered items. It is important that split-half reliability be determined for particular scales, not for entire questionnaires comprising different scales. For example, if a questionnaire assesses both anxiety and depression, the split-half reliability of the two measures will need to be evaluated separately.
  - **The Kuder-Richardson Formula 20 (KR-20)** [100]. The KR-20 can be used to provide an estimate of internal consistency for scales calling for binary (dichotomous) responses (e.g., "yes"/"no," "true"/"false," "agree"/"disagree," "symptomatic"/"asymptomatic"). Unlike the split-half method (described above), which is based only on a single splitting of items, the KR-20 computes split-half reliability based on all combinations of splittings and produces an estimate of the mean correlation of the items comprising the measure. Values

can range from 0.00 to 1.00 (sometimes expressed as whole numbers, 1–100). A high KR-20 coefficient (i.e., >0.90) indicates a homogeneous measure or scale. A variant, the KR-21, is computationally simpler (it is based only on the assessment mean, variance, and number of items on the scale), but tends to produce lower reliability estimates.

- ***Cronbach's Alpha*** [101] is the best known, and most commonly used, measure of internal consistency. Like the KR-20, Cronbach's alpha conceptually represents the mean of all split-half reliability estimates for a scale [76] and is computed by calculating pair-wise correlations between items in a scale; however, Cronbach's alpha can be used with scales that include several ordinal response options (e.g., 1 = "strongly agree" through 5 = "strongly disagree" or 0 = "not limited by heart failure symptoms" through 3 = "severely limited by heart failure symptoms") as well as those that include binary response options, making it more flexible than the KR-20. Values of 0.70 or above are widely viewed as acceptable, and values of approximately 0.90 are considered to be excellent [102]; however, extremely high reliability estimates (i.e., ≥0.95) suggest that some of the items may be redundant, contributing no additional information than that furnished by other items on the scale. "Alpha if item is deleted" is a widely used index that can be useful for deleting nonhomogenous or redundant items during the process of scale development. Nonetheless, when using standardized scales, all items (including those that reduce alpha) should be retained to permit meaningful comparison with previous as well as future assessments employing the same instrument.
- ***Alternate (Equivalent, Parallel) Form Reliability***. An investigator may be concerned that repeated measurement using the same instrument might threaten the internal validity of an intervention study because (as noted in Chap. 5) exposure to the first assessment can influence the results of subsequent assessment by providing an opportunity for practice or learning independent of the intervention. This threat to internal validity ("testing effects") can be minimized (though not entirely eliminated) by using alternate forms of measurement of the same construct or content domain before and after the intervention. One commonly used approach to creating these alternate forms is to generate a large pool of items, each of which addresses the construct being studied, and randomly dividing the items to create two functionally equivalent instruments of similar difficulty and length. Other methods include changing the wording or order of the questions in the two instruments. (The same approach is used to discourage cheating on high stakes achievement or aptitude tests.) After the alternate forms are created, they are administered to the same sample, and the results are correlated. If they produce similar results for the same subjects (i.e., they yield correlation coefficients >0.80), they are considered to be equivalent forms and can be used interchangeably [62]. (The reader will note that the methodology for establishing alternate form reliability, when based on division of a related item pool, is analogous to that used for estimating split-half reliability. The primary difference is that with split-half reliability, items within a single scale or measure are divided solely for the purpose of determining internal consistency, whereas with the alternate form approach, the objective is to construct two equivalent instruments that can be used independently of one another.)

Ethical and Legal Aspects of Survey Methods

Given below is a brief précis of some ethical and legal issues involved in survey research. Any investigator should carefully review the policies of his or her institution to ensure compliance.

If the investigator has a professional license, that licensing body may also have relevant rules and regulations governing survey research.

1. **General participation**. In all cases, respondents must know that they are free to *not* participate, to skip questions, and to stop the survey at any time.
2. **Sensitive questions**. If sensitive questions are asked, provision should be made for debriefing, and respondents should be provided with information about relevant services, as appropriate. For example, if an investigator asks a subject about illicit drug use, information may need to be provided about available treatment facilities.
3. **Privacy**. Especially when sensitive information is discussed, substantial efforts should be made to keep identifying information private. One solution is to use code numbers rather than names and, if necessary, to store a link of code numbers to names in a separate and secure location.
4. **Snowball (chain-referral) sampling**. Sometimes, when a sampling characteristic is relatively rare within a population, or when a population is "concealed" from society at large, an investigator may have difficulty locating an adequate number of subjects for a survey. This can occur when the population of interest comprises individuals who exhibit illegal or otherwise stigmatized behaviors (e.g., illicit drug use or prostitution). One approach that sometimes is used to increase sample size under these conditions is to recruit a relatively small number of subjects who possess the desired sampling attribute and ask each subject to bring in additional subjects from among their acquaintances ("social network") who possess the same attribute. These, in turn, may be called upon to recruit similar additional subjects for the study. Thus, the sample grows metaphorically like a "snowball." Though snowball sampling can reduce subject search costs and provide access to subjects who would otherwise be inaccessible, the investigator must take great care to adequately protect the potentially sensitive and damaging information given by respondents during the chain referral process, as disclosures from the investigator could compromise privacy of the subject and confidentiality of their data, destroy the relationships within the chain, and militate against further recruitment [103].
5. **Focus groups**. Focus groups pose ethical special problems, because members of the focus group share information that can, potentially, be used by one participant against another. As a hypothetical example, suppose a focus group of medical students were convened to evaluate specific academic programs and one member of the focus group identified a certain faculty member as incompetent. If another focus group member knew the identity of the participant expressing this view, he or she could be threatened or even blackmailed. As another example, if a focus group member acknowledged having HIV or some other stigmatized condition or admitted to engaging in illicit behavior (such as abuse of prescription or nonprescription drugs), similar problems could ensue.
6. ***Children and other special populations***. Additional rules apply when conducting self-report surveys involving children and other special populations (e.g., prisoners, individuals with mental disabilities). These populations may have limited ability to supply informed consent, either due to lack of comprehension (e.g., young children and individuals with mental disabilities) or because of feelings of duress (e.g., prisoners). (A listing of these rules can be found in the Code of Federal Regulations, Title 45 Public Welfare, Department of Health and Human Services [104].)

Summary: A General Guide to Constructing a Measure

This chapter has highlighted the complexities of constructing a self-report measure. If the investigator believes that the need for a new measure outweighs the effort required to develop it, the following provides an outline of the essential steps involved, adapted from those suggested by

DeVellis [40] and Fowler [39]. (Further details of these steps can be found in their writings.)

1. **Determine precisely what must be measured.** It is not sufficient to have a vague idea of what it is to be measured—one needs to be fairly precise. If the study is analytic, how well does the new measure facilitate testing of the research hypothesis? If the study is performed to generate a hypothesis, how well will the anticipated responses achieve this objective? Will the measure assess knowledge, attitudes, behaviors, or a combination of these areas? What areas must be covered? How will the new measure differ from existing measures? What theory will guide the development of the new measure? How specific versus general should the measure be? As is the case for all forms of research, time spent clarifying objectives at the outset will save a great deal of time later on.
2. **Define the population of interest.** State, as precisely as possible, whom you wish to study. Often, the choice will be a compromise between optimal versus available subjects. An investigator may be interested in all humans with a disease, but it is never possible to study all such individuals. It also is very difficult, if not impossible, to obtain a random sample of such individuals from around the world. Early in the design of the study, the investigator should identify the age group and gender(s) of interest, the geographic location of potential respondents, their racial or ethnic characteristics, etc.
3. **Select the type of self-report to be used.** Decide whether the information being sought is best obtained via a mailed self-completed questionnaire, an in-person or telephone interview, or a computer-based method. Each approach has advantages and disadvantages, as noted above.
4. **Generate the item pool.** Initially, a large pool of items should be generated, covering as many different parts of the construct of interest as possible from different perspectives. Brainstorm. At this stage, the creator of the survey instrument should not fear redundancy or a long list of items—these can be narrowed later in the process. It is not uncommon for the initial pool to contain four times as many items as the number of items comprising the final scale.
5. **Determine the measurement format.** As previously indicated, questions and responses can be framed in numerous ways. The preferred format should be considered at the same time that the item pool is generated to maintain consistency. For example, will the survey be unstructured, semistructured, or structured? If the questions call for closed-ended responses, how many response categories will there be? What type of scaling will be used? Will the time frame to which the questions refer be specified or implied, etc.?
6. **Develop "validation items."** Validation items are of two types: (a) those that do not directly measure the construct under study, but which may be useful for detecting flaws (biases) in the measurement process, and (b) those which assist in assessing the construct validity of the new measure. Including a social desirability scale can help to determine which items tend to be influenced by this positive bias and serve as a basis for eliminating them. The inclusion of items from a putatively related measure can be used to buttress a claim of construct validity or identify poorly performing items [40].
7. **Pretest.** Once a large pool of items has been defined, it can be reduced to a manageable number and screened for omissions, errors, and related problems. Independent review by content-matter experts, colleagues, and key decision makers can be helpful for establishing both the face and content validity of the preliminary instrument and for obtaining feedback regarding specific items. Reviewers can be asked:
   - How relevant each item is to the construct being measured
   - How clear the items are
   - If there are ways to make the items more concise
   - If key items are missing (there should be at least one question for every variable of interest)

- If items are superfluous or redundant
- If items are difficult to read or answer (e.g., are ambiguous or otherwise unclear)

It also is helpful to solicit review of the drafted items from individuals who are similar to the intended respondents. This can be done within a focus group or as a series of one-on-one "cognitive interviews" conducted among a small number of individual respondents. Both approaches allow exploration of how well the items are understood and are particularly useful when the intended respondents differ greatly from the individuals writing the survey instrument. Specific questions should be asked about how respondents interpreted the questions, how they thought the various questions differed from each other, how readable they were, and what their responses meant. At this stage, questions can be open-ended, as one of the goals of pretesting is to identify response options that may have been overlooked (a prespecified list of responses options will, by force, constrain the respondent to think like the survey developer). Feedback from the pretest can be use to add, delete, and otherwise refine questions to be included in the preliminary instrument and to frame appropriate response options.

8. **Pilot test**. Pilot testing is crucial to development of a valid and useful scale. No matter what care is taken in developing and screening items, some will be misinterpreted by respondents. Pilot testing involves administering the preliminary questionnaire (including the cover letter and directions) to respondents who, again, are as similar as possible to members of the target population. The pilot should be performed, to the extent possible, under conditions that mirror the conditions under which the final survey will be conducted. It should ask respondents to find flaws in the survey (e.g., Were directions and skip patterns (if any) clear? Was the survey too long? Was the format appropriate? Were any of the questions confusing or otherwise unclear? Did any not apply? Were any overly intrusive? Were any redundant? Did they flow well?). Statistical methods (e.g., evaluation of distributional characteristics, examination of missing answers, item-to-item and item-to-scale correlations) can be applied to responses obtained in the pilot to detect poorly performing or redundant items and to evaluate their impact on internal consistency when retained or deleted. It is difficult to find guidance regarding the minimal number of participants to be included in a pilot. Some workers in the field have suggested 300 [105]; others [40] have recommended that for single scales comprising relatively few (e.g., 20) items, a smaller number may suffice. A cautionary note is in order. If too few respondents are chosen, it may not be possible to evaluate the items properly; if the sample is not representative, items may have different meanings to the pilot sample versus the target population, and the relationships among the items may be different as well [40].
9. **Edit**. Invariably, once a measure is pilot tested, revision will be required. Directions may need to be clarified. Confusing, overly intrusive, or unanswered questions will need to be deleted or reworded (though reworded items may need to be retested). If revisions are extensive, a second round of pilot testing may be required. Once poorly performing items are eliminated, the length of the instrument should be evaluated. Too short a measure will not fully explore the construct of interest. However, one that is too long may bore or frustrate the respondents.
10. **Assess reliability and validity**. Before an instrument can be used for formal research purposes, its reliability and validity must be assessed in the population of interest. As noted above, the most common test for reliability is Cronbach's alpha; for validity, the appropriate method depends on the degree of development of substantive knowledge and the existence of (a) other measures of the same construct, (b) measures of similar but different constructs, and (c) the availability of a "gold standard."

Take-Home Points

- A self-report (a.k.a. survey) is a measure where the respondent supplies information about him or herself.
- Self-reports are important in medical research because some variables (e.g., attitudes, beliefs, self-judged ability) only can be assessed from information directly furnished by the patient or other subject.
- A self-report is obtained by questionnaire, interview, or related methods.
- Questionnaires are written documents that can be self-completed without interviewer involvement or read aloud as part of an interview; interviews usually (but not always) are administered orally; both can be structured (comprise closed-ended questions), unstructured (comprise open-ended questions), or semistructured (comprise a mix of both question types).
- If answers to a research question can be obtained only via self-report, the investigator should first determine whether an instrument already exists that is reliable, valid, and otherwise suitable for the population of interest.
- In situations where a new instrument must be developed, the investigator must clearly define the question(s) of interest; identify the population to be surveyed; select the preferred type of self-report/format of measurement; consider inclusion of validation questions; pretest, pilot test and edit the measure; and test the final battery of questions for reliability and validity.
- When developing or implementing a survey, the investigator must be certain to observe all ethical and legal aspects of survey methodology.

References

1. Polit DF, Beck CT. Nursing research: principles and methods. 7th ed. Philadelphia: Lippincott, Williams and Wilkins; 2004.
2. Kish L. Survey sampling. New York: Wiley; 1995.
3. Groves RM, Fowler FJ, Couper MP, Lepkowski JM, Singer E. Survey methodology. New York: Wiley; 2004.
4. Cochran WG. Sampling techniques. 3rd ed. New York: Wiley; 1977.
5. Derogatis LR. BSI: Brief Symptom Inventory: administration, scoring and procedures manual. Minneapolis: National Computer Systems; 1993.
6. Ware JE, Snow KK, Kosinski M, Gandek B. SF-36 health survey: manual and interpretation guide. Lincoln: RI, QualityMetric, Inc.; 2000.
7. Skevington SM, Bradshaw J, Saxena S. Selecting national items for the WHOQOL: conceptual and psychometric considerations. Soc Sci Med. 1999;48: 473–487.
8. Rector TS, Cohn JN. Assessment of patient outcome with the Minnesota Living with Heart Failure Questionnaire: reliability and validity during a randomized, double-blind, placebo-controlled trial of pimobendan. Pimobendan Multicenter Research Group. Am Heart J. 1992;124:1017–25.
9. Morisky DE, Green LW, Levine DM. Concurrent and predictive validity of a self-reported measure of medicine adherence. Med Care. 1986;24:67–72.
10. Strauss AL, Corbin JM. Basics of qualitative research: techniques and procedures for developing grounded theory. 2nd ed. Thousand Oaks: Sage; 1998.
11. Cohen MZ, Ley C, Tarzian AJ. Isolation in blood and marrow transplantation. West J Nurs Res. 2001;25:37–48.
12. Fadiman A. The spirit catches you and you fall down: a Hmong child, her American doctors, and the collision of two cultures. New York: Farrar, Straus and Giroux; 1998.
13. Drever E. Using semi-structured interviews in small-scale research, a teacher's guide. ERIC. Edinburgh: SCRE; 1995.
14. Benson J, Britten N. Respecting the autonomy of cancer patients when talking with their families: qualitative analysis of semistructured interviews with patients. BMJ. 1996;313:729–731.
15. O'Dea JA. Consumption of nutritional supplements among adolescents: usage and perceived benefits. Health Educ Res. 2003;18:98–107.

16. Allan G. A note on interviewing spouses together. J Marriage Fam. 1980;42:205–210.
17. Kalischuk RG, Davies B. A theory of healing in the aftermath of youth suicide. J Holist Nurs. 2001;19: 163–186.
18. Dolezal C, Mellins C, Brackis-Cott E, Abrams EJ. The reliability of reports of medical adherence from children with HIV and their adult care givers. J Pediatr Psychol. 2003;28:355–361.
19. Dym B, Berman S. The primary health care team: family physician and family therapist in joint practice. Fam Syst Med. 1986;4:9–21.
20. Morrison-Beedy D, Côté-Arsenault D, Feinstein NF. Maximizing results with focus groups: moderator and analysis issues. Appl Nurs Res. 2001;14:48–53.
21. Quatromoni PA, Milbauer M, Posner BM, Carballeira NP, Brunt M, Chipkin SR. Use of focus groups to explore nutrition practices and health beliefs of urban Caribbean Latinos with diabetes. Diabetes Care. 1994;17:869–873.
22. Hicks LK, Lin Y, Robertson DW, Robinson DL, Woodrow SI. Understanding the clinical dilemmas that shape medical students' ethical development: questionnaire survey and focus group study. BMJ. 2001;322:709–710.
23. Flanagan JC. The critical incident technique. Psychol Bull. 1954;51:327–358.
24. Coté CJ, Notterman DA, Karl HW, Weinberg JA, McClosky C. Adverse sedation events in pediatrics: a critical incident analysis of contributing factors. Pediatrics. 2000;105:805–14.
25. Branch W, Pels RJ, Arky R. Becoming a doctor. Critical-incident reports from third-year medical students. N Engl J Med. 1993;329:1130–1132.
26. Allery LA, Owen PA, Robling MR. Why general practitioners and consultants change their clinical practice: a critical incident study. BMJ. 1997;314: 870–874.
27. Faithfull S. The diary method for nursing research. Eur J Cancer Care. 2007;1:13–18.
28. Bruijnzeels NA, Foets M, van der Wooden JC, Prins A, van den Houvel WJ. Measuring morbidity of children in the community: a comparison of interview and diary data. Int J Epidemiol. 1998;27: 96–100.
29. White MM, Howie-Esquivel J, Caldwell MA. Improving heart failure symptom recognition: a diary analysis. Cardiovasc Nurs. 2010;25:7–12.
30. Woodfield R, Goodyear-Smith F, Arroll B. N-of-1 trials of quinine efficacy in skeletal muscle cramps of the leg. Br J Gen Pract. 2005;55(512):181–185.
31. Aitken L, Mardegan KJ. Thinking aloud: data collection in the natural setting. Western J Nurs Res. 2000;22:841–853.
32. Fonetyn M, Fisher A. Use of think aloud method to study nurse's reasoning and decision making in clinical practice settings. J Neurosci Nurs. 1995;27: 124–128.
33. Ericsson K, Simon H. Protocol analysis: verbal reports as data. London: MIT Press; 1993.
34. Murphy LL, Spies RA, Plake BS, editors. Tests in print VII. Lincoln: Buros Institute of Mental Measurements; 2006.
35. Geisinger KF, Spies RA, Carlson JF, Plake BS, editors. The seventeenth mental measurements yearbook. Lincoln: Buros Institute of Mental Measurements; 2007.
36. Goldman BA, Mitchell DF, Egelson PE, editors. Directory of unpublished experimental mental measures. Washington, DC: American Psychological Association; 2007.
37. Bieri D, Reeve R, Champion GD, Addicoat L, Ziegler JB. The Faces Pain Scale for the self-assessment of the severity of pain experienced by children: development, initial validation and preliminary investigation for ratio scale properties. Pain. 1990;41:139–150.
38. Choi BCK, Pak AWP. A catalog of biases in questionnaires. Prev Chronic Dis. 2005;2:1–13.
39. Fowler FJ. Improving survey questions. Thousand Oaks: Sage; 1995.
40. DeVellis RF. Scale development: theory and applications. Newbury Park: Sage; 1991.
41. Chang AM, Chau JPC, Holroyd E. Translation of questionnaires and issues of equivalence. J Adv Nurs. 2010;29:316–322.
42. Healey B, Gendall P. Asking the age question in mail and online surveys. Austral and New Zeal Marketing Acad (ANZMAC) Conference 2007. Dunedin; 2007.
43. Heise DR. The semantic differential and attitude research. In: Summers GF, editor. Attitude measurement. Chicago: Rand McNally; 1970.
44. Aiken LR. Rating scales and checklists. New York: Wiley; 1996.
45. DeLoach LJ, Higgins MS, Caplan AB, Stiff JL. The visual analog scale in the immediate postoperative period: intrasubject variability and correlation with a numeric scale. Anesth Analg. 1998;86:102–106.
46. Brealey SD, Atwell C, Bryan S, Coulton S, Cox H, Cross B, Fylan F, Garratt A, Gilbert FG, Gillan MGC, Hendry M, Hood K, Houston H, King D, Morton V, Orchard J, Robling M, Russell IT, Torgerson D, Wadsworth V, Wilkinson C. Improving response rates using a monetary incentive for patient completion of questionnaires: an observational study. BMC Med Res Methodol. 2007;7:12–16.
47. Asch D, Jedrziewski MK, Christakis N. Response rates to mail surveys published in medical journals. J Clin Epidemiol. 1997;50:1129–1136.
48. Diment K, Garrett-Jones S. How demographic characteristics affect mode preference in a postal/web mixed survey of Australian researchers. Soc Sci Comput Rev. 2007;25:410–417.
49. Shih TH. Comparing response rates from web and mail surveys: a meta-analysis. Field Methods. 2008;20:249–271.
50. O'Toole J, Sinclair M, Leder K. Maximising response rates in household telephone surveys. BMC Med Res Methodol. 2008;8:71.

51. Tourangeau R, Smith TW. Asking sensitive questions: the impact of data collection mode, question format and question context. Public Opin Q. 1996;60: 275–304.
52. Turner CF, Al-Tayyib AA, Rogers SM, Eggleston MA, Villarroel MA, Roman AM, Chromy JR, Cooley PC. Improving epidemiological surveys of sexual behavior conducted by telephone. Int J Epidemiol. 2009;38:1118–1127.
53. Couper MP, Nicholls II WL. The history and development of computer assisted survey information collection methods. In: Couper MP et al., editors. Computer assisted survey information collection. New York: Wiley; 1998.
54. Vataja R, Pohjasvaara T, Leppävuori A, Mäntylä R, Aronen HJ, Salonen O, Kaste M, Erkinjuntti T. Magnetic resonance imaging correlates of depression after ischemic stroke. Arch Gen Psychiatry. 2001;58:925–31.
55. Schackman BR, Dastur Z, Rubin DS, Berger J, Camhi E, Netherland J, Ni Q, Finkelstein R. Feasibility of using audio computer-assisted self-interview (ACASI) screening in routine HIV care. AIDS Care. 2009;21:992–999.
56. Oetting ER, Beauvais F. Adolescent drug use. J Consult Clin Psychol. 1990;58:385–394.
57. Fidler DS, Kleinknec RE. Randomized response versus direct questioning: two data-collection methods for sensitive information. Psychol Bull. 1977;84: 1045–1049.
58. Lensvelt-Mulders GJLM, Hox JJ, van der Heijden PGM, Maas CJM. Meta-analysis of randomized response research. Sociol Method Res. 2005;33: 319–348.
59. Edwards P, Roberts I, Clarke M, DiGuisseppi C, Pratap S, Wentz R, Kwan I. Increasing response rates to postal questionnaires. BMJ. 2002;324:1183–91.
60. Brennan M, Charbonnau J. Improving mail survey response rate using chocolate and replacement questionnaires. Public Opin Q. 2009;73:368–378.
61. Merriam-Webster Online. Available at http://www.m-w.com/. Accessed 27 July 2010.
62. Waltz CF, Strickland OL, Lenz ER. Measurement in nursing and research. New York: Springer Publishing Inc; 2005.
63. Cook DA, Beckman TJ. Current concepts in validity and reliability for psychometric instruments: theory and application. Am J Med. 2006;119(2):166.e7–166.e16.
64. Litwin MS. How to measure survey reliability and validity. Thousand Oaks: Sage; 1995.
65. Beck AT, Steer R, Brown GK. Manual for the Beck Depression Inventory-II. San Antonio: Psychological Corporation; 1996.
66. Williams RA. Women's health content validity of the family medicine in-training exam. Fam Med. 2007;39:572–577.
67. Ware JE, Sherbourne CD. The MOS 36 item short form health survey. Med Care. 1992;30:473–483.
68. Feldman AB, Haley SM, Coryell J. Concurrent and construct validity of the pediatric evaluation of disability inventory. Phys Ther. 1990;70:602–610.
69. Lin JM, Brimmer DJ, Maloney EM, Nyarko E, BeLue R, Reeves WC. Further validation of the Multidimensional Fatigue Inventory in a US adult population sample. Popul Health Metr. 2009; 7:18 doi:10.1186/1478-7954-7-18.
70. McHorney CA, Ware Jr JE, Raczek AE. The MOS 36-item Short-Form Health Survey (SF-36): II. Psychometric and clinical tests of validity in measuring physical and mental health constructs. Med Care. 1993;31:247–263.
71. Management Sciences for Health. Creating a climate that motivates staff and improves performance. The Manager. 2003;11:1–22.
72. Tennant R, Hiller L, Fishwick R, Platt S, Joseph S, Parkinson J, Secker J, Stewart-Brown S. The Warwick-Edinburgh Mental Well-Being Scale (WEMWBS): development and UK validation. Health and Quality of Life Outcomes 2007; 5:63doi:10.1186/1477-7525-5-63.
73. Cooper SM, Baker JS, Tong RJ, Roberts E, Hanford M. The repeatability and criterion related validity of the 20 m Multistage Fitness Test as a predictor of maximal oxygen uptake in active young men. Br J Sports Med. 2005;39:e19.
74. Reuben DB, Siu AL, Kimpau S. The predictive validity of self-report and performance-based measures of function and health. J Gerontol. 1991;47: M106–M110.
75. Heather N, Rollnick S, Bell A. Predictive validity of the readiness to change questionnaire. Addiction. 1993;88:1667–1677.
76. Portney LG, Watkins MP. Foundations of clinical research. Applications to practice. Upper Saddle River: Prentice Hall Health; 2000.
77. Guyatt G, Walter S, Norman G. Measuring change over time: assessing the usefulness of evaluative instruments. J Chronic Dis. 1987;40:171–178.
78. Hays RD, Hadorn D. Responsiveness to change: an aspect of validity, not a separate dimension. Qual Life Res. 1992;1:73–75.
79. Beaton DE, Bombadier C, Katz JN, Wright JG. A taxonomy for responsiveness. J Clin Epidemiol. 2001;54:1204–1217.
80. Husted JA, Cook RJ, Farewell VT, Gladman DD. Methods for assessing responsiveness: a critical review and recommendations. J Clin Epidemiol. 2000;53:459–468.
81. Roach KE. Measurement of health outcomes: reliability, validity and responsiveness. JPO. 2006; 18:8–12.
82. Liang MH, Fossel AH, Larson MG. Comparison of five health status instruments for orthopedic evaluation. Med Care. 1990;28:632–642.
83. Angst F, Verra ML, Lehmann S, Aeschlimann A. Responsiveness of five condition-specific and generic outcome assessment instruments for chronic

pain. BMC Med Res Methodol 2008;8:26 (published online 2008 April 25 doi:10.1186/1471-2288-8-26).
84. Tavris C, Aronson E. Mistakes were made, but not by me. Orlando: Harcourt Books; 2008.
85. Crowne DP, Marlowe D. A new scale of social desirability independent of psychopathology. J Consult Psychol. 1960;24:349–354.
86. Strahan R, Kerbasi K. Short homogenous version of the Marlowe-Crowne Social Desirability Scale. J Cin Psychol. 1972;28:191–193.
87. Furnham A, Henderson M. The good, the bad and the mad: Response bias in self-report measures. Pers Indiv Differ. 1982;3:311–320.
88. Leary MR, Kowalski RM. Impression management: a literature review and two-component model. Psychol Bull. 1990;107:34–47.
89. Lenski GE, Leggett JC. Caste, class, and deference in the research interview. Am J Sociol. 1960;65: 463–467.
90. Krosnick JA, Alwin DF. An evaluation of cognitive theory of response order effects in survey measurement. Public Opin Q. 1987;51:201–219.
91. Toner B. Impact of agreement bias on the rating of questionnaire response. J Soc Psychol. 1987;127: 221–222.
92. Nelson NW, Parsons TD, Grote CL, Smith CA, Sisung II JR. The MMPI-2 Fake Bad Scale: concordance and specificity of true and estimate scores. J Clin Exp Neuropsychol. 2006;28:1–12.
93. Thorndike EL. A constant error in psychological rating. J Appl Psychol. 1920;4:25–29.
94. Roeckelein J. Elsevier's dictionary of psychological theories. Amsterdam: Elsevier BV; 2006.
95. Feldt LS, Brennan RL. Reliability. In: Linn RL, editor. Educational measurement. 3rd ed. New York: American Council on Education and Macmillan; 1989.
96. Downing SM. Validity: on the meaningful interpretation of assessment data. Med Educ. 2003;37: 830–837.
97. Landis JR, Koch GG. The measurement of observer agreement for categorical data. Biometrics. 1977;33: 159–174.
98. Shrout PE, Fleiss JL. Intraclass correlations: uses in assessing rater reliability. Psychol Bull. 1979;86: 420–428.
99. McDowell I, Newell C. Measuring health. A guide to rating scales and questionnaires. 2nd ed. New York: Oxford University Press; 1996.
100. Kuder GF, Richardson MW. The theory of the estimation of test reliability. Psychometrika. 1937;2: 151–60.
101. Cronbach LJ. Coefficient alpha and the internal structure of tests. Psychometrika. 1951;16:297–334.
102. George D, Mallery P. SPSS for Windows step by step. Boston: Allyn & Bacon; 2003.
103. Faugier J, Sargeant M. Sampling hard to reach populations. J Adv Nurs. 1997;26:790–797.
104. Code of Federal Regulations, Title 45 Public welfare, department of Health and Human Services, Revised 15 Jan 2009, (Effective 14 July 2009).
105. Nunnally JC. Psychometric theory. New York: McGraw-Hill; 1978.

9 Selecting and Evaluating Secondary Data: The Role of Systematic Reviews and Meta-analysis

Lorenzo Paladino and Richard H. Sinert

Sorting through the body of available literature is a daunting task. MEDLINE, only one of many databases, indexed 902,346 articles in 2010. This number reflects a continuing increase over 2009 (854,506) and 2008 (821,834). How can clinicians have any chance of keeping up with the literature or use it for guiding research or for formulating clinical practice decisions if their primary sources are restricted to individual studies? The answer is that it is difficult, if not increasingly impractical. Reliance on individual studies is further complicated when current beliefs and standards of practice are challenged by new studies. For clinicians to make informed decisions, they must analyze multiple studies for both their quality and relevance to the patient population of interest. This is a principal reason for the long lag time before clinical research is incorporated into standard practice. A representative example is the 20-year delay between initial reports suggesting the utility of thrombolytic therapy for myocardial infarctions in the late 1970s and its adoption in the 1990s [1]. For these reasons, secondary sources such as narrative reviews, systematic reviews, and meta-analyses are an important means for physicians to translate clinical research into standard practice and help reconcile conflicting studies in the literature.

Difference Between a Narrative Review, Systematic Review, and Meta-analysis

A narrative review (sometimes termed a traditional literature review) is a summary of primary published studies in which conclusions are drawn by the reviewer, guided by his or her own interpretations of the studies, rather than by external criteria. Narrative reviews are well suited for general topics or broad coverage of a field as they usually cover a wide range of issues within a given topic [2], e.g., "Update on Multiple Sclerosis." Typically, they are written by experts in the specific field of study rather than by experts on research methodology. As such, narrative reviews do not necessarily explicitly state or follow the rules of evidence-based search strategies (including selection criteria for articles and abstracts found) or assess the quality or validity of the included studies. This deficit leads to lack of transparency and reproducibility and is likely to reflect a biased selection of the total evidence available (selection bias). A common bias in narrative reviews is failure to include research that conflicts with the beliefs or opinions of the expert. Nonetheless, the majority of published reviews are narrative rather than systematic.

L. Paladino, MD • R.H. Sinert, DO (✉)
Department of Emergency Medicine,
SUNY Downstate Medical Center,
450 Clarkson Avenue, 1228, Brooklyn,
NY 11203, USA
e-mail: Lorenzopaladino@yahoo.com;
Richard.sinert@downstate.edu

P.G. Supino and J.S. Borer (eds.), *Principles of Research Methodology: A Guide for Clinical Investigators*,
DOI 10.1007/978-1-4614-3360-6_9,

In contrast, systematic reviews (in medicine, written most commonly about treatment or diagnostic research) focus on a specific question within a topic (e.g., "Are steroids effective in controlling flares of multiple sclerosis?" "Does positron emission tomography have strong positive predictive value for breast cancer?"), rendering them amenable to an explicit search strategy. This characteristic makes them excellent tools to explore clinically relevant topics. Systematic reviews identify the databases searched and, thus, present clear and reproducible search strategies. A comprehensive literature search is conducted, and all identified studies identified are assessed for relevance and methodology. Selection is based on predefined inclusion and exclusion criteria, quality is assessed, and data are abstracted in a standardized format. By explicitly stating how the evidence was found, how it was appraised or validated, and which studies were excluded (and why), systematic reviews eliminate many of the biases inherent in narrative reviews.

A meta-analysis (sometimes termed a "quantitative review") often, but not always, is included as a component of a systematic review. First used for medicine in 1904 by renowned statistician Karl Pearson to examine the preventive effect of serum innoculations against enteric fever [3] and later formalized by contemporary statistician and educational researcher, Gene V. Glass (who coined the term in 1976) [4], meta-analysis currently is employed in many disciplines as a statistical methodology to combine the results of several studies about a topic as if they were from one large study. In studies of treatment (the most common focus of meta-analysis in clinical medicine), its principal purposes are to enable detection of overall and subgroup effects (as statistical power may be suboptimal due to limitations in sample size of individual trials), to improve estimates of the magnitude of these effects, and to aid in the resolution of uncertainty due to inconsistent findings (i.e., interstudy differences) [5]. The studies included in a meta-analysis should be found using the same rigorous search methodology as that used for systematic reviews.

Well-constructed systematic reviews and meta-analyses have many of the characteristics of effective research described by Tuckman [6] and reviewed in Chap. 1. They are **systematic** because information gathering is done in a structured and rigorous way and the data contained within them are interpreted. They are **logical** in that their methodologies employ tools for assessing the studies' bias (internal validity) and procedures to discern the effects of varying populations on study results (external validity). They are **replicable** both because they demonstrate whether the results of individual studies are congruent and also because the methodology employed in the review, if properly performed and reported, is sufficiently explicit to be permit reproduction. **They are transmittable** because, by "digesting" available information and coming to a conclusion, they effectively summarize what is currently known on a specific topic and, when published, enable clinicians to learn about the conclusions of research. In addition, meta-analyses, specifically, gather, compare, and pool the **empirical** products (data) of the studies collected and are **reductive** to a clinical conclusion. As noted above, meta-analyses increase sample size by pooling the subjects of smaller studies when appropriate. This larger N increases the **generalizability** of the results. When the results cannot be pooled, they often shed light on reasons why results may not be generalizable.

Searching for a Systematic Review or Meta-analysis

Almost all of the of the databases described in Chap. 2 can be used to search for meta-analyses and systematic reviews. The *Clinical Queries* link on the PubMed interface for MEDLINE can be used to apply search filters to focus on systematic reviews [7]. A variety of databases also are available that specialize in systematic reviews and meta-analyses. The *Cochrane Library* (www.thecochranelibrary.com), developed under the auspices of the *Cochrane Collaboration* (an international network dedicated to promoting well-informed health-care decision-making), maintains an online collection of systematic reviews on intervention and treatment. The *Database of*

Promoting Health Effectiveness Reviews (DoPHER) is a registry of systematic and nonsystematic reviews of public health. BestBETs (www.bestbets.org), *ACP Journal Club* (www.acpjc.org), and the *TRIP Database* (www.tripdatabase.com/index.html) are other sources of systematic reviews for clinical questions. The *Database of Abstracts of Reviews of Effectiveness* (DARE) (www.crd.york.ac.uk/CMS2Web) contains abstracts of systematic reviews that have been assessed for their quality.

Steps in Writing a Systematic Review

There are several steps in writing a systematic review. Below is a brief outline that may serve as an overview (discussion of these steps is provided below):

1. Formulate the question.
2. Define the literature searching strategy.
3. Select the studies to be included.
4. Summarize results across studies.
5. Assess heterogeneity.
6. Consider appropriateness of pooling results for meta-analysis.

Formulating the Question

As is true for all well-designed primary studies, the first step in conducting a systematic review is definition of a clear searchable question. The importance of this initial step often is underestimated, leading to frustrating and unsuccessful searches. The process is best guided by the often-used four-part "PICO" method, originally defined by the McMaster University Centre for Evidence-Based Medicine (Hamilton Ontario) 1992 recommendations for asking focused clinical questions [8]. The PICO method can help translate a question into terms that will allow whichever search engine is selected to retrieve the most appropriate literature. Its components are described below:

- "P" denotes the patient population or problem. The reviewer needs to carefully define the population from among many available options. What is the age group of interest? Should the search be focused on males or females only? For which specific diseases is information sought (eg., diabetes or acute myocardial infarction or acute myocardial infarctions in diabetics)? An overly broad search typically will yield an excessive quantity of information, whereas an overly narrow search (e.g., females 30–35 years of age) will result in too few or no results.
- "I" denotes the intervention. In the setting of clinical medicine, the term intervention commonly is considered to be therapy (e.g., medical or surgical treatment or a risk-reduction initiative such as a smoking-cessation or weight-reduction program). However, this component of the PICO is somewhat of a misnomer as it also can pertain to diagnostic testing. When the PICO method is applied to analyze questions about progression of disease, the "intervention" (more appropriately termed "factor of interest" as it is not purposively applied) would be presence of a prognostic factor such as age, gender, morbidity, lifestyle, or family.
- "C" denotes the comparator, that is, to what the intervention in question will be compared. A clinician might argue, "I don't want to compare two drugs, I just want to know if giving aspirin is beneficial to my patients?" This question, however, by its very nature, must include a comparator, that is, giving aspirin versus giving nothing, in which case the target of the search likely will include studies that involve administering a placebo as a comparison. In diagnostic questions such as "Is a ultrasound a good study for detection of common bile duct stones?" the comparator optimally is the best available or "gold" standard test (i.e., endoscopic retrograde cholangiopancreatography [ERCP]). (In questions about prevention and prognosis, the optimal comparators are, respectively, absence of a preventive initiative or a given prognostic factor or factors.)
- The "O" (outcome) denotes the component that often spurs the research question. For example, will this therapy decrease morbidity or mortality? This element of the PICO typically requires refinement (consider the

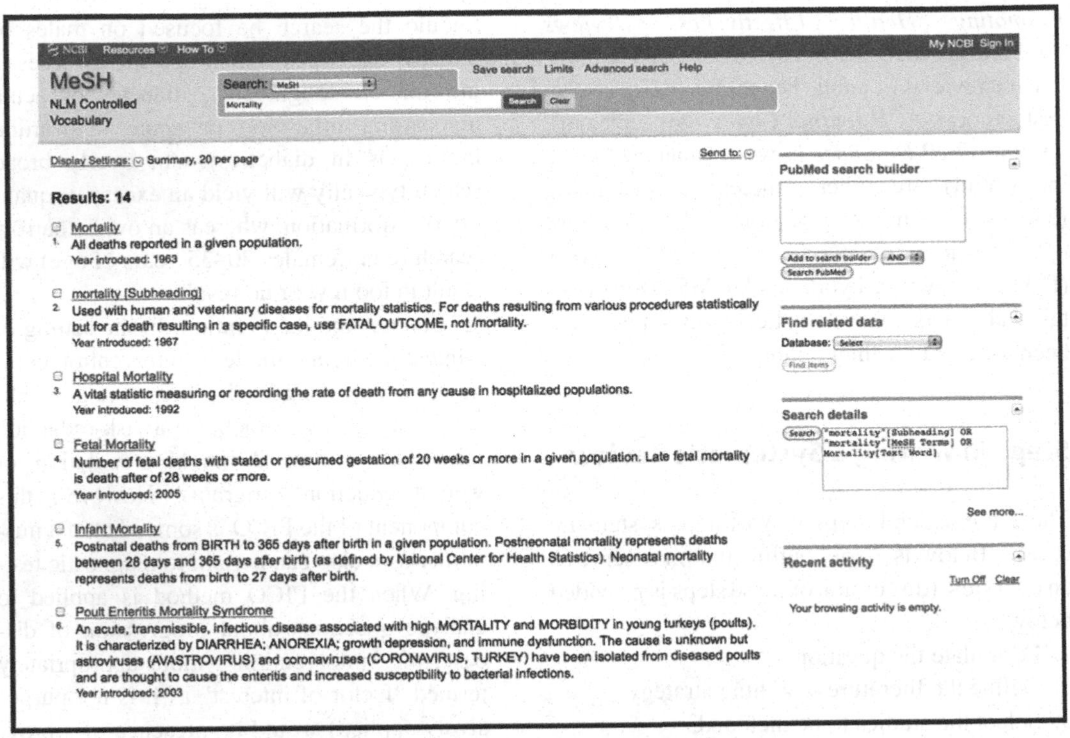

Fig. 9.1 MeSH for mortality on PubMed. Available at http://www.ncbi.nlm.nih.gov/mesh?term=mortality

concept of mortality reduction: what period of time is clinically meaningful? 30 days? 6 weeks? 6 months? 1 year?).

Defining the Literature Search Strategy: Keywords, MeSH, and Boolean Operators

An organized literature search will increase the likelihood of finding answers to the question of interest. The PICO question described above can be subdivided into its four components for entry into the database's search engine. We recommend that the reviewer search broadly at first and then search more narrowly ("cone down"). The more limited the initial search, the more likely it will miss relevant articles. Each component of the question should be searched by keywords, probable synonyms, and, if using PubMed, its MeSH (medical subject headings) terms (also called "descriptors"). MeSH is the US National Library of Medicine's (NLM) controlled vocabulary thesaurus that is used for indexing articles; it is hierarchically arrayed to facilitate searching at varying levels of specificity [9]. Use of all of these tools invariably will yield a more inclusive search.

Consider the example: "Does drawing blood cultures (intervention) change mortality (outcome) in adult patients with pneumonia (population)?" (The comparison implied by the question is *not* drawing blood cultures.) In some literature, blood culture may be classified as "microbiological culture," "microbial culture," or "microbial testing"; pneumonia as "lung infection" or "respiratory infection"; and mortality as "death" or "survival." MeSH terms can help expand the search by including many or all of these synonyms under one umbrella (Fig. 9.1). However, they should not be solely relied upon because inclusion or exclusion of an item under a specific MeSH is determined subjectively by those performing the NML indexing.

During the search, the selected terms are connected by the Boolean operators "AND," "OR," and "NOT" (see Venn Diagram,

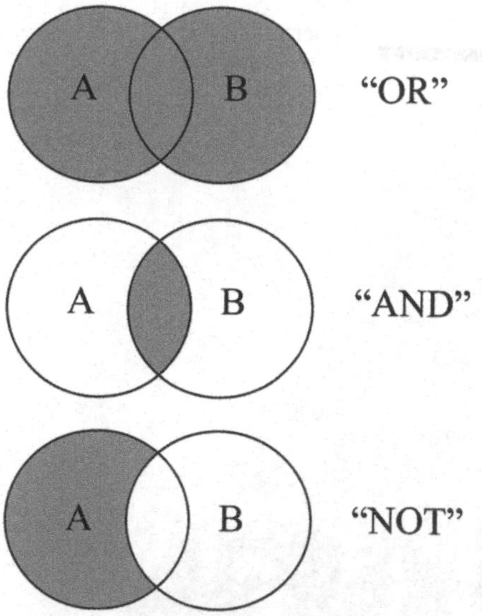

Fig. 9.2 Boolean terms OR, AND, and NOT

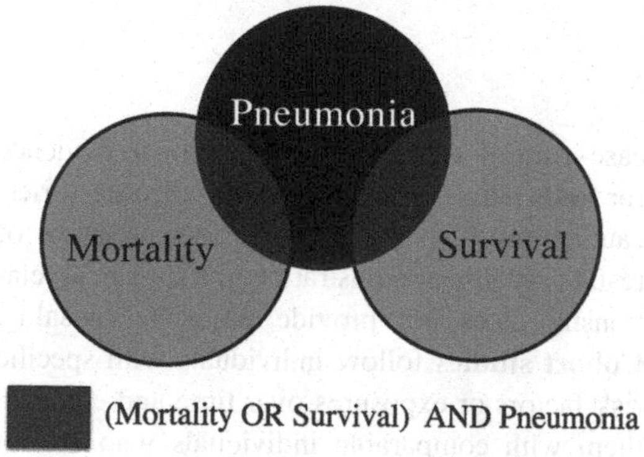

Fig. 9.3 (Mortality OR survival) AND pneumonia

Fig. 9.2). The meaning of these operators are self-explanatory; however, the implications of their additions to a search deserves outlining. The "OR" operator expands the search to include *any* of the selected terms, whereas "AND" limits it to those that contain *all* selected terms.

To start a search broadly, the keywords in the query should be connected by the "OR" operator (e.g., mortality OR survival). This strategy provides the sum of all words as if they were searched individually. By adding AND pneumonia, the search will yield articles only about both mortality (OR survival) and pneumonia. This concept is illustrated by the Venn diagram given in Fig. 9.3.

Though, as noted, the Boolean "NOT" operator is available, to optimize inclusiveness, it is better to search positively (i.e., to *join* desired concepts) rather than to search by exclusion.

An inclusive search should not miss any relevant information. Unfortunately, the literature is not centralized, and many databases (e.g., MEDLINE, EMBASE, and others listed in Chap. 2) must be queried to assure a complete search. The bibliographies of relevant papers should be checked for articles missed by the initial search, a methodology often refered to as "snowballing." Repeating this process on the additional papers can lead to greater retrieval. Citation searches using the *Web of Science* or *SciVerse-Scopus* also may yield additional papers. New keywords found on these papers can be added to augment the original search terms. Consulting a research librarian to perform expert searches also should be done for completeness. Unpublished studies can be found by searching clinical trials registries and by contacting experts and individual authors in the field. The Cochrane Library maintains a registry of controlled clinical trials, *Cochrane Library Cochrane Central Register of Controlled Trials* (CENTRAL) as does Clinicaltrials.gov. These important steps help to prevent the reviewer from missing relevant yet unpublished research, common with negative studies (see below: "Detecting Publication Bias").

Selecting Articles

Having formed the search question, the next step in constructing the systematic review is consideration of the types of literature available to answer the question. Selection should be based on several key factors, the most important of which are listed below.

Levels of Evidence

Medline and other databases contain literature that is very heterogenous with regard to the strength of evidence provided. The varying types of studies contained within the literature are represented here as a pyramid (Fig. 9.4), with the weakest evidence for answering clinical

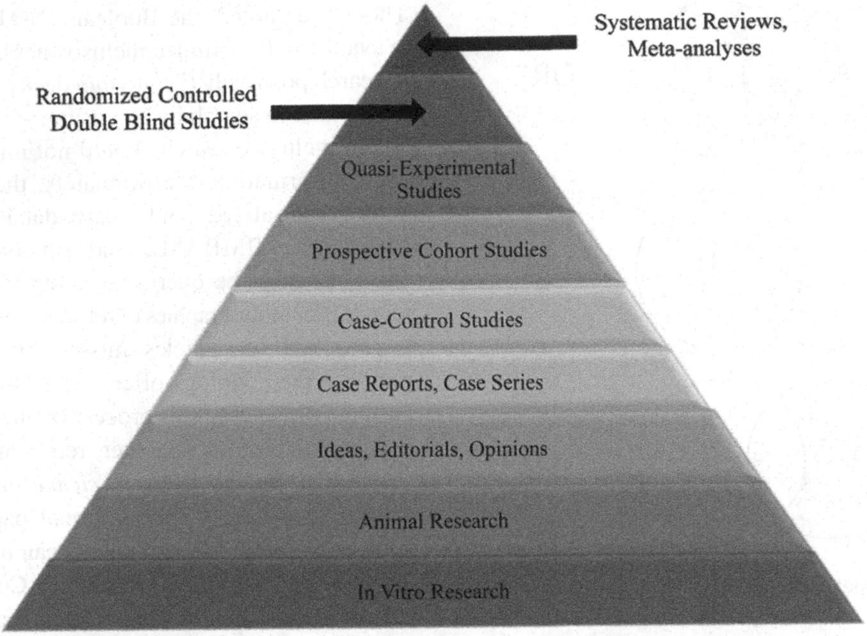

Fig. 9.4 Pyramid of evidence

questions shown at the bottom and the strongest evidence shown at the top. Bias decreases as we move up the pyramid, in direct contrast to the amount of literature available on a given topic.

In vitro and animal studies, although important for hypothesis generation, cannot be applied directly for clinical care or provide a direct answer to a clinical research question, as can case reports, series, case–control, cohorts, and randomized controlled clinical trials (RCTs). As noted in previous chapters, a **case report** describes the presentation and/or treatment of an individual patient, whereas **a case series** consists of a collection of reports on several individual patients. Because they do not have control groups with which to compare outcomes, neither has validity for drawing conclusions about associations or cause and effect. **Case–control studies** are always retrospective studies in which subjects who already have a specific condition are compared with those who do not. These studies are well suited to test associations between risks or toxic exposures and diseases, especially when the latter are relatively rare. Data collection typically is based on the medical record and/or patient recall. Though case–control studies provide stronger evidence for association than case reports or case series, caution must be exercised in interpretation of results because demonstration of a statistical relationship does not provide proof of causality. **Cohort studies** follow individuals with specific risk factors or exposures over time and compare them with comparable individuals who do not have the risk factor or exposure being studied to evaluate differences in outcomes. Though cohort studies (particularly those that are prospective in nature) provide better evidence of association than case–control studies, they (like case–control studies) are observational and, as such, are subject to more bias than studies in which an intervention has been purposely applied; their greatest utility in clinical epidemiology is for defining prognosis of a disease. **Quasi-experimental studies** contain some of elements of true experiments (parallel control groups and/or repeated assessments) but (as noted in Chap. 5), due to lack of random allocation to treatment group, are not fully protected from all threats to internal validity. In contrast, **randomized controlled clinical trials (RCTs)** study the effects of a

Table 9.1 Criteria for calculating the Jadad score (Reprinted with permission from Jadad et al. [12])

Criteria		Yes (1 point)	No (0 points)
1. Was the study described as randomized?			
2. Was the randomization process described, and was it appropriate?			
3. Was the study described as double blind?			
4. Was the method for double blinding appropriate?			
5. Were the withdrawals and drops out of the study enumerated?			
Interpretation			
Score 0–2	Low-quality study		
Score 3–5	High-quality study		

purposively applied therapy by comparing an intervention group and control group to which subjects have been randomly allocated. They also incorporate additional methodologies such as blinding (masking) and analysis by "intention-to-treat" that reduce the potential for a variety of threats to internal validity, though they may suffer from limitations in generalizability (external validity). In theory, as syntheses of prior research, systematic reviews and meta-analyses, though relatively few in number, are at the top of the pyramid, providing the strongest evidence for associations or cause-and-effect relationships. However, for this to be true, both must meet stringent methodological quality criteria (described below) and the elements of the meta-analysis (i.e., the included studies), specifically, must have sufficiently similar study design characteristics to permit pooling of results, a criterion that is not always met in practice. When it does not, a meta-analysis, if performed, will be more useful for hypothesis generation than for hypothesis testing [10].

Standardizing Selection of Articles

The list of abstracts generated from the PICO search query is next screened for selection of relevant articles. Although inclusion criteria (e.g., nature of the patient population, specific outcomes and summary measures) optimally are predefined, the process is not immune to subjectivity and bias. The list should be screened independently by two reviewers to minimize subjectivity. Any discrepancies should be compared and discussed to reach a consensus. The reviewers' interrater reliability should be measured and reported. The predefined inclusion and exclusion criteria should be reported in the methods section and the search strategy in the appendix, to facilitate replication of results.

Assessing the Quality of Primary Studies

Assessment of bias in the methodology of the individual studies is a core component of a systematic review; therefore, tools for appraising the quality of the individual studies should be integrated. Unfortunately, no gold standard exists to evaluate the methodology of therapeutic trials or assessments of diagnostic test performance even though their quality and methods for synthesis are thought by some to be superior to that of other forms of clinical research (e.g., prognostic studies) [11]. Consensus and working groups continually reevaluate and improve upon assessment tools; thus, the preferred methods or systems change over time. Below is a listing and brief discussion of a cross section of tools for detecting bias in these types of studies. We present these to introduce the topic rather than to advocate a specific scoring system. (For the author of a primary study, they can be used as a check list to ensure a sufficiently comprehensive methods section.)

Therapeutic Testing Articles Appraisal

A variety of assessment tools for therapeutic articles exist such as the Jadad scale [12], shown in Table 9.1. Common to all is evaluation of key areas prone to bias. Inclusion and exclusion criteria should be reviewed to decide whether the patients included in the identified study meet the requirements of the "P" of the PICO. As indicated earlier, the highest quality studies optimally will use randomized treatment assignment with concealment of allocation, double blinding, and intention-to-treat analyses. Follow-up should be complete and transparent. In addition, readers should look for an explanation as to why participants may have dropped out of an investigation, as differential attrition from a study may impact conclusions regarding the effectiveness of the investigational treatment (e.g., if the sickest patients dropped out of the treatment arm receiving an investigational new drug, the drug might appear to be more effective than it is.)

Studies about treatment, optimally, will express the impact of therapy quantitatively as the number needed to treat (NNT) or the number needed to harm (NNH). The NNT is the number of patients that need to be given the intervention for one patient to benefit, thus expressing the effectiveness of an intervention in a clinically meaningful manner. It is calculated as the reciprocal of the difference in outcomes of the intervention and control groups (absolute risk reduction) derived from a therapeutic trial. The closer the NNT is to 1, the greater the efficacy of the intervention; the further from 1, the lesser its efficacy. As an example, in the landmark study ISIS-2 [13], the efficacy of (1) 1 h of IV infusion of 1.5 MU streptokinase (SK), (2) 1 month of 160 mg of enteric-coated aspirin (ASA) taken daily for 30 days, and (3) both active agents versus placebo was evaluated through 35 days after a suspected acute myocardial infarction (AMI) among 17,187 patients. Analysis revealed that the absolute reductions in risk of vascular mortality associated with SK and ASA and their combination versus placebo, respectively, were 2.8%, 2.4%, and 5.2%, yielding NNTs of 36 (SK), 42 (ASA), and 19 (SK+ASA). These NNTs (not calculated in the original study) indicated that 36 patients would need to be treated with SK and 42 patients with ASA aspirin to prevent one vascular death, whereas the same result could be achieved with combination therapy in 19 patients. A closely related parameter is the number needed to harm (NNH), calculated as the inverse of the absolute risk increase (again expressed as a proportion) and interpreted as the number of patients one would need to treat to expect an adverse outcome. The NNT must be weighed with the baseline risk, NNH, benefit magnitude and/or cost to have comprehensive meaning to the clinician. It may be more acceptable in clinical practice to apply a treatment that is inexpensive, easy to use, and of almost no adverse risk but has higher NNT than one that has a lower NNT but is expensive, dangerous, and has only a marginal clinical benefit. For example, while the NNT was relatively higher with aspirin than with SK in ISIS-2, there was no reported bleeding requiring transfusion or confirmed cerebral hemorrhage associated with aspirin (a very low cost, easy-to-manage intervention), whereas there was a very small (though statistically significant) excess occurence of these events with SK (0.5% vs. 0.2% with placebo [major bleeds], equivalent to a NNH=333; 0.1% (SK) vs. 0.0% with placebo [cerebrovascular hemorrhage], equivalent to a NNH=1,000).

Diagnostic Testing Articles Appraisal

Diagnostic accuracy studies investigate how well the results from an index test (test being evaluated) agree with the results of the reference standard. (As noted above, the reference standard or gold standard is considered the best available method to determine the presence or absence of a condition.) Diagnostic studies have unique design features which differ from therapeutic testing; therefore, different methods exist for detecting bias and variability.

The Quality Assessment of Diagnostic Accuracy Studies (QUADAS) tool [14] is one such method. The tool comprises 14 items, defined by expert consensus, that examine a variety of important biases and other methodological concerns specific to the evaluation of diagnostic tests (Table 9.2), though it it does not address the issue of intra- or interobserver reliability. Responses are framed as binary "yes/no" questions, or if not enough information is supplied, "unclear." The Cochrane Collaboration offers a similar tools for assesing diagnostic studies [15].

In the past, calculations of the sensitivity, specificity, and predictive values of a diagnostic were considered sufficient for evaluation of its utility. In this era, a high-quality diagnostic

Table 9.2 The development of QUADAS: a tool for the quality assessment of studies of diagnostic accuracy included in systematic reviews (Reproduced with permission from Whiting et al. [14])

Item	Yes	No	Unclear
1. Was the spectrum of patients representative of the patients who will receive the test in practice?	( )	( )	( )
2. Were selection criteria clearly described?	( )	( )	( )
3. Is the reference standard likely to correctly classify the target condition?	( )	( )	( )
4. Is the time period between reference standard and index test short enough to be reasonably sure that the target condition did not change between the two tests?	( )	( )	( )
5. Did the whole sample or a random selection of the sample, receive verification using a reference standard of diagnosis?	( )	( )	( )
6. Did patients receive the same reference standard regardless of the index test result?	( )	( )	( )
7. Was the reference standard independent of the index test (i.e. the index test did not form part of the reference standard)?	( )	( )	( )
8. Was the execution of the index test described in sufficient detail to permit replication of the test?	( )	( )	( )
9. Was the execution of the reference standard described in sufficient detail to permit its replication?	( )	( )	( )
10. Were the index test results interpreted without knowledge of the results of the reference standard?	( )	( )	( )
11. Were the reference standard results interpreted without knowledge of the results of the index test?	( )	( )	( )
12. Were the same clinical data available when test results were interpreted as would be available when the test is used in practice?	( )	( )	( )
13. Were uninterpretable/intermediate test results reported?	( )	( )	( )
14. Were withdrawals from the study explained?	( )	( )	( )

study also will define thresholds values for their diagnostic test using receiver operator characteristic (ROC) curves which are plots of the true positive rate (sensitivity) versus the false positive rate (1-specificity) (Fig. 9.5). The area under the curve reflects the relationship between sensitivity and specificity for a given test. As a curve asymptotically approaches the upper left-hand corner, the area under the curve approaches 1 (100% sensitivity and specificity). A random guess would generate a point along the diagonal bisecting the graph, also called the line of no discrimination. Points above the diagonal represent better results (greater diagnostic accuracy), while points below the line are poor (lower diagnostic accuracy). (For further discussion of the use of ROC curves for determination of diagnostic accuracy, the reader is referred to Chap. 11.)

Once thresholds for a positive and negative diagnostic test are defined by ROC curves, then an evidence-based operating characteristic of the test can be defined by its likelihood ratios (*LR*). The *LR* is the probability that a given test result would be expected in a patient with the target disorder divided by the probability (P) that that same result would be expected in a patient without the target disorder. LRs can be calculated both for positive (*LR*+) and negative (*LR*–) test results, as shown below.

$$LR+ = \frac{\text{sensitivity}}{1-\text{specificity}} \quad \frac{\rightarrow P(\text{Test} + | \text{ Disease } +)}{\rightarrow P(\text{Test} + | \text{ Disease}-)}$$

$$LR- = \frac{1-\text{sensitivity}}{\text{specificity}} \quad \frac{\rightarrow P(\text{Test}- | \text{ Disease}+)}{\rightarrow P(\text{Test}- | \text{ Disease}-)}$$

High $LR+$ values ($LR+ > 10$) significantly increase the probability of disease and low $LR-$ values ($LR- < 0.1$) significantly decrease the probability of disease. The extent to which the results of a diagnostic test changes the probability that the patient has a disease (posttest probability) can be estimated using a graphical tool known as the Fagan nomogram [16] by

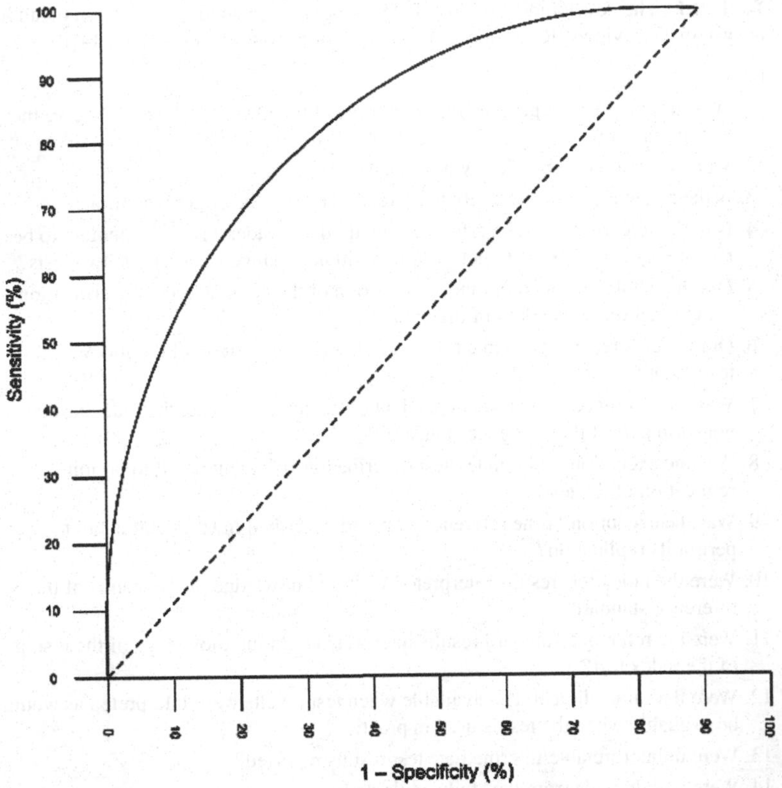

Fig. 9.5 Receiver operator characteristic curve

using a straight edge to draw a line from the pretest probability through the calculated *LR* (Fig. 9.6).

Summarizing the Results: The Role of Meta-analysis

As noted earlier, sometimes the size of an individual clinical trial may be too small to detect a treatment effect or to estimate its magnitude reliably. Meta-analysis is a method to increase the power of statistical analyses and precision of estimates by pooling the results of related trials (i.e., those that address a similar hypothesis) to obtain a quantified synthesis. Not all systematic reviews lead to a meta-analysis. The trials may be so varied in their methodology, end points, or results that combining them may not be appropriate.

In a conventional meta-analysis (sometimes known as "aggregate-level" meta-analysis, a summary statistic (e.g., a risk ratio, a difference between outcome means) for the observed effect is abstracted or recalculated from each included study. (A less common approach, not reviewed in this chapter, combines original or patient-level data from prior studies; for an excellent discussion of the pros and cons of this method, known as "Individual Patient Data [IPD]" meta-analysis, the reader is referred to Stewart and Tierney 2002) [17].) Next, a *pooled effect estimate* is calculated as a weighted average by sample size of the intervention effects reported in the individual studies. By pooling results, the standard error of the weighted average effect size of the included studies and its associated confidence interval are reduced, typically affording greater statistical power to detect an effect than would be possible from any one consitutent study. Reduction of the confidence intervals also increases precision of the estimated population effect size [18]. In assigning weights for generating the pooled

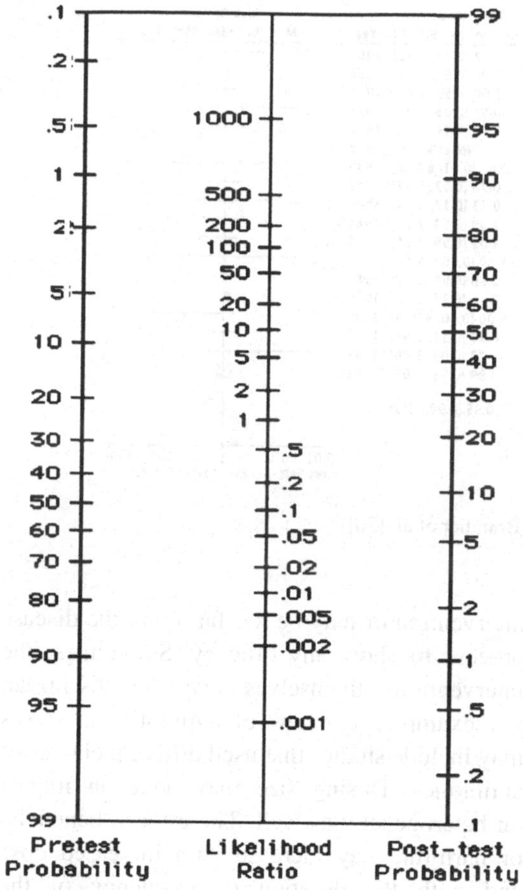

Fig. 9.6 The Fagan nomogram (Reproduced with permission from Fagan [16])

estimate, the evaluator needs to consider whether it is more appropriate to use a fixed versus a random effects model as these make different assumptions about the nature of the included studies. A fixed effects model assumes that all of the studies contained within the meta-analysis have attempted to measure a single "true effects value" and that variation in observed effect sizes is due only to chance. An assumption underlying such a model is that all of the studies have been conducted under similar conditions with similar subjects, differing only in their power to detect the outcome of interest. (This rarely, if ever, is the case.) In contrast, a random effects model assumes that the true effect size can vary from study to study along a distribution due to differences in the nature of the populations, dosing, timing, and measurable differences other than sampling variability (see also assessment of heterogeneity below). Athough more data are required for random effects models to achieve the same statistical power as with fixed effects models, the former represents a more conservative assumption. Unless the author of a meta-analysis has guidance from a statistician indicating that a fixed model is appropriate, a random effects model typically is preferrable.

Most meta-analyses summarize their findings graphically using a *forest plot* [19]. A forest plot illustrates the relative effects of multiple studies addressing the same question or hypothesis. The studies are listed in the left-hand column, typically in chronological order. The measured effect for each of these studies is represented by a square, whose area is related to the relative sample size of the individual study. The effect may be an odds ratio, risk difference, or a correlation coefficient. The confidence intervals (CI) are represented by horizontal lines bisecting the square. The width of the CI is related to the power and variability of the study. The combined results of the meta-analysis usually are represented by a diamond, the width of which is the CI for the pooled data. A vertical line is placed at 1 for ratios (odds or risks) and correlation coefficients, or at 0 for differences, representing no effect. If the CI of an individual study or the pooled data crosses this line, the null hypothesis is accepted. Figure 9.7 illustrates a forest plot used in a meta-analysis of the effects of administration of beta blockade on in-hospital mortality rates among patients with acute coronary syndrome [20].

Assessment of Heterogeneity: Methods of Investigation

Heterogeneity in meta-analysis refers to the variation in outcomes among included studies. As noted above, a certain degree of variability should be expected when comparing multiple studies (hence, the rationale for suggesting the more conservative random effects model for pooling data). "Clinical variability" occurs when there are differences in the study population, interventions,

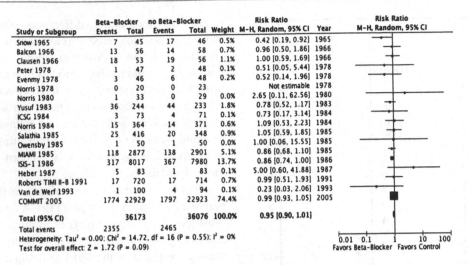

Study or Subgroup	Beta-Blocker Events	Beta-Blocker Total	no Beta-Blocker Events	no Beta-Blocker Total	Weight	Risk Ratio M-H, Random, 95% CI	Year
Snow 1965	7	45	17	46	0.5%	0.42 [0.19, 0.92]	1965
Balcon 1966	13	56	14	58	0.7%	0.96 [0.50, 1.86]	1966
Clausen 1966	18	53	19	56	1.1%	1.00 [0.59, 1.69]	1966
Peter 1978	1	47	2	48	0.1%	0.51 [0.05, 5.44]	1978
Evenmy 1978	3	46	6	48	0.2%	0.52 [0.14, 1.96]	1978
Norris 1978	0	20	0	23		Not estimable	1978
Norris 1980	1	33	0	29	0.0%	2.65 [0.11, 62.56]	1980
Yusuf 1983	36	244	44	233	1.8%	0.78 [0.52, 1.17]	1983
ICSG 1984	3	73	4	71	0.1%	0.73 [0.17, 3.14]	1984
Norris 1984	15	364	14	371	0.6%	1.09 [0.53, 2.23]	1984
Salathia 1985	25	416	20	348	0.9%	1.05 [0.59, 1.85]	1985
Owensby 1985	1	50	1	50	0.0%	1.00 [0.06, 15.55]	1985
MIAMI 1985	118	2877	138	2901	5.1%	0.86 [0.68, 1.10]	1985
ISIS-1 1986	317	8017	367	7980	13.7%	0.86 [0.74, 1.00]	1986
Heber 1987	5	83	1	83	0.1%	5.00 [0.60, 41.88]	1987
Roberts TIMI II-B 1991	17	720	17	714	0.7%	0.99 [0.51, 1.93]	1991
Van de Werf 1993	1	100	4	94	0.1%	0.23 [0.03, 2.06]	1993
COMMIT 2005	1774	22929	1797	22923	74.4%	0.99 [0.93, 1.05]	2005
Total (95% CI)		**36173**		**36076**	**100.0%**	**0.95 [0.90, 1.01]**	
Total events	2355		2465				

Heterogeneity: $Tau^2 = 0.00$; $Chi^2 = 14.72$, df = 16 ($P = 0.55$); $I^2 = 0\%$
Test for overall effect: $Z = 1.72$ ($P = 0.09$)

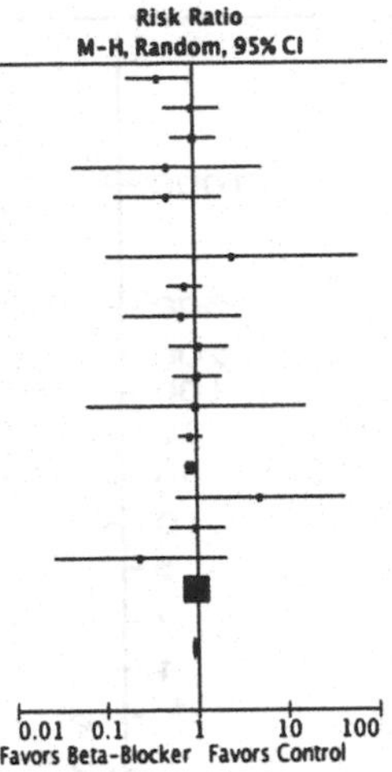

Fig. 9.7 The forest plot (Reproduced with permission from: Brandler et al. [20])

or outcomes measured. "Methodological variability" occurs when there are differences in study design. Not suprisingly, clinical or methodological differences will cause variations in the effect measured. Heterogeneity refers to this difference in effect size (or direction) between studies. Of course, like all statistical tests, the heterogeneity of the effect size in pooled studies may occur by chance.

Assessment of clinical and methodological heterogeneity includes both qualitative and quantitative elements. One begins by comparing the study populations. Are the studies similar in age, sex, or even type of disease? If not, is it appropriate to pool them together? Are the interventions the same? Some studies may include co-interventions which may be a source of confounding. Studies also may exhibit variability in terms of the timing of the intervention; thus, imposition of an intervention at different stages during the disease process may cause differences in degree of efficacy. For example, a study on the impact of oncologic surgery would likely exhibit differences in efficacy if conducted early after cancer detection as opposed to after metastases had developed. The question of timing overlaps the issue of population differences as patients may be sicker at one stage of the disease than another. This can magnify the effects or negate them. An ill population may exaggerate the beneficial effects of an intervention or may be too far along the disease process to show any efficacy. Sometimes, the interventions themselves may be dissimilar. For example, a review of antibiotics in sepsis may include studies that used different classes of antibiotics. Dosing size may have an impact on heterogeneity as well. The effects, beneficial or harmful, may increase with increased dose and with the duration or frequency of the intervention.

Clearly, outcome measures also must be similar to permit appropriate comparison. Thus, 6-month mortality after cardiac intervention in one study should not be compared to left ventricular ejection fraction at 6 months in another. Length of follow-up of a trial may have an influence on the estimate of treatment effect. Like applying the intervention at disparate times, follow-up at different stages of the disease likely will impact outcomes. This issue should have be resolved during the study selection stage of a review so that studies lacking the desired outcome measure were excluded. One should also be critical of surrogate marker use as an outcome measure, especially when being compared to a direct outcome. Different study methods will have different degrees of bias. Those conducting meta-analyses should consider whether it is appropriate to compare RCTs with blinding and concealment to unblinded cohort studies.

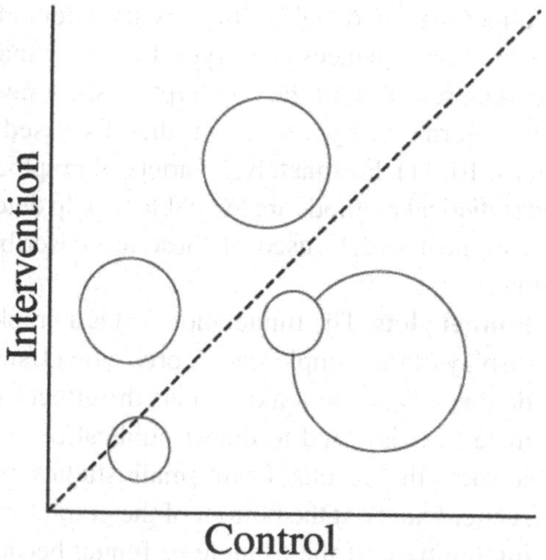

Fig. 9.8 The L'Abbé plot

Heterogeneity of the effect size can be analyzed graphically or statistically. The following are some of the commonly accepted methods:

- **The forest plot** (described above) can be visually analyzed to determine whether the effects of the individual studies are scattered about on both sides of the "no difference/association line" or whether they are grouped together (i.e., are on one side or another of the this line). If there is very little or no overlap of the confidence intervals, then significant heterogeneity exists and pooling of the results may not be appropriate. If a meta-analysis is carried out, the authors should address the cause of the heterogeneity, whether clinical, methodological, or both, and provide a justification for continuation.
- The L'Abbé plot (Fig. 9.8) also can be used to explore the heterogeneity of effect estimates [21]. The proportion of events in the intervention group (y-axis) is plotted against that in the control group (x-axis). The no effects line runs between them at 45°. The symbol size is proportional to sample size.
- **The Cochran chi-square (Cochran Q)** is a common test for quantifying heterogeneity in meta-analyses. It assumes the null hypothesis that all the variability among the individual study results is due to chance. The Cochran Q test generates a *p* value, based on a chi-square distribution with N − 1 degree of freedom (df), that indicates whether the individual effects are farther away from the common effect, beyond what would be expected by chance. A p value < 0.10 indicates significant heterogeneity. (The level of significance for Cochran Q often is set at 0.1 due to the low power of the test to detect heterogeneity.) If the Cochran Q is not statistically significant, but the ratio of Cochran Q and the degrees of freedom (Q/df) is >1, the result is interpreted to indicate possible heterogeneity. If the Cochran Q is not statistically significant and Q/df is <1, then heterogeneity is much less likely. A limitation of the Cochran Q test is that it is underpowered to detect heterogeneity if there are few studies in the meta-analysis. Conversely, it is overpowered (i.e., may detect negligible variability) when the number of studies is large. An additional limitation is that the Cochran Q test evaluates only the presence or absence of heterogeneity rather than its magnitude.

Table 9.3 Assessing heterogeneity with I2 statistic

I^2	Degree of heterogeneity
<0.25	Low
0.25 to 0.50	Moderate
>0.50	High

- **The I^2 statistic** represents the percentage of variation across studies due to heterogeneity. I^2 is an index that quantifies the degree of heterogeneity in a meta-analysis and can be used as a complement to the Cochran Q test. I^2 is calculated from the Cochran *Q* according to the formula: $I^2 = 100 \times (Q - df)/Q$, where df = degrees of freedom. Values may range from 0% to 100%, with a value of 0% indicating no observed heterogeneity (Table 9.3). Although negative values are possible from the equation, they are equivalent in meaning to 0.
- **Sensitivity analysis.** A sensitivity analysis tests whether the results of the meta-analysis are affected by restrictions and alterations in the included studies. Examples include removing an outlier (i.e., the study with the largest effect size in either direction) or removing the largest study to test if this

changes the magnitude or direction of the pooled effect size or its statistical significance. This analysis helps to determine whether the pooled result is influenced heavily by a particular trial. Other permutations include using only blinded, higher quality trials (or excluding lower quality trials) or performing the analysis under fixed and random effects assumptions. If the results are consistent, the sensitivity analysis provides stronger evidence of an effect and of generalizability.

Pooling Results for Meta-analysis: Considerations

Heterogeneity (whether defined graphically or statistically) should be considered alongside a qualitative assessment of the combinability of studies. When significant methodological differences *and* heterogeneity are detected, a meta-analysis probably should not be performed as it may be misleading. Under these circumstances, the systematic review should report the results descriptively using text and tables and not pool the data. However, if effect sizes are similar despite variability of clinical and methodological differences, the results probably are robust and generalizable. A cost-free program for producing the tables and graphs and performing the statistics for a meta-analysis is available from the Cochrane group, RevMan 5 (Review Manager, Version 5.0, The Cochrane Collaboration, Copenhagen, Denmark).

Detecting Publication Bias

The literature tends to be biased toward positive findings—a phenomenon known as "publication bias" [22]. Studies with large sample sizes have a greater probability of achieving statistical significance and, therefore, achieving publication. This holds true for studies demonstrating large treatment effects as well, even if the sample size is small. Indeed, many smaller or negative trials are never published. "Publication Bias" produces a positive relationship between sample or effect size and publication, with potentially adverse consequences (i.e., type I error or inappropriate rejection of the null hypothesis in favor of the alternative hypothesis, further discussed in Chaps. 10, 11). Fortunately, a variety of graphical and statistical methods are available to help detect it. The most widely used of these are described below:

- **Funnel plots.** The funnel plot [23] is a graphic display of the sample size or precision (1/standard error) on the y-axis versus the effect estimate (x-axis) used to detect publication bias. Ideally, the results from small studies will scatter widely at the bottom of the graph forming the base of the triangle or funnel because they have less precision, with the spread narrowing around the summary effects line at the apex for larger studies. This pattern occurs when publication bias is absent or unlikely. Asymmetry indicates systematic differences, errors of measurement, or publication bias; as noted, small studies with positive results are more likely to be published, whereas negative studies of similar size are not and, therefore, not found during execution of the search strategy. The absence of these "balancing" studies are made visually obvious in the asymmetry of the plot (Fig. 9.9). Although funnel plots usually are employed to test for publication bias, there are other causes of asymmetry such as systematic differences and errors of measurement. When found, the causes of the asymmetry should be investigated and explained to justify the continued grouping of these studies for meta-analysis.
- **Fail-safe N.** The inability to locate every unpublished study about a subject might be unnerving to authors of a meta-analysis. As a method of compensation for what may be unknown, Rosenthal [24] developed formulae based on the desired level of significance (p value), later named the fail-safe *N* by Cooper [25]. Orwin [26] adapted the fail-safe N to adjust for small ($d=0.2$), medium ($d=0.5$), or large ($d=0.8$) effect sizes [27]. The formula calculates the number of studies that would be needed to confirm the null hypothesis and, thereby, reverse a conclusion that a significant

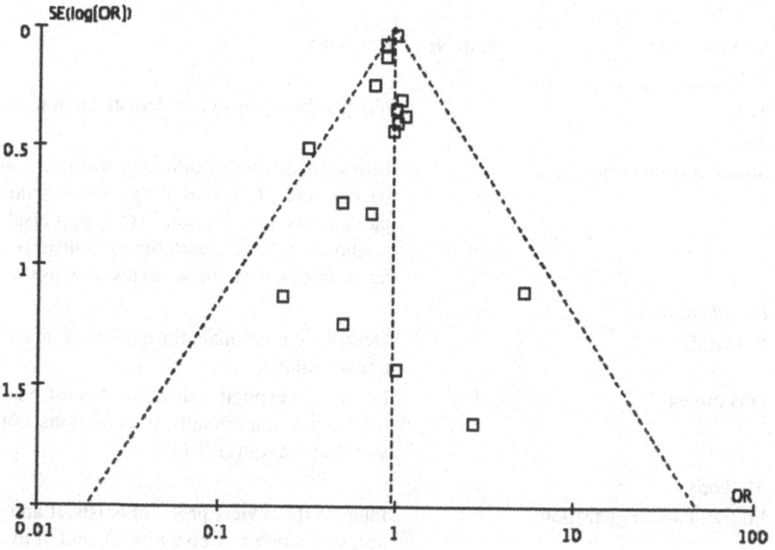

Fig. 9.9 The funnel plot

relationship exists. The formula for Orwin's fail-safe N [26] is given below:

$$N_{fs} = \frac{N(\overline{d} - \overline{d}_c)}{d_c}$$

where N=the number of studies in the meta-analysis, $\overline{d}$ = the average effect size for the studies synthesized, and d_c = the criterion value selected that d would equal when some knowable number of hypothetical studies (N_{fs}) were added to the meta-analysis. If the fail-safe N is sufficiently high, it may provide reassurance that a few missing studies would not alter the conclusion.

Assessing Quality of Systematic Reviews and Meta-analyses

Systematic reviews and meta-analysis are powerful informational tools. However, unless properly conducted and reported, they can produce erroneous conclusions that potentially could impact the public health [28, 29]. Thus, as there are tools for assessing the quality of individual trials, there also are guidelines for assessing the quality of systematic reviews and meta-analysis. In 1996 (published in 1999) [30], the QUOROM (quality of reporting of meta-analyses) statement was issued to address standards for improving the quality of reporting of meta-analyses of clinical randomized controlled trials. Since that time, many additions, updates, and expansions of this statement for broader applicability have led to the development of the PRISMA. ("Preferred Reporting Items for Systematic Reviews and Meta-analyses") statement, which provides guidelines designed to "reduce the risk of flawed reporting of systematic reviews and improve the clarity and transparency in how reviews are conducted" [31]. Included are a 27-item checklist (Table 9.4) and 4-phase flowchart (Fig. 9.10) [32].

Though not part of current current checklists, conflicts of interest such as financial funding of individual trails should be reported in the systematic review or meta-analysis.

Limitations of Systematic Reviews and Meta-analyses

The major limitations of narrative reviews have been described above. The reader should be aware that caution also must be exercised when conducting or interpreting a systematic review or meta-analysis. Of note, an evaluation of 300 systematic reviews conducted by Moher et al. in 2007 found that the quality of these reviews was inconsistent [33], a finding that led to the above-mentioned 2009 PRISMA statement. Other criticisms are based on poor methodology including

Table 9.4 PRISMA checklist for reporting systematic reviews with (or) without meta-analyses (Reproduced with permission from Moher et al. [32]

Section/topic	Item No	Checklist item	Reported on page No
Title			
Title	1	Identify the report as a systematic review, meta-analysis, or both	
Abstract			
Structured summary	2	Provide a structured summary including, as applicable, background, objectives, data sources, study eligibility criteria, participants, interventions, study appraisal and synthesis methods, results, limitations, conclusions and implications of key findings, systematic review registration number	
Introduction			
Rationale	3	Describe the rationale for the review in the context of what is already known	
Objectives	4	Provide an explicit statement of questions being addressed with reference to participants, interventions, comparisons, outcomes, and study design (PICOS)	
Methods			
Protocol and registration	5	Indicate if a review protocol exists, if and where it can be accessed (such as web address), and, if available, provide registration information including registration number	
Eligibility criteria	6	Specify study characteristics (such as PICOS, length of follow-up) and report characteristics (such as years considered, language, publication status) used as criteria for eligibility, giving rationale	
Information sources	7	Describe all information sources (such as databases with dates of coverage, contact with study authors to identify additional studies) in the search and date last searched	
Search	8	Present full electronic search strategy for at least one database, including any limits used, such that it could be repeated	
Study selection	9	State the process for selecting studies (that is, screening, eligibility, included in systematic review, and, if applicable, included in the meta-analysis)	
Data collection process	10	Describe method of data extraction from reports (such as piloted forms, independently, in duplicate) and any processes for obtaining and confirming data from investigators	
Data items	11	List and define all variables for which data were sought (such as PICOS, funding sources) and any assumptions and simplifications made	
Risk of bias in individual studies	12	Describe methods used for assessing risk of bias of individual studies (including specification of whether this was done at the study or outcome level), and how this information is to be used in any data synthesis	
Summary measures	13	State the principal summary measures (such as risk ratio, difference in means).	
Synthesis of results	14	Describe the methods of handling data and combining results of studies, if done, including measures of consistency (such as I^2 statistic) for each meta-analysis	
Risk of bias across studies	15	Specify any assessment of risk of bias that may affect the cumulative evidence (such as publication bias, selective reporting within studies)	
Additional analyses	16	Describe methods of additional analyses (such as sensitivity or subgroup analyses, meta-regression), if done, indicating which were pre-specified	
Results			
Study selection	17	Give numbers of studies screened, assessed for eligibility, and included in the review, with reasons for exclusions at each stage, ideally with a flow diagram	

(continued)

Table 9.4 (continued)

Section/topic	Item No	Checklist item	Reported on page No
Study characteristics	18	For each study, present characteristics for which data were extracted (such as study size, PICOS, follow-up period) and provide the citations	
Risk of bias within studies	19	Present data on risk of bias of each study and, if available, any outcome-level assessment (see item 12).	
Results of individual studies	20	For all outcomes considered (benefits or harms), present for each study (a) simple summary data for each intervention group and (b) effect estimates and confidence intervals, ideally with a forest plot	
Synthesis of results	21	Present results of each meta-analysis done, including confidence intervals and measures of consistency	
Risk of bias across studies	22	Present results of any assessment of risk of bias across studies (see item 15)	
Additional analysis	23	Give results of additional analyses, if done (such as sensitivity or subgroup analyses, meta-regression) (see item 16)	
Discussion			
Summary of evidence	24	Summarize the main findings including the strength of evidence for each main outcome; consider their relevance to key groups (such as health care providers, users, and policy makers)	
Limitations	25	Discuss limitations at study and outcome level (such as risk of bias), and at review level (such as incomplete retrieval of identified research, reporting bias)	
Conclusions	26	Provide a general interpretation of the results in the context of other evidence, and implications for future research	
Funding			
Funding	27	Describe sources of funding for the systematic review and other support (such as supply of data) and role of funders for the systematic review	

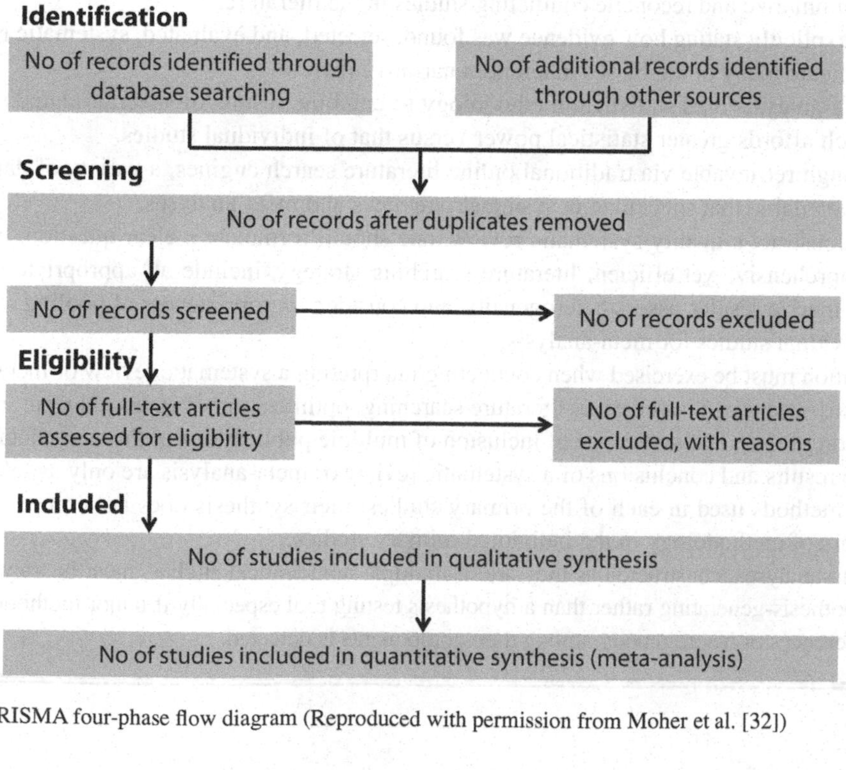

Fig. 9.10 PRISMA four-phase flow diagram (Reproduced with permission from Moher et al. [32])

nonadherence to proper searching strategies, lack of statistical rigor, and introduction of bias (intentional or unintentional) in which studies were "cherry picked" to suit the personal agenda of the reviewer/analyst. Unfortunately, not all of the limitations can be minimized by strict methodology. A fundamental limitation of meta-analysis, specifically, is that it is comprised of studies performed under different protocols and at different times; for purposes of the analysis, it is assumed that the differences in protocol and study design of the elements are obviated by the large number of observations ultimately available. This assumption is highly questionable. As noted above, if clinical and methodological diversity across studies is such that substantial heterogeneity is determined, it may be better not to combine them in a meta-analysis (if a meta-analysis is performed under these circumstances, as noted earlier, it should be considered for hypothesis generation only). In addition, the increased power gained by pooling the results of individual studies that is advantageous for decreasing type II errors also may allow small biases to be interpreted erroneously as an effect, increasing type I errors. (Again, see Chaps. 10 and 11 for further elaboration of these fundamental concepts.) On occasion, the same dataset may be published multiple times, making the results *not* independent. If this is not recognized, the dataset will be weighed more than once in the analysis, artificially inflating the results. Finally, the results and conclusions of a systematic review or meta-analysis are only as reliable as the methods used in each of the primary studies. The methodology used for their qualitative or quantitative synthesis does not compensate for flaws or errors in the individual primary studies.

Take-Home Points

- For clinicians to make informed decisions for patient management and research, they must analyze multiple studies for quality and relevance to the population of interest.
- Secondary sources of information (especially systematic reviews and meta-analyses) help to summarize and reconcile conflicting studies in the literature.
- By explicitly stating how evidence was found, selected, and evaluated, systematic reviews eliminate many of the biases inherent in narrative reviews.
- Meta-analysis uses statistical methodology to combine results of several related studies, which affords greater statistical power versus that of individual studies.
- Though retrievable via traditional online literature search engines, a variety of databases are available that specialize in systematic reviews and meta-analyses.
- To construct a quality systematic review, one should formulate a clear question, define a comprehensive yet efficient literature searching strategy, include all appropriate studies, summarize results, assess heterogeneity, and consider appropriateness of pooling results if individual studies for meta-analysis.
- Caution must be exercised when conducting/interpreting a systematic review or meta-analysis to: ensure inclusiveness of literature searching, optimization of statistical rigor, minimization of bias, and avoidance of inclusion of multiple publications of the same dataset.
- The results and conclusions of a systematic review or meta-analysis are only as reliable as the methods used in each of the primary studies; their synthesis does not compensate for errors of methodology in the individual primary studies.
- Meta-analyses, constructed as they are of multiple nonidentical studies, must be viewed as a hypothesis-generating rather than a hypothesis testing tool especially if major methodological differences or heterogeneity among their components is detected.

References

1. Lau J, Antman EM, Jimenez-Silva J, Kupelnick B, Mosteller F, Chalmers TC. Cumulative meta-analysis of therapeutic trials for myocardial infarction. N Engl J Med. 1992;327:248–54.
2. Collins JA, Fauser BCJM. Balancing the strengths of systematic and narrative reviews. Hum Reprod Update. 2005;11:103–4.
3. Pearson K. Report on certain enteric fever inoculation statistics. Br Med J. 1904;3:1243–6.
4. Glass GV. Primary, secondary, and meta-analysis of research. Educ Res. 1976;5:3–8.
5. Sacks HS, Berrier J, Reitman D, Ancona-Berk VA, Chalmers TC. Meta-analyses of randomized controlled trials. N Engl J Med. 1987;316:450–5.
6. Tuckman BW. Conducting educational research. 3rd ed. New York: Harcourt Brace Jovanovich; 1972.
7. Wilczynski NL, Haynes RB, Lavis JN, Ramkissoonsingh R, Arnold-Oatley A, HSR Hedges Team. Optimal search strategies for detecting health services research studies in MEDLINE. CMAJ. 2004;171:1179–85.
8. Oxman AD, Sackett DL, Guyatt GH. Users' guides to the medical literature. I. How to get started. The Evidence-Based Medicine Working Group. JAMA. 1993;270:2093–5.
9. Fact Sheet. Medical Subject Headings (Mesh®). U.S. National Library of Medicine. http://www.nlm.nih.gov/pubs/factsheets/mesh.html. Accessed 16 Aug 2011.
10. Yu CH, Beattie WS. The effects of volatile anesthetics on cardiac ischemic complications and mortality in CABG: a meta-analysis. Can J Anaesth. 2006;53:906–18.
11. Centre for Reviews and Dissemination. Systematic reviews: CRD's guidance for undertaking reviews in healthcare. York: University of York NHS Centre for Reviews & Dissemination; 2009.
12. Jadad AR, Moore RA, Carroll D, Jenkinson C, Reynolds DJM, Gavaghan DJ, McQuay HJ. Assessing the quality of reports of randomized clinical trials: is blinding necessary? Control Clin Trials. 1996;17:1–12.
13. ISIS-2 (Second International Study of Infarct Survival) Collaborative Group. Randomised trial of intravenous streptokinase, oral aspirin, both, or neither among 17,187 cases of suspected acute myocardial infarction: ISIS-2. Lancet. 1988;2:349–60.
14. Whiting P, Rutjes AW, Reitsma JB, Bossuyt PM, Kleijnen J. The development of QUADAS: a tool for the quality assessment of studies of diagnostic accuracy included in systematic reviews. BMC Med Res Methodol 10 Nov 2003;3:25. http://www.biomedcentral.com/1471-2288/3/25. Accessed 16 Sep 2011.
15. Deeks JJ, Bossuyt PM, Gatsonis C, editors. Cochrane handbook for systematic reviews of diagnostic test accuracy version 1.0. The cochrane collaboration, 2010. http://srdta.cochrane.org/. Accessed 16 Sep 2011.
16. Fagan TJ. Letter: nomogram for Bayes theorem. N Engl J Med. 1975;293:257.
17. Stewart LA, Tierney JF. To IPD or not to IPD? Advantages and disadvantages of systematic reviews using individual patient data. Eval Health Prof. 2002;25:76–97.
18. Matt GE, Cook TD. Threats to the validity of research synthesis. In: Cooper H, Hedges LV, editors. The handbook of research synthesis. NewYork: Russell Sage; 1994.
19. Lewis S, Clarke C. Forest plots: trying to see the wood and the trees. BMJ. 2001;322:1479–80.
20. Brandler E, Paladino L, Sinert R. Does the early administration of beta-blockers improve the in-hospital mortality rate of patients admitted with acute coronary syndrome? Acad Emerg Med. 2010;17:1–10.
21. L'Abbe KL, Detsky AS, O'Rourke K. Meta-analysis in clinical research. Ann Intern Med. 1987;107:224–33.
22. Easterbrook PJ, Berlin JA, Gopalan R, Matthews DR. Publication bias in clinical research. Lancet. 1991;337:867–72.
23. Egger M, Smith DG, Schneider M, Minder C. Bias in meta-analysis detected by a simple, graphical test. BMJ. 1997;315:629–34.
24. Rosenthal R. The "file drawer problem" and tolerance for null results. Psychol Bull. 1979;86:638–41.
25. Cooper HM. Statistically combining independent studies: a meta-analysis of sex differences in conformity research. J Pers Soc Psychol. 1979;37:131–46.
26. Orwin RG. A fail-safe N for effect size in meta-analysis. J Educ Stat. 1983;8:157–9.
27. Cohen J. Statistical power analysis for the behavioral sciences. New York: Academic; 1969.
28. Monami M, Bigiarini M, Rotella CM, Mannucci E. Inaccuracy in meta-analysis on rosiglitazone and myocardial infarction. Nutr Metab Cardiovasc Dis. 2011;21:e7–8. Epub 2010 Dec 25.
29. Claggett B, Wei JL. Analytical issues regarding rosiglitazone meta-analysis. Arch Intern Med. 2011;171:179–80. author reply 180.
30. Moher D, Cook DJ, Eastwood S, Olkin I, Rennie D, Stroup DF. Improving the quality of reports of meta-analyses of randomized controlled trials: the QUOROM statement. Lancet. 1999;354:1896–900.
31. Liberati A, Altman DG, Tetzlaff J, Mulrow C, Gøtzsche PC, Ioannidis JP, Clarke M, Devereaux PJ, Kleijnen J, Moher D. The PRISMA statement for reporting systematic reviews and meta-analyses of studies that evaluate health care interventions: explanation and elaboration. Ann Intern Med. 2009;151:W65–94.
32. Moher D, Liberati A, Tetzlaff J, Altman DG, The PRISMA Group. 2009. Preferred reporting items for systematic reviews and meta-analyses: The PRISMA statement. http://www.plosmedicine.org/article/info%3Adoi%2 F10.1371%2Fjournal.pmed.1000097. Accessed 14 Sep 2011.
33. Moher D, Tetzlaff J, Tricco AC, Sampson M, Altman DG. Epidemiology and reporting characteristics of systematic reviews. PLoS Med. 2007;4:e78. doi:10.1371/journal.pmed.0040078.

Sampling Methodology: Implications for Drawing Conclusions from Clinical Research Findings

10

Richard C. Zink

Introduction

It is our inherent curiosity that drives us to understand the world around us. We design experiments, observe and collect data, and perform analyses in the hopes that our findings will provide insight into the problem at hand. Perhaps the most difficult subject to understand is the human being. Our bodies are extraordinarily complex, affected by our environment, diet, physical conditioning, and genetic background. Further, research involving human beings is guided by ethical principles that limit our means of investigation. We also live complicated lives, making it difficult to add study participation to our busy schedules. Finally, people are at times unreliable, forgetting to take medications, not exercising consistently, or failing to attend scheduled study visits. Ideally, all of these factors should be considered in the design and reporting of any clinical investigation.

In clinical research, we obtain conclusions that (hopefully) address the study hypothesis. These findings certainly apply to the sample of individuals under study. However, we generally wish to extend our conclusions beyond our study to the larger population. Careful selection of the study sample is important to reduce *bias*, the difference between what our sample tells us about the population and the truth [1]. This chapter will address these topics and provide insight into the concept of sampling.

Throughout this chapter, we will illustrate many concepts using the clinical development program for entecavir. Entecavir is an antiviral agent indicated for the treatment of chronic hepatitis B infection, a disease that ultimately can lead to liver cirrhosis and hepatocellular carcinoma. The goal of any effective medication against the hepatitis B virus (HBV) is to reduce and suppress viral load, while simultaneously limiting the possibility of viral mutation which can lead to the reemergence of the virus due to drug resistance [2–4]. We refer to two phase III clinical trials by Chang et al. [5] and Lai et al. [6] comparing entecavir to lamivudine, the standard of care at the time, in the treatment of antiviral-naïve subjects with one of two subtypes of HBV, hepatitis B e antigen-positive (HBeAg+) or hepatitis B e antigen-negative (HBeAg-) disease. Though the primary endpoint of both trials was histologic improvement, reduction of viral load was a key secondary endpoint and an important factor for long-term liver health [4]. We will refer to viral load, the count of the number of viral particles per milliliter of blood, throughout the remainder of this chapter.

A second example is employed to illustrate some of the more complex sampling designs. Data on diarrheal disease was examined from four prevalence surveys in Africa and Asia to

R.C. Zink, PhD (✉)
JMP Life Sciences, SAS Institute, Inc,
SAS Campus Drive, Cary, NC 27513, USA
e-mail: richard.zink@jmp.com

P.G. Supino and J.S. Borer (eds.), *Principles of Research Methodology: A Guide for Clinical Investigators*, DOI 10.1007/978-1-4614-3360-6_10, © Phyllis G. Supino and Jeffrey S. Borer 2012

determine the levels of household and village clustering [7]. The goal of the research was to identify the risk factors and understand the patterns of disease transmission. Careful study of factors at the household and village level ultimately could lead to an optimal strategy for intervention. Within each survey, villages were randomly selected for inclusion into the study, and all households within each village that had at least one child within the appropriate age range were included.

Populations and Samples

As noted in Chap. 2, all research begins with a question. For example, in developing a new antiviral for chronic hepatitis B infection, we could ask whether entecavir is more efficacious than lamivudine. Here, we might assume that our population of interest is all individuals with chronic HBV infection. However, most clinical trial protocols are written with a number of inclusion or exclusion criteria in order for subjects to participate. For example, subjects generally need to be of a certain age with a well-defined and specific disease severity, and we may wish to focus on a particular subtype of the disease, such as those positive or negative for HBeAg [5, 6]. Further, subjects with other coexisting diseases or medications that may interfere or complicate interpretation of the results, or that could pose an unreasonable safety risk, would be excluded from participation in the trial. Therefore, it is more appropriate to define our population as all individuals with chronic hepatitis B infection meeting the inclusion and exclusion criteria of the study. We can refer to the larger population and those eligible for the study as the "population with the condition" and the "study population," respectively [8].

For reasons of time and money, it is generally impractical to consider the entire study population to address the research hypothesis. Money is an obvious limitation, but time can be an important factor as well, as the disease under study may naturally change over time. For example, antiviral treatment can lead to mutations that enable resistance to therapy [2, 3]. Minimizing heterogeneity of the disease is important for careful study and can be accomplished using the study inclusion/exclusion criteria and designing studies of appropriate sample size and duration. Due to the above limitations, a sample of individuals is selected from the study population. Data are collected from this sample; summary statistics, confidence intervals, and statistical tests are computed, and conclusions are generated. Inferences about the study population are made from the sample findings, and the quality of this inference is related to how representative the sample is to the study population.

Suppose, for example, that there was interest in estimating the average viral load for subjects chronically infected with HBV meeting study entry criteria—our study population. Typically, viral load is measured on the $\log_{10}$ scale since values often are skewed to the right (i.e., there is a long tail of large viral load counts). The $\log_{10}$ transformation is applied to make the viral loads appear more normally distributed. For the study population, the average $\log_{10}$(viral load) is denoted by μ, and the spread of $\log_{10}$(viral load) from this average value is represented by σ, so that roughly 95% of the values are within $\mu \pm 2\sigma$. The unknown parameters μ and σ are referred to as the mean and standard deviation of $\log_{10}$(viral load) in the study population, and if normally distributed, we can describe the distribution of $\log_{10}$(viral load) values as $N(\mu,\sigma^2)$.

If we select a sample of size n from the study population, we can use the sample mean $\bar{x} = \frac{\sum_{i=1}^{n} x_i}{n}$ and sample variance $s^2 = \frac{\sum_{i=1}^{n} (x_i - \bar{x})^2}{n-1}$ as estimates for μ and σ^2, respectively. The sample mean $\bar{x}$ will be distributed $N(\mu,\sigma^2/n)$, and we can use this fact to compute confidence intervals and hypothesis tests to generate inference for the population mean μ. Figure 10.1 plots several normal distributions for the sample mean of $\log_{10}$(viral load) for varying sample sizes with $\mu = 9.6$ and $\sigma = 2$ (similar to summary statistics from Lai et al. [6]). Note that as the sample size n increases, the

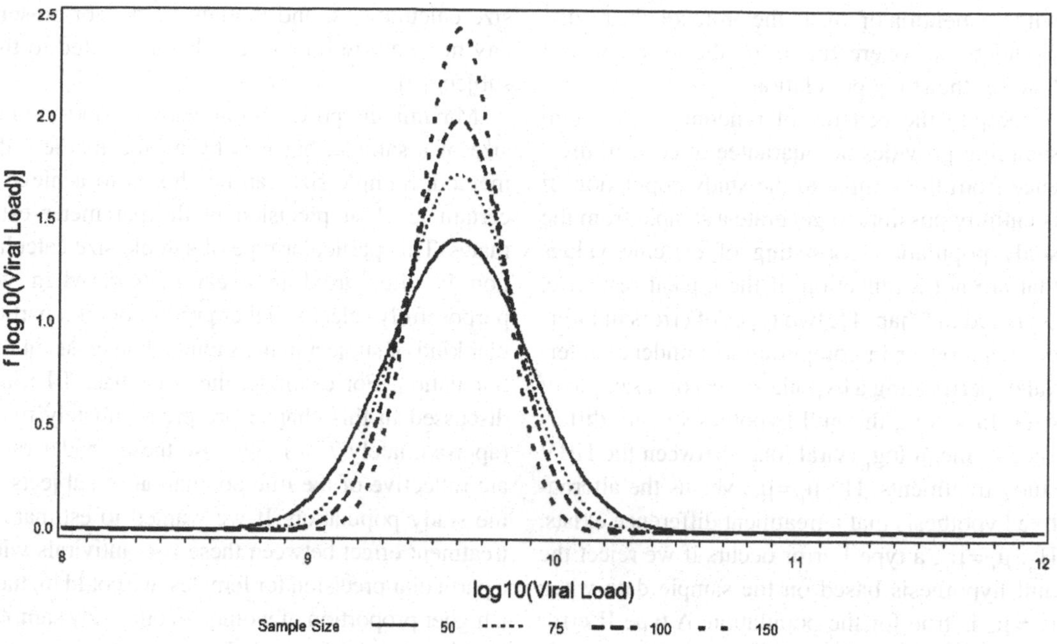

Fig. 10.1 Plot of normal distributions

distribution of $\overline{x}$ becomes narrower, allowing for more precise inference for describing μ, the average $\log_{10}$(viral load) of the study population. We will return to the discussion of sample size later.

How then does one choose a sample? Samples can be selected by probabilistic or nonprobabilistic means. Probabilistic or random sampling assigns each individual in the study population a chance of being selected into the sample. Based on some random process, which typically is performed using computer software or from tables of random numbers, individuals are chosen for participation in the sample. Of course, participation in the study is always a choice left to the individual, and nonresponse should be considered when interpreting the study results since if nonresponders vary systematically from those who participate in the study, we will obtain a biased estimate of the population parameters. A random sample generally will provide a representative snapshot of the characteristics known to be important or influence the outcome, so that estimates from this sample are representative of the study population. An additional benefit of random sampling is that the sample should achieve an accurate representation of factors that may be unknown to have an impact on the outcome or those factors that are not being measured for the current study. However, one difficulty of random sampling is enumerating all of the individuals in the study population, the *sampling frame*.

Nonprobability or nonrandom sampling, as the name implies, does not have this element of randomness in selecting the study sample. Individuals may be selected based on convenience or based on certain characteristics they exhibit. Nonprobability sampling usually is employed when it is not possible or practical to identify every individual within the study population to assign them a chance of entry into the sample. Though straightforward to apply, nonprobability sampling does raise a concern, namely, that important characteristics of the study population may not be represented in the sample. Therefore, any conclusions reached in the sample may provide a biased or misleading representation of the study population. Returning to our example above, if a physician was interested in the average viral load for subjects with HBV and selected only the sickest individuals for study with no mention of this in the protocol, the results would be an overestimate of the average viral load for the study population.

Despite the benefits of randomness, random sampling provides no guarantee of correct inference from the sample to the study population. It is entirely possible to generate a sample from the study population consisting of extreme values that are not a reflection of the typical response. As noted in Chap. 11, two types of errors in inference can occur in computing a confidence interval or performing a hypothesis test on a sample of data. In testing the null hypothesis of no difference in mean $\log_{10}$(viral load) between the HBV study treatments, H_0: $\mu_E = \mu_L$, versus the alternative hypothesis that a treatment difference exists, H_A: $\mu_E \neq \mu_L$, a type I error occurs if we reject the null hypothesis based on the sample data when $\mu_E = \mu_L$ is true for the population. A type II error occurs when we fail to reject the null hypothesis when the null hypothesis is false. In the context of our clinical trial example, a type I error could lead one to conclude that entecavir had better efficacy than lamivudine, when in actuality there is no difference between the two antivirals. A type II error would have the sponsor conclude that the two antivirals have similar efficacy, when entecavir is the more potent drug.

Sample Size

As further discussed in Chap. 11, the probability of making a type I or type II error is referred to as α and β, respectively. Typically, the sample size for a clinical trial is chosen to minimize the probability of these errors occurring, subject to available resources. Appropriate values for α and β depend on the scientific question at hand, but typical practice in clinical trials has α fixed at 0.05, with β chosen between 0.1 and 0.2. Alternatively, we could choose sample size to maximize the probability $1-\beta$, which is called *power*. Power is the probability of rejecting the null hypothesis, given the null hypothesis is false, and *powering* a study means allocating sufficient sample size to have a high likelihood of rejecting the null hypothesis in favor of the specified alternative. Formulae exist for many types of sample size calculations, and though we do not present any here, entire books have been devoted to the subject [9].

Maximizing power is one way of choosing the size of a sample, but it is by no means the only method. Sample size can be chosen to achieve a certain level of precision in the parameter estimates. This particular type of sample size calculation is often used in *oversampling*, when we purposefully select a higher proportion of a particular kind of subject in the sample than exists in the population. For example, the two phase III trials discussed in this chapter are predominately male (approximately 75%). Suppose these gender rates are reflective of the true population of subjects in the study population. If we wanted to estimate a treatment effect between these two antivirals with a particular precision for females, we could include a higher proportion of women in our study sample. In this scenario, our overall treatment effect could be biased if gender has an important impact on the characteristics of the disease. To obtain an unbiased estimate, we could employ survey weights to downplay the contribution of females to obtain overall estimates for the various endpoints that are reflective of the study population.

A final comment on sample size is worth mentioning in the conduct of clinical trials. While it is important to have sufficient sample size to have a representative sample and achieve high levels of power for testing the null hypothesis, the trial designer should realize that every subject enrolled in the trial potentially is exposed to some unknown safety risk attributable to the medications under investigation. Therefore, it is of paramount importance that the trial designers study enough subjects to achieve their goals, without exposing unnecessary additional individuals to an experimental treatment with an unknown or limited safety profile.

Probability Sampling

As alluded to above, probability sampling identifies the individuals within the study population and assigns every subject a chance of being selected into the sample. The easiest method of selecting a sample assigns every individual the same chance of being selected into the study. This method of sampling subjects is referred to as *simple random sampling*, and within clinical research, it generally is performed *without replacement*. "Without replacement sampling" implies that once a particular subject is selected for inclusion into the study, the subject is not returned to the pool for further sampling. The practical implication of this approach is that each subject is counted exactly once within a single clinical investigation. In contrast, "with replacement sampling" returns the sampled observation to the study population for further sampling.

While simple random sampling is straightforward to apply, it does have some disadvantages. First, sampling from particularly large populations can be cumbersome since it requires enumeration of all possible subjects to define the sampling frame. Such data may not exist or could be expensive to generate. Second, while we expect the average sample to be representative of the population, it is possible to generate a sample where important characteristics related to the study outcome are under- or overrepresented by random chance. These deficiencies can be addressed using methods described below.

In *stratified random sampling*, mutually exclusive subcategories (strata) of the study population are defined prior to sampling. Then, within each stratum, a separate random sample is selected. By defining the sampling scheme in this manner, it is possible to maintain the appropriate proportions of important disease characteristics within the study sample. Suppose, in lieu of the two separate clinical trials for HBeAg+ and HBeAg− subjects described above, sufficient funding was available for only a single study to obtain an overall estimate of $\log_{10}$(viral load) for the study population of HBV subjects. Further, suppose that HBeAg− disease accounts for roughly one-third of all HBV infection [6]. If we applied simple random sampling to select subjects from the study population, we could by random chance obtain a sample where the proportion of HBeAg− subjects differs substantially from 33%. Since the $\log_{10}$(viral load) of HBeAg− subjects tends to be lower than HBeAg+ subjects [6], the overall estimate of viral load would be biased for the study population, and the magnitude of this bias would depend on how far the proportion of HBeAg− subjects in the sample is from one-third of the total sample. However, employing a stratified random sampling scheme, we can select separate samples from each stratum such that 67% and 33% of the total sample size come from HBeAg-positive and HBeAg-negative subjects, respectively. Thus, we maintain the appropriate proportions of this important disease characteristic within our sample.

Stratified random sampling has a number of additional benefits. First, stratified sampling can lead to more efficient statistical testing through a reduction in the variability of the sample estimates. Second, distinct methods for sampling can be employed within each of the strata. For example, individuals located in more populated areas may be sampled at the individual level, while subjects in more remote areas might be sampled as part of a cluster (described below) [10]. While the aforementioned example could have financial benefits in sampling distant individuals, it actually may be *necessary* due to the nature of the information available to define the sampling frame within each stratum.

Though stratified random sampling is advantageous, there are a number of difficulties associated with its use. First, it is possible to stratify only for characteristics known to influence the disease in question, and the ability to identify these characteristics quickly and easily is important for generating the sample. Second, if there are multiple endpoints under investigation, it may be difficult to select strata that are beneficial for every endpoint. Stratification can result in efficient statistical testing when the strata are correlated with the outcome of interest (such as HBeAg status and viral load). However, strata that do not have this property may contribute to additional complexity and cost in the study design.

If it is possible to order a sampling frame, a *systematic random sample* can be generated by selecting every *k*th value in the list after randomly selecting a starting observation. Sampling proceeds in this manner until the required sample size is obtained. One benefit of systematic random sampling is that it can naturally account for the presence of strata, by sorting the frame by the stratification variables. However, an important drawback of systematic sampling can occur if the sampling frame has periodicity present. For example, suppose we attempt to replace our two phase III trials of HBeAg-positive and HBeAg-negative subjects with a single study. Further, suppose that the sampling frame is ordered such that positive and negative subjects alternate within the list. Choosing an even value for k would result in a sample that was either entirely positive or negative in terms of HBV infection. Though this is an extreme example, it illustrates the importance of understanding how the sampling frame is ordered prior to sampling.

The methods described above assume that a sampling frame exists for the selection of individual subjects. However, it is often difficult or expensive to generate such lists, or such information may not readily be available. One alternative to selecting at the subject level is to randomly select groups or clusters of observations for study—*cluster random sampling*. For example, as described in a study of diarrheal disease in Africa and Asia [7], villages were randomly selected for inclusion into the samples of four separate population surveys. Once a village was selected, all households within the village that met the study criteria were included in the sample. A benefit of sampling clusters of observations is that it can simplify the data collection process. For example, in a situation where hundreds of villages may exist, randomly selecting villages reduces the number of villages to which it may be necessary to travel. A simple random sample of subjects across all villages may require traveling to a majority of the villages to collect the necessary information. However, one downside of cluster sampling is that it typically requires a larger sample size than a simple random sample to obtain the same power or precision of sample estimates. This is because individuals within clusters tend to be more alike than individuals across clusters, and this often leads to an increase in the variability of the estimated parameters. In the example above, the reduced travel costs may more than make up for the additional subjects needed for study.

By employing the selection of clusters of observations, it is possible to refine the above design for diarrheal disease into a *multistage sampling* design. Suppose that many of the villages or townships were large and that sufficient information was available to describe each household within each village. In the first stage, we could randomly select villages. In the second stage, we could select a random sample of households from within each sampled village and include every individual within the chosen households meeting study criteria. Another option would be to apply a simple random sample of individuals within each of the randomly selected villages, but this approach would rely on each village having a list of all its citizens. To further complicate the design, stratification could be applied to allow for different sampling schemes within each stratum (the four countries described in the manuscript could be considered strata). Ultimately, there is no one-size-fits-all solution to define an appropriate sampling scheme. Based on the available information, study design is a careful balance of costs, statistical efficiency, and operational complexity.

An important note about selecting clusters: Cluster sizes may vary greatly, and as noted above, it is quite reasonable to expect that individuals are more similar within the cluster than between clusters. Because of this, it may be more appropriate to select clusters with *probability proportional to the size* of the cluster. For example, suppose that our population consisted of five villages with 100, 150, 200, 250, and 300 inhabitants and that we select one village to generate an estimate for the subjects of all villages. If we sample the smaller village of 100 inhabitants, the estimate of our endpoint may not fully reflect the individuals within the larger villages. Rather than give each village an equal likelihood of being in the sample (in this case, 1/5 or 20%), we can define the selection probability for each cluster as equal to the total size of the village divided by the total population of all villages combined. For our example, the villages would be selected with probabilities 100/1,000, 150/1,000, 200/1,000, 250/1,000, and 300/1,000 or 10%, 15%, 20%, 25%, and 30%, respectively. By sampling in this manner, we give larger clusters a greater chance of being selected into the sample, though this choice also increases the expected sample size of the study.

Nonprobability Sampling

Recall, nonprobability sampling does not employ random selection; it often is chosen when it is not practical to identify every individual within the study population to assign them a chance of entry into the sample. Though these sampling methodologies are frequently employed, particularly in the preliminary stages of research, great care should be used before applying the study findings to other related groups of individuals.

A commonly used method is *convenience sampling*. In short, the researcher enrolls subjects that are readily available. Perhaps, for the purposes of a graduate research project, the researcher will sample subjects from classes he/she attends, or from a frequently visited location, such as the student center, to describe a larger population of students. The benefit of convenience sampling is that it is cost-effective and that subjects are typically plentiful and readily available. Should the researcher have entry criteria that perhaps limit the number of subjects from whom data can be collected, *snowball or chain sampling* may be employed (see also Chap. 8). In this particular sampling design, additional subjects are recruited from the friends, family, and acquaintances of the individuals the researcher identifies. In this way, the researcher is able to readily identify additional people with the necessary characteristics for inclusion into the study, often with additional aid from those currently under study.

If it is necessary to divide the population into mutually exclusive groups (like strata) and recruit a specified number of each type, this is referred to as *quota sampling*. A typical example is recruiting sufficient males or females to evaluate gender-related differences. Unlike the examples above, the investigator has identified a characteristic that may be important to the endpoints of interest. *Judgment sampling* chooses individuals based on the knowledge or expertise of an expert, while *extreme or deviant case sampling* selects individuals that are particularly notable to learn about a particular topic or phenomenon.

Some limitations of nonprobability sampling are evident. Certain methods are purposefully biased, such as deviant case sampling. While such a method may provide interesting examples for the purposes of illustration, the sampled subjects should not be interpreted as representing the average subject in the study population. The potential bias of other methods may be less obvious. If the goal of the researcher is to describe characteristics of the student body, selecting individuals from her classes may not provide an accurate representation of individuals with majors that differ substantially from the researcher. Sampling from the student center may not include students whose courses are typically located at a distance, or it may underrepresent students who live off campus or attend part-time. One could argue that the appropriate study population consists of students who visit the student center. Even so, other important factors could arise based on how sampling is performed. For example, if the researcher obtains samples every morning prior to classes, she could miss an entire group of individuals that visit the student center later in the day. These concerns may or may not be important to the final conclusions of the study; however, it is important to consider such factors when designing a study and interpreting results.

Returning to Our Clinical Trial Example

After trumpeting the importance of random sampling, it may be somewhat surprising to the reader to hear that clinical research often is conducted using nonprobability sampling methods. For our clinical trial example, we suggested that the study population be defined as subjects with the appropriate disease characteristics meeting the eligibility requirements of the trial. Ideally, to describe this study population, a random sample of subjects would be selected for participation into the study. However, this typically is not the manner in which subjects are enrolled in a clinical trial. In general, a pharmaceutical company identifies clinicians who are interested in participating in research and may have access to patients appropriate for the study. Of particular importance is identifying not only clinicians with the expertise to aid in the design of the trial (e.g., which tests to perform, what endpoints to measure, and the appropriate disease characteristics for inclusion and exclusion criteria) but also those influential persons whose participation may entice other physicians to become involved (and eventually write prescriptions).

The clinician may have a number of patients who regularly attend his or her practice for disease management who could be included in the study, and in the course of his or her day-to-day job, s(he) may gauge these individuals' interest in participating in a trial for a new medical therapy. Additionally, the clinician may choose to advertise the clinical trial to attract additional patients from medical practices not participating in the trial, or those individuals who may not, for one reason or another, have routine exams with their doctor. Should the patients meet eligibility criteria and consent to study procedures, they would be randomized to one of the available treatment arms of the study.

However, as the statistician Senn points out, clinical trials are concerned with the comparative inference of the drugs under study among the subjects under study; rarely are they concerned with being representative of the study population [11]. In other words, the primary goal of the trial is to illustrate the effectiveness of a new medication against concurrent and comparable controls. Subjects are randomized to treatments to minimize bias in measuring the treatment effect since on average over all randomizations, the treatment groups would be considered equal at baseline. This is not to say that representative samples are never used within clinical research, but how a researcher samples an individual from a population should be tied to the ultimate goals of the study. This raises important questions: How can one safely apply the results of a clinical investigation to other subjects? To what study population do the subjects ultimately belong?

Perhaps the most straightforward way of identifying the individuals to whom these results may apply to is to review the table of summary statistics for baseline demographic and disease characteristics and the eligibility criteria from the study manuscript or drug label.

Subjects who are quite characteristically different than described should have the study results applied cautiously. Additionally, in reviewing the study materials, consider these additional questions: Are important geographical considerations overlooked? How are subjects who did not consent to study procedures different from those who did? Are subjects who do not seek routine care sicker than those who do? What important disease features differ in subjects who cannot stop taking medications that are prohibited within the study? How are subjects who are not local to participating clinicians different than those who are? How might subjects who took the drug at the time of the trial be different from those who will take it when it becomes approved? These questions may never be answered satisfactorily, and ultimately a leap of faith may be needed to apply sample findings to the population with the condition [8].

Conclusions

We are often in such a hurry to collect and analyze data that we neglect the importance of careful study design, and how we select individuals for study is a critical feature. Through many of the examples described above, we have learned that whom we select, where and how we select them, and even at what time they are selected may have serious implications on the study findings and how they may be interpreted or applied. This is true for samples of convenience as well as for any complex probabilistic survey sample. Without knowing the characteristics of the subjects under study and how they were chosen, the researcher has an incomplete grasp of the conclusions of the study. In fact, there may be a number of shortcomings that become obvious only once the sampling scheme is understood. Finally, it is important to remember that not all studies are designed to comprehensively reflect the population with the condition. Particularly for clinical researchers and physicians prescribing new medications, it is important to first understand the subjects under investigation and how they may differ from other populations available for treatment. Understanding these key points ensures a more successful application of new knowledge.

Take-Home Points

- Generating a random sample from a population is important to minimize the bias of sample estimates in describing the population parameters.
- Despite the benefits of random sampling for generating appropriate inference, clinical research often relies instead on samples of convenience.
- Baseline characteristics and study inclusion and exclusion criteria can help identify the study population from which the sample was drawn.
- It is important to understand the factors that differ between the study sample and the larger population and the potential impact these differences may have on the conclusions of the study and how appropriate it is to apply study results to the larger population.

References

1. Durham TA, Turner JR. Introduction to statistics in pharmaceutical clinical trials. London: Pharmaceutical Press; 2008.
2. Allen MI, Deslauriers M, Andrews CW, Tipples GA, Walters KA, Tyrrell DL, Brown N, Condreay LD. Identification and characterization of mutations in hepatitis B virus resistant to lamivudine. Hepatology. 1998;27:1670–7.
3. Liaw YF, Chien RN, Yeh CT, Tsai SL, Chu CM. Acute exacerbation and hepatitis B virus clearance after emergence of YMDD motif mutation during lamivudine therapy. Hepatology. 1999;30:567–72.
4. Liaw YF, Sung JJY, Chow WC, Farrell G, Lee CZ, Yuen H, Tanwandee T, Tao QM, Shue K, Keene ON, Dixon JS, Gray F, Sabbat J; Cirrhosis Asian Lamivudine Multicentre Study Group. Lamivudine for patients with chronic hepatitis B and advanced liver disease. N Engl J Med. 2004;351:1521–31.
5. Chang TT, Gish RG, de Man R, Gadano A, Sollano J, Chao YC, Lok AS, Han KH, Goodman Z, Zhu J, Cross A, DeHertogh D, Wilber R, Colonno R, Apelian D. A comparison of entecavir and lamivudine for HBeAg-positive chronic hepatitis B. N Engl J Med. 2006;354:1001–10.
6. Lai CL, Shouval D, Lok AS, Chang TT, Cheinquer H, Goodman Z, DeHertogh D, Wilber R, Zink RC, Cross A, Colonno R, Fernandes L. Entecavir versus lamivudine for patients with HBeAg-negative chronic hepatitis B. N Engl J Med. 2006;354:1011–20.
7. Katz J, Carey VJ, Zeger SL, Sommer A. Estimation of design effects and diarrhea clustering within households and villages. Am J Epidemiol. 1993;138:994–1006.
8. Friedman LM, Furberg CD, DeMets DL. Fundamentals of clinical trials. 4th ed. New York: Springer; 2010.
9. Chow SC, Wang H, Shao J, editors. Sample size calculations in clinical research. 2nd ed. Boca Raton: Chapman & Hall/CRC; 2008.
10. Kish L. Survey sampling. New York: Wiley; 1995.
11. Senn S. Statistical issues in drug development. 2nd ed. Chichester: Wiley; 2007.

Introductory Statistics in Medical Research

11

Todd A. Durham, Gary G. Koch, and Lisa M. LaVange

Introduction

Statistics is a discipline concerned with the collection, analysis, and interpretation of quantitative information. As discussed by Senn (2003) [1], "modern" statistics and probability in medical research date back to the 1700s and include investigations into the sex ratio at birth, causes of death, and an early clinical trial for scurvy. Since the early 1900s, there have been significant developments in statistical methodology and an increasing number of applications for statistics in medical research. Statistical methods are applicable to a wide range of medical investigations including case control studies, cohort studies, and therapeutic clinical trials. As discussed in other chapters, each of these types of studies has its own strengths and limitations, which should be considered when interpreting the results obtained from them.

The objective of this chapter is to introduce readers to some common statistical methods encountered in medical research, with selected examples for illustration. The presentation of technical details has purposely been kept to a minimum. It is an ambitious objective to cover a wide range of statistical topics in a single chapter. Given the brief coverage of this material, suggested reading is provided for readers to delve in to particular topics of interest. General references that cover similar material in this chapter include Campbell et al. (2007) [2], Durham and Turner (2008) [3], Bowers, House and Owens (2006) [4], Schork and Remington (2000) [5], and Woolson and Clarke (2002) [6].

Descriptive Statistics and Exploratory Data Analysis

All studies are limited in size for reasons of time, money, or logistics and are conducted on a sample of subjects, a subset of a larger population of subjects of interest. In accordance with a study's objectives, a number of characteristics are measured for individual subjects that comprise the study sample, and these characteristics typically vary from subject to subject (e.g., age or weight). In statistics, any characteristic which varies among subjects is a variable, and it becomes a random variable through its representation in a sample. Random variables may be quantitative (e.g., height in inches) or qualitative (e.g., gender) and are symbolically represented as X. Realized values of a random variable are called observations. There are a number of ways for researchers to characterize a group of individual

T.A. Durham, MS (✉)
Axio Research, LLC, 2601 4th Avenue, Suite 200, Seattle, WA 98121, USA
e-mail: todd.a.durham@gmail.com

G.G. Koch, PhD • L.M. LaVange, PhD
Department of Biostatistics, University of North Carolina at Chapel Hill Gillings School of Global Public Health, Chapel Hill, NC, USA
e-mail: bcl@bios.unc.edu; Lisalavange@yahoo.com

P.G. Supino and J.S. Borer (eds.), *Principles of Research Methodology: A Guide for Clinical Investigators*, DOI 10.1007/978-1-4614-3360-6_11, © Phyllis G. Supino and Jeffrey S. Borer 2012

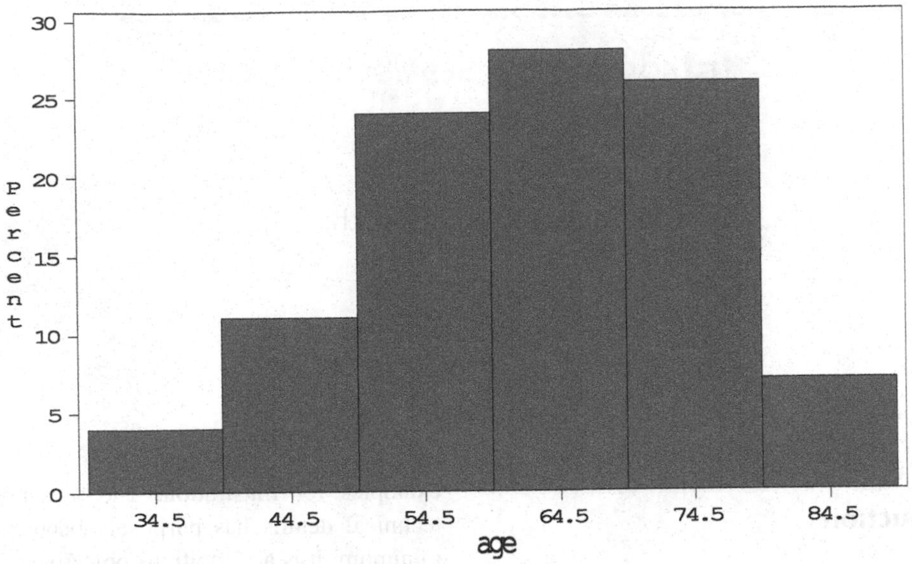

Fig. 11.1 Histogram of the relative frequency of 100 age values

observations (e.g., age values of participants in a medical study), such as the relative frequency of each value, the typical value in the group, and the extent to which individual observations vary from subject to subject. When statistical techniques are used simply to summarize random variables from the sample, the results obtained from them are said to be descriptive statistics.

The number of observations which comprise a sample is referred to as the sample size, denoted by the symbol n. One way to describe a sample of observations with respect to a quantitative random variable is to display the frequency of values of the random variable graphically. One type of graphical display is the frequency histogram. A histogram is constructed by:

- Defining 3–10 mutually exclusive (nonoverlapping) categories of equal width for the variable of interest.
- Tabulating the number of observations that fall into each category.
- Calculating the relative frequency of observations in each category as the count of observations in each category divided by the sample size.
- Displaying a bar for each category contiguously on the x-axis with a bar height equal to the relative frequency of each category on the y-axis. Bars are typically centered about the midpoint of the interval.

A sample histogram of 100 ages from a clinical trial is provided in Fig. 11.1. By examining a frequency histogram, one can see which values of the variable are more or less common. A graphical representation or mathematical expression of the relative frequency of values of a random variable is referred to as a distribution. For the construction of a histogram, the width of each category should be the same for all categories. However, it is important to note that the number of categories used can affect the shape of the distribution. Care should be taken so that valuable information is not lost through the use of too few categories. If the overall sample size is large, more than 10 categories may be used.

Histograms are useful since they enable one to inspect the shape of the distribution. Distributions which have more values in the middle and fewer values on the extremes are said to be unimodal, and they are symmetric when the extremes have similar representation. Distributions which have more values at one extreme than at the middle or the opposite extreme are said to be asymmetric or skewed. As evident in Fig. 11.1, the most common age values are in the category of 60–69 (midpoint of 64.5). There were very few observations with ages less than 50 or more than 79. For Fig. 11.1, the shape of the distribution of age values in the sample is reasonably symmetric.

Identification of a typical value or a measure of central tendency from the sample is frequently of interest. There are a number of measures of central tendency, some of which include the arithmetic mean, the median, and the mode. The arithmetic mean, typically referred to simply as the mean, is calculated as the sum of the individual values (indexed by the subscript i below) divided by the sample size:

$$\bar{x} = \frac{\sum_{i=1}^{n} x_i}{n}$$

The mean is always defined for a sample of numeric values. If the relative frequency of values or the distribution is at least somewhat symmetric, the sample mean is a reasonable choice as a measure of central tendency. One disadvantage of the mean is sensitivity to extreme values. For example, heart rate values of 60, 61, 63, 58, and 98 beats per minute have a mean of 68, which poorly represents a typical value.

When there are a few extreme values or a skewed distribution, the median can be a more appropriate measure of central tendency. The median is the middle value after all observations have been sorted from lowest to highest. If the sample size is odd, the median is the $((n+1)/2)th$ value after sorting (e.g., the third largest value from a sample of 5). If the sample size is even, the median is calculated as the mean of the two middle values, the $(n/2)th$ value and the $((n/2)+1)th$ value. For example, if there are 20 observations in a sample, the median is calculated as the mean of the 10th and 11th values. The median is always defined for a sample of numeric values.

Another measure of central tendency is the mode, defined as the most common value. The mode is 1 among the following rating scores: 0, 0, 1, 1, 1, 1, 1, 2, 2, 2, and 3. If all values of the random variable are unique, the mode is not defined. However, if there are multiple values which are equally as common, there is not one mode, but multiple modes. The modes are 43 and 81 for the following ages of participants in a clinical trial: 37, 39, 43, 43, 56, 57, 63, 81, 81, and 85.

For quantitative variables, the mean is the preferred measure of central tendency if the distribution is relatively symmetric. If the distribution is asymmetric, the median and mode are appropriate measures. For qualitative variables (e.g., gender), the mode is the most appropriate measure of central tendency.

In addition to measures of central tendency, the extent to which values of a characteristic vary from observation to observation, i.e., the dispersion or variety of values, is also of interest. If two groups from a study have similar mean numbers of lesions, but one group has more variation in the number of lesions across subjects, one may suspect that the two groups are different in some way. There are a number of measures of dispersion, and the appropriate choice among them depends on what one would like to say about the variation and, to some extent, on the shape of the distribution (i.e., symmetric vs. skewed). All measures of dispersion are nonnegative, and dispersion of zero indicates no variation in the random variable from observation to observation.

The simplest measure of dispersion is the range, defined as the difference between the maximum and minimum values. Quartiles can also be used to describe dispersion. Just as the median represents the middle value, through the value below and above which approximately 50% of the values lie, the 25th percentile (or first quartile) is the value below which approximately 25% of the values lie. Similarly, the 75th percentile (or third quartile) is the value below which approximately 75% of the values lie. The interquartile range, another measure of dispersion, is defined as the difference between the third and first quartiles. It also represents the dispersion of values that encompasses the middle 50% of values.

A graphical display which features a number of measures of central tendency and dispersion is a box plot. There are a number of different types of box plots, but typically box plots are used to display the values of the mean, median, 25th percentile, and 75th percentiles. Extreme values may also be plotted and often include the

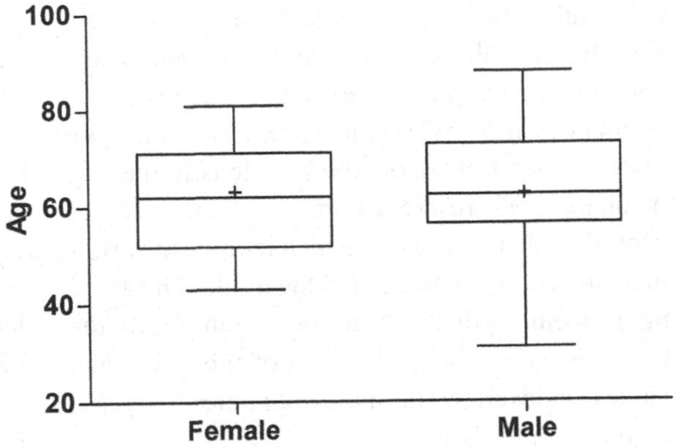

Fig. 11.2 Box plot of age by gender

minimum and maximum values. Box plots can be displayed side by side for the comparison of characteristics of distributions among levels of the experimental factor (e.g., cases and controls, treatments in a clinical trial, or time points in an observational study). Box plots of age values for males and females in a cohort study are displayed in Fig. 11.2. In this figure, the 25th percentile and 75th percentile are represented by the box, the median by the line bisecting the box, the mean by the crosses, and the minimum and maximum value by the lines extending from the box.

A measure of dispersion of values about the mean is the variance. The sample variance, denoted by the symbol s^2, is calculated by summing squared differences between each value and the mean (to obtain a positive value), and dividing the result by $n-1$:

$$s^2 = \frac{\sum_{i=1}^{n}(x_i - \bar{x})^2}{n-1}$$

It is difficult to interpret the variance since it is expressed in squared units (e.g., age^2). As a result, the square root of the variance is taken to obtain the standard deviation, which is often denoted by the symbol s. A small value of the standard deviation indicates that most values are close to the sample mean. A large value of the standard deviation indicates many values are far from the sample mean. Other words which are used to convey the concept of the standard deviation are "spread" and "scale."

The coefficient of variation is a unit-less measure of dispersion, defined as the standard deviation divided by the mean:

$$CV = \frac{s}{\bar{x}}$$

The coefficient of variation is helpful when used to compare two or more random variables with regard to their dispersion. It is used as a measure of precision in assay development, but may also be used to compare dispersion between two unrelated random variables each with different scales (e.g., dispersion of heart rate vs. systolic blood pressure).

Descriptive analyses such as those described above may be used as part of a preplanned analysis (e.g., as prescribed in a study protocol or analysis plan) or for exploratory purposes. Results from exploratory analyses often generate new hypotheses to test in future research. Descriptive statistical analyses provide insight into the nature of the data, as well as provide a rationale for the statistical methods used to make inferences about the population from which the sample arose.

Estimation, Confidence Limits, and Hypothesis Testing

One important goal of statistics is to use data from a sample (e.g., a limited number of participants in a clinical trial) to draw a conclusion about a larger set of subjects, a population.

Statistical procedures for which the aim is to make inferences about a relevant population are called inferential statistical methods. A population of interest in a clinical trial may be all patients who will ever be diagnosed with a particular viral infection. A population of interest in a cohort study may be all Americans exposed to a carcinogen in the environment. A population from a case control study may be adults who have and have not been diagnosed with coronary heart disease. Statistical inferences about these populations are necessary since they can be used to justify important policy decisions, such as making a new medical therapy available for use or revising educational material about lifestyle changes that reduce the risk of adverse health events.

However, as noted in Chap. 10, it is not feasible to study every person who may be a member of the population. As a result, research is conducted on a small number of them, a sample, and statistical methods are used to make inferences about the population of interest. One note of caution is that the validity of the statistical inference depends not only on the appropriate use of statistics but also on the selection of an appropriate sample on which the inference will be based. A general conceptual description of inferential statistics is provided in this section.

A parameter is a quantitative characteristic from a population, the value of which is considered fixed but unknown. For a case control study, one may be interested in the value of the population odds ratio, an estimate of the relative risk of an event. An example of a relevant population parameter from a randomized clinical trial is the difference in population mean response. Summary statistics (e.g., proportions of subjects exposed to some risk factor among cases and controls or the difference in sample means between the treated and control groups in a clinical trial) are calculated from the sample as estimates of the unknown population parameter of interest. The purpose of statistical inference is to evaluate how well a sample statistic estimates an unknown population parameter. The general process of making statistical inferences is as follows:

- Select a sample from a population of interest.
- Collect data from the sample.
- Calculate appropriate sample statistics as estimates of the population parameter.
- Make a statistical inference about the population parameter.
- Make a conclusion about the population itself.

The value of the summary statistic from a sample is called a point estimate, and it represents the estimate of the population parameter that is reasonably well supported by the sample data. If one were to repeat an experiment or study with a new sample of the same size from the same population, a different point estimate would be obtained. When each sample has an equal chance of being selected from the population, the sample is called a simple random sample. The extent to which point estimates vary from sample to sample (of the same size) represents sampling variability and can be quantified. If one were to select a sample of size n from the population of interest, calculate a sample statistic or point estimate (e.g., the sample mean), record it, and repeat the process a large number of times, the relative frequency of values of the sample statistic over all samples of size n would constitute the sampling distribution of the sample statistic.

In the previous section, the term standard deviation was defined and represented the "typical" spread of observations about the sample mean. If one were to calculate the standard deviation of values of the sample statistics (i.e., the standard deviation of the sampling distribution), the result represents the typical spread of sample statistics about the population parameter. This quantity is known as the standard error. The standard error of an estimate is a measure of how precisely the sample statistic has estimated the population parameter or, stated another way, the extent to which use of the sample has misestimated the true population parameter. The larger the sample is, the smaller the standard error will be, indicative of less uncertainty about the population parameter. It is important to note that there is not just one standard error. For every estimator, or mathematical rule used to calculate a sample statistic, there is a standard error. The remainder of this section will define the standard error for one estimator, the sample mean. Later sections mention standard errors for other estimators, but details of their derivation will not be included. As will be seen, the standard error of an estimate can be calculated from the sample.

Since a single point estimate from a sample will likely vary from sample to sample, a more useful way of estimating the population parameter of interest is an interval estimate, with a lower limit (*LL*) and an upper limit (*UL*). The general conceptual approach with interval estimation is to define an interval so that the proportion of random samples that enclose the parameter θ within the lower and upper limits is $(1-\alpha)$. Using some notational shorthand, we would like to estimate values, *LL* and *UL*, such that $P(LL < \theta < UL) = 1-\alpha$, where *P* expresses the proportion of random samples. The lower and upper limits are random variables, the values of which depend on the point estimate, the standard error of the estimate (a measure of the error attributed to sampling), and a precision coefficient.

A precision coefficient is a measure of how consistently a sample statistic estimates the population parameter, and it is obtained from well-defined distributions of standardized random variables. To illustrate, consider a random variable that has a particular distribution known as the normal distribution. Normal distributions are symmetric about their means with a bell shape, the downward slope determined by the standard deviation. For any random variable, *X*, that has a normal distribution (mean μ and standard deviation σ), the following can be said about the probability of observing certain values of the random variable:

$$P(\mu - 1.04\sigma < X < \mu + 1.04\sigma) = 0.70$$
$$P(\mu - 1.96\sigma < X < \mu + 1.96\sigma) = 0.95$$
$$P(\mu - 2.58\sigma < X < \mu + 2.58\sigma) = 0.99$$

In other words, 70% of values are within 1.04 standard deviations of the mean; 95% of values are within 1.96 standard deviations of the mean; and 99% of values are within 2.58 standard deviations of the mean. It is possible to standardize any normally distributed random variable by subtracting the population mean from each value and dividing by the standard deviation:

$$Z = \frac{X - \mu}{\sigma}$$

The resulting random variable has a standard normal distribution with mean 0 and standard deviation 1. A random variable that follows the standard normal distribution is often denoted by Z and called a *Z* score. Using the expressions above:

$$P(-1.04 < Z < 1.04) = 0.70$$
$$P(-1.96 < Z < 1.96) = 0.95$$
$$P(-2.58 < Z < 2.58) = 0.99$$

The precision coefficient is specific to the parameter being estimated. Precision coefficients can be obtained from tabled values or from statistical software. If a random variable follows a standard normal distribution, one can use the known distribution of Z scores to state that 95% of all Z scores lie between −1.96 and 1.96. The value 1.96 is the precision coefficient needed for an interval estimate with 95% confidence. Stated simply, a precision coefficient is the number of standard deviations within which $100(1-\alpha)\%$ of the values of the random variable fall from the population parameter. The symbol α represents one's willingness to estimate the underlying population parameter incorrectly. In most fields of research, an α level of 0.05 is considered reasonable, but there may be times when a higher or lower α level is acceptable.

In general, the standard error gets smaller as the sample size increases. The standard error for the sample mean is defined as the standard deviation divided by the square root of the sample size:

$$SE(\overline{x}) = \frac{s}{\sqrt{n}}$$

Greater confidence for an interval estimate requires a larger precision coefficient. These observations hold for standard errors of other estimators and for other distributions used in the construction of intervals. The construction of a confidence interval follows a general form of:

Point estimate ± (precision factor) (standard error of the estimate).

Given this general form, the following observations are worth noting. All other things being equal, confidence intervals are:

- Narrower with larger sample sizes than smaller sample sizes
- Wider when more confidence is required than when less confidence is required

Although somewhat of a simplification, confidence intervals represent a plausible range of values of the population parameter given the sample estimate and uncertainty attributed to the sampling process.

Since population parameters (e.g., the population standard deviation) are not known, there are related standardized scores which utilize only data from the sample.

The *t*-statistic is perhaps the best known of these, and it will be used as an example of a confidence interval for a population mean. When the sample size is small (particularly <30) and the population standard deviation is unknown, the ratio of a standard normal random variable to its standard error has a *t* distribution for which the shape is determined by the number of degrees of freedom ($n-1$). The statistic,

$$T = \frac{\overline{x} - \mu}{s / \sqrt{n}}$$

follows a *t* distribution ("Student's *t*"). The *t* distribution is symmetric about its mean (zero) and looks like a normal distribution with, in cases of sample sizes less than 200, heavier "tails." As was the case with the normal distribution, the shape of the *t* distribution can be used to find two values which define a central area under the density curve of size $(1-\alpha)$. It can be shown that once a value of T associated with an area of interest (translated as a probability) is determined, the sample mean $\overline{x}$ is within $T(s/\sqrt{n})$ of the population mean, μ. This enables one to calculate a confidence interval for the population mean when the sample size is small and the population variance is unknown.

The interval estimate of the population mean, the two-sided $(1-\alpha)$% confidence interval for the population mean, is

$$\overline{x} \pm t_{1-\alpha/2,n-1}(s/\sqrt{n})$$

Note that the precision coefficient, $t_{1-\alpha/2,n-1}$, is the $100(1-\alpha)$th percentile of the *t* distribution with $n-1$ degrees of freedom. Since the *t* distribution is symmetric about zero, $t_{1-\alpha/2}$ is the precision coefficient that defines a central area of $(1-\alpha)$.

As an example, consider an observational study of 25 patients with primary biliary cirrhosis (PBC). Among these 25 patients, the mean alkaline phosphatase (U/L) value was 1,983 U/L and the standard deviation was 2,140 U/L. Researchers are interested in a 95% confidence interval for the population mean alkaline phosphatase. In this case, the precision factor is the value from the *t* distribution with 24 degrees of freedom that defines a central area of 95%. From a table of values, one finds this value to be 2.06. The 95% confidence interval is then

$$\begin{aligned} 1983 \pm 2.06(2140/5) &= 1983 \pm 881.7 \\ &= (1101.3, 2864.7) \end{aligned}$$

The statistical interpretation of this result is that we are 95% confident that the interval (1,101.3, 2,864.7 U/L) includes the population mean alkaline phosphatase value among patients with PBC.

A statistical concept that is closely related to the construction of confidence intervals is hypothesis testing. Hypothesis testing involves the following steps:

- Posing a null hypothesis about the value of the population parameter of interest
- Stating the alternative hypothesis about the value of the population parameter
- Identifying an appropriate test statistic against which the null hypothesis will be evaluated
- Describing the distribution of the test statistic when the null hypothesis is true; identifying values of the test statistic that occur less than 100 α% of the time under the null hypothesis (the rejection or critical region)
- Calculating the test statistic
- Making a conclusion about the null and alternative hypotheses on the basis of the test statistic compared to the rejection region

Since the inference is being made from a sample, the hypothesis test can result in two types of errors: rejecting the null hypothesis when it should not have been rejected (a type I error) or failing to reject the null hypothesis when it should have been rejected (a type II error). Making an erroneous conclusion at the end of a study is undesirable. Hence, studies are designed to limit the probability of either of these errors occurring. The probability of a type I error is denoted by alpha (α), previously referred to as the significance level, and that for a type II error is denoted by beta (β). Its complement, $(1-\beta)$, is called the power of a test and is the probability of correctly rejecting the null hypothesis. For clinical trials, study design considerations include specification of α and $(1-\beta)$ since these affect the ability of a study sponsor to address study objectives (e.g., to claim an effect of an investigational drug).

The process of hypothesis testing can be illustrated with data from the previous example. Suppose researchers would like to know if, as they suspect, the mean alkaline phosphatase value among patients with primary biliary cirrhosis is different from otherwise normal subjects. The mean among normal volunteers is around 80 U/L. The null hypothesis is that the mean alkaline phosphatase among patients with PBC is 80 U/L. If there is sufficient evidence to reject the null hypothesis, the following alternative hypothesis will be concluded: the mean alkaline phosphatase among patients with PBC is not 80 U/L. Using statistical notation:

$$H_0 : \mu = 80 \quad \text{versus} \quad H_A : \mu \neq 80$$

Note that rejection of the null hypothesis could occur because the mean PBC level was less than or greater than the hypothesized value. Since there are two sides to the alternative hypothesis, the test is considered two-sided. In advance, the researchers will have decided upon a value of α, the "size" of the test, which represents the probability that they will reject the null hypothesis erroneously. The choice of the size of the test depends on one's willingness to commit a type I error. For example, if the implication of committing a type I error is not very important as in early studies in drug development, a researcher may be satisfied with an α level of 0.10 or 0.20. A common value for α in confirmatory research settings is 0.05, but there may be instances in which smaller values are desirable. The test statistic is calculated as the difference between the sample mean and the hypothesized value divided by the standard error of the mean:

$$t = \frac{\overline{x} - \mu_0}{s / \sqrt{n}}$$

If this value is close to zero, there will be insufficient evidence to reject the null hypothesis. If the value is far from zero, the evidence is considered sufficient to reject the null hypothesis. The rejection region is represented by those values of the test statistic that occur with probability α or less when the null hypothesis is true. If the null hypothesis is rejected, either the population mean alkaline phosphatase is not 80 U/L or a type I error has occurred.

For the results obtained, the calculated value of the test statistic is

$$t = \frac{1983 - 80}{2140 / \sqrt{25}} = \frac{1903}{428} = 4.45$$

Using tabled values of the t distribution with 24 degrees of freedom, one obtains a rejection region of $t < -2.06$ or $t > 2.06$. Since the test statistic is in the rejection region, the null hypothesis is rejected at the $\alpha = 0.05$ level. The conclusion from the hypothesis test is that the difference between the sample estimate and the hypothesized value is greater than would be expected by chance (due to sampling) alone. The population mean alkaline phosphatase value for patients with PBC is different from 80 U/L.

It is possible that two people would not agree on the appropriate value of α, so another probability, the p value, is often used to reflect the "extremeness" of the value of the test statistic. A p value is the probability of observing the actual value of the test statistic or one more extreme (i.e., favoring the alternative hypothesis) when the null hypothesis is true. If a p value is $\leq \alpha$, one rejects the null hypothesis. A p value of 0.02 means that the value of the observed test statistic and all other values more extreme (i.e., contradictory of the null hypothesis) occurs with probability of 0.02 under the null hypothesis. One major drawback of p values as a measure of evidence is that they are highly dependent on the sample size

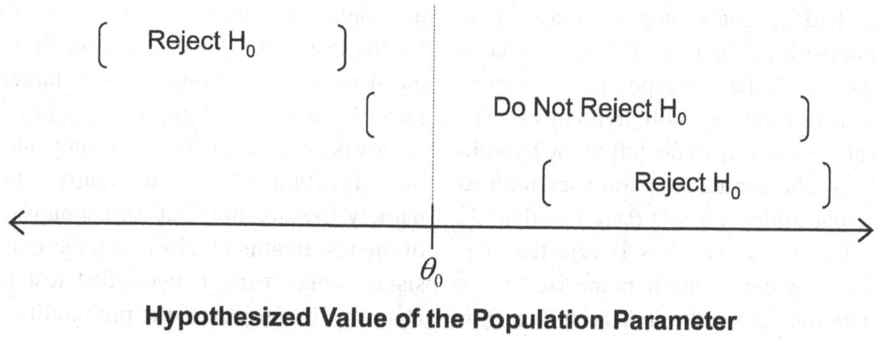

Fig. 11.3 Relationship between confidence intervals and hypothesis tests

as it relates to the standard error of the estimator and, thereby, the power to contradict the null hypothesis. The sample size for a study typically is estimated in advance to ensure there is adequate power to detect an effect of interest.

The sample size required to provide power of $(1-\beta)$ to reject the null hypothesis that the mean μ is not different from a specified value μ_0 while maintaining a type I error of α is

$$n = \frac{\left(Z_\alpha + Z_\beta\right)^2 \sigma^2}{\Delta^2}$$

where $\Delta = (\mu - \mu_0)$ is the applicable difference and Z_α and Z_β are precision coefficients for $(1-\alpha)$ and $(1-\beta)$ of the standard normal distribution. Note that the variance, σ^2, and the true difference, Δ, must be defined specifically for the type of outcome (e.g., means, proportions) being evaluated. The true difference is often regarded as a clinically meaningful difference or the difference one would like to detect. Estimates of the variance are typically obtained from previous studies. The sample size expression can be rewritten using algebra as

$$\frac{\sigma^2}{n} = \left(\frac{\Delta}{Z_\alpha + Z_\beta}\right)^2$$

The quantity $\frac{\sigma^2}{n}$ is the required squared standard error for $(1-\beta)$ power to contradict μ_0 as the null hypothesis with type I error of α when the true mean μ differs from μ_0 by Δ.

Another algebraic manipulation of the sample size expression yields the following:

$$n = \frac{\left(Z_\alpha + Z_\beta\right)^2}{(\Delta / \sigma)^2}$$

The expression (Δ / σ) is called the effect size. In the case where Δ is defined as the difference between two means with a common standard deviation, σ, Cohen (1992) [7] has characterized effect sizes around 0.2 as "small," around 0.5 as "moderate," and 0.8 or greater as "large." Another use of effect sizes is that they may be compared across studies for comparative purposes, or when appropriate, combined across similarly designed studies as a "meta-analysis," as described in Chap. 9.

Confidence intervals and hypothesis tests are closely related inferential procedures. In the case of a two-sided $100(1-\alpha)\%$ confidence interval, the lower and upper limits represent the range of plausible values of the unknown population parameter. A hypothesis test may be carried out by positing a number of values of the population parameter in the null hypothesis. All values outside of the limits of the two-sided $100(1-\alpha)\%$ confidence interval would be rejected by a two-sided hypothesis test of size α. Conversely, values within the two-sided $100(1-\alpha)\%$ confidence interval would not be rejected. Thus, a confidence interval can be used to test a number of values of the population parameter.

A graphical representation of the relationship between a two-sided $100(1-\alpha)\%$ confidence interval about the population parameter, θ, and a two-sided hypothesis test of the null hypothesis, $H_0: \theta = \theta_0$, is presented in Fig. 11.3. In Fig. 11.3, three hypothetical confidence intervals (with lower and upper limits indicated by the brackets) are displayed with the corresponding statistical conclusion regarding the null hypothesis. The first interval lies entirely to the left of the hypothesized value of the population parameter, indicating that the plausible values of θ are less than θ_0. Therefore, the null hypothesis is rejected. The second interval encloses the hypothesized value of the population parameter, indicating that θ_0 is among the plausible values of θ. Therefore, the null hypothesis is not rejected. The third interval lies entirely to the right of the hypothesized value of the population parameter, indicating plausible values of θ are greater than θ_0. Hence, the third confidence interval is also consistent with rejection of the null hypothesis.

The formulation of the confidence interval depends on the population parameter being estimated, which depends on the null hypothesis, which in turn depends on the research question of interest. Medical research includes observational studies (prospective and retrospective) and clinical trials which are intended to evaluate the effects of a medical intervention, such as a pharmaceutical agent, a surgical procedure, use of a device, or implementation of an educational or counseling program. Pharmaceutical agents are evaluated for their usefulness, among other things, on the basis of their efficacy and safety [3]. In the context of pharmaceutical development, the objective of a clinical trial can be to demonstrate that a test treatment is:

- Superior to an inactive or active control
- Not unacceptably worse than (not inferior to) an active control
- Equivalent to an active control

The following statistical hypotheses correspond to a clinical trial intended to demonstrate the superiority of a test treatment compared to a control with respect to a continuous outcome:

$$H_0 : \mu_{\text{test}} - \mu_{\text{control}} = 0 \quad \text{versus}$$
$$H_A : \mu_{\text{test}} - \mu_{\text{control}} \neq 0$$

The null hypothesis of interest could be rejected if the difference in mean response is far from zero in the negative direction (i.e., mean for the control group is much larger than the mean for the test group) or the positive direction (i.e., mean for the test group is much larger than the mean for the control group). In many instances, sponsors of clinical trials are only interested in one direction of the alternative hypothesis, namely, the direction that corresponds to a benefit of the test treatment. However, the null hypothesis is tested using a two-sided test of size α. Hence, if it is rejected, the probability of erroneously claiming a benefit of the treatment is $\alpha/2$ and the probability of erroneously detecting a harm of the treatment is $\alpha/2$.

Test products which are intended to be similar to an existing product in terms of the clinical response are evaluated in equivalence trials. The objective of an equivalence trial is to demonstrate that the difference in response between the test treatment and the active control does not exceed an acceptable margin. New pharmaceutical products which are shown to be equivalent to an active control may have other advantages to justify their use such as better safety, more convenient dosing, or lower cost. Bioequivalence studies are intended to demonstrate that the pharmacokinetic properties of two formulations of a treatment are equivalent.

The following statistical hypotheses correspond to a clinical trial intended to demonstrate the equivalence of a test treatment to an active control with respect to the difference in population means of a continuous outcome:

$$H_0 : |\mu_{\text{test}} - \mu_{\text{control}}| \geq \delta_{\text{equivalence}} \quad \text{versus}$$
$$H_A : |\mu_{\text{test}} - \mu_{\text{control}}| < \delta_{\text{equivalence}}$$

The quantity $\delta_{\text{equivalence}}$ is called the equivalence margin, and it must be specifically defined in advance of the study analysis. In the case of pharmaceutical studies, the equivalence margin must be agreed upon by regulatory authorities if the study is to be used for registration purposes.

The null hypothesis in equivalence trials is typically tested using a confidence interval about the difference in population parameters (e.g., means or proportions). If the confidence interval excludes the equivalence margin (by being entirely within it), the null hypothesis is rejected.

An important consideration in equivalence trials is that rejection of the null hypothesis can be interpreted as meaning that the test and control are both efficacious or neither is. The credibility of such a result depends on the ability to demonstrate that the active control would have been efficacious if an inactive control were used in the study. The ability of a study to differentiate an efficacious treatment from an inefficacious treatment is called assay sensitivity. One way assay sensitivity can be established is by the use of historical data for the inactive control to demonstrate that the active control would have been superior to the inactive control if it had been studied. Another way to establish assay sensitivity is to include an inactive control group in addition to the active control, although such a design may not be ethical. Interested readers may refer to Chow and Liu (2004) [8] for further information on equivalence and noninferiority clinical trials.

Another objective of some clinical trials is to demonstrate that a test treatment is not unacceptably inferior to the control. Studies with such an objective are called noninferiority studies, and they may be used when it is unethical or logistically difficult to use an inactive control. If the test treatment is considered not unacceptably worse than the active control, it may have other advantages such as better safety or greater convenience. The following statistical hypotheses correspond to a clinical trial intended to demonstrate the noninferiority of a test treatment to an active control with respect to the difference in population means of a continuous outcome. In this formulation of the hypotheses, a larger value of the mean is favorable:

$$H_0 : \mu_{\text{test}} - \mu_{\text{control}} \le \delta_{\text{non - inferiority}} \quad \text{versus}$$
$$H_A : \mu_{\text{test}} - \mu_{\text{control}} > \delta_{\text{non - inferiority}}$$

As with equivalence trials, the noninferiority margin must be specified in advance. The null hypothesis is tested using a confidence interval. If the noninferiority margin is enclosed within the confidence interval, the null hypothesis is not rejected. If the noninferiority margin is below the lower limit of the confidence interval, the null hypothesis is rejected, and the conclusion is that the test treatment is not inferior to the active control. Similar to equivalence trials, interpreting this statistical conclusion also depends on the ability of the study to establish assay sensitivity.

As seen in this section, both hypothesis tests and confidence intervals are used to draw conclusions about a quantitative characteristic of a population. In the remaining sections, specific statistical methods are described.

Differences Between Means and Proportions

A common statistical analysis involves making an inference about the equality of two means when the observations are independent, meaning the value of one observation does not depend on another. In many medical studies, observations can be considered independent because the observations are single values from different study subjects. However, medical studies frequently involve repeated tests for the same individual (e.g., heart rate taken at a number of times for the same individual) or related tests within the same individual (e.g., presence of a characteristic in more than one skin location within an individual study subject). Such observations are considered dependent.

In the case of independent observations, the hypothesis tested for the equality of two population means is

$$H_0 : \mu_1 - \mu_2 = 0$$

If this null hypothesis is rejected, the following alternative hypothesis will be favored:

$$H_A : \mu_1 - \mu_2 \ne 0$$

The test statistic to test the null hypothesis is

$$t = \frac{\bar{x}_1 - \bar{x}_2}{s_p \sqrt{\frac{1}{n_1} + \frac{1}{n_2}}}$$

where the numerator is the difference in sample means, an estimate of the difference in population means, and the denominator is the standard error of the difference in sample means. The quantity $s_p = \sqrt{\frac{(n_1 - 1)s_1^2 + (n_2 - 1)s_2^2}{n_1 + n_2 - 2}}$ is the pooled standard deviation and represents the weighted average of the standard deviation across the two samples with sample sizes of n_1 and n_2. This test is called Student's t test or the independent groups t test because the test statistic follows a t distribution under the null hypothesis.

The assumptions required for the use of the two-sample t test are that the distribution of the random variable is approximately normal, the two groups represent simple random samples from the two populations of interest, and the population variances are equal (although likely unknown). Under the null hypothesis (i.e., assuming the two population means are equal), the test statistic follows a t distribution with $n_1 + n_2 - 2$ degrees of freedom. For a two-sided hypothesis test of size α, the rejection region is defined as any value of the test statistic $t > t_{1-\alpha/2, n_1+n_2-2}$ or $t < t_{\alpha/2, n_1+n_2-2}$, i.e., the values from the t distribution with $n_1 + n_2 - 2$ degrees of freedom that lie outside of a central area of $(1-\alpha)$. Note that since the t distribution is symmetric, $\left|t_{\alpha/2, n_1+n_2-2}\right| = t_{1-\alpha/2, n_1+n_2-2}$.

Consider the following example. One may be interested in whether or not there is a difference in the mean LDL cholesterol between adults with coronary heart disease (CHD) and adults without CHD. To answer such a research question, two samples corresponding to the populations of interest (i.e., adults with a diagnosis of CHD and adults with no diagnosis of CHD) would be studied. LDL cholesterol levels were ascertained for 25 subjects from each group. The sample means were 134 mg/dL and 118 mg/dL for the CHD and non-CHD subjects, respectively. The sample standard deviations were 14 mg/dL and 12 mg/dL, respectively. The statistical hypotheses are

$$H_0 : \mu_{\text{CHD}} - \mu_{\text{non-CHD}} = 0 \quad \text{versus}$$
$$H_A : \mu_{\text{CHD}} - \mu_{\text{non-CHD}} \neq 0$$

The size of the test will be α=0.05. Given the sample sizes in each group, the rejection region is any value of the test statistic t<−2.01 or t>2.01, which corresponds to values of the t distribution with 48 degrees of freedom which define areas in the left-hand tail of 0.025 and in the right-hand tail of 0.025, respectively. The values that define the rejection region can be obtained from tables of the distribution or from statistical software.

The pooled standard deviation is calculated as

$$s_p = \sqrt{\frac{(25-1)14^2 + (25-1)12^2}{25+25-2}} = 13$$

The test statistic is calculated as

$$t = \frac{134 - 118}{13\sqrt{\frac{1}{25} + \frac{1}{25}}} = 5.1$$

Since the value of the test statistic, 5.1, is in the rejection region (t>2.01), the null hypothesis is rejected. The evidence from the study suggests that the population mean LDL is different between adults with CHD and those without CHD. Since the difference between the sample statistic and the hypothesized value of the population parameter differs much more than what would be expected by chance alone, such a difference is often called "statistically significant." A corresponding confidence interval for the difference between two group means can be written as

$$(\bar{x}_1 - \bar{x}_2) \pm \left(t_{1-\alpha/2, n_1+n_2-2}\right) s_p \sqrt{\frac{1}{n_1} + \frac{1}{n_2}}$$

Note that this confidence interval follows the general form described previously. In this case, the quantity $s_p \sqrt{\frac{1}{n_1} + \frac{1}{n_2}}$ is the standard error of the difference in sample means.

For this particular example, the corresponding 95% confidence interval is

$$(134-118) \pm 2.01\left(13\sqrt{\frac{1}{25}+\frac{1}{25}}\right)$$
$$= 16 \pm 7.4 = 8.6, 23.4$$

The interpretation of this result is that we are 95% confident that the interval (8.6, 23.4) encloses the true difference in population mean LDL. Note that the hypothesized value of the difference, zero, is outside of the calculated interval which is consistent with the rejection of the null hypothesis of no difference.

A similar method can be used when the difference in population means represents dependent observations, such as a subject's systolic blood pressure (SBP) before and after treatment with an antihypertensive. The null and alternative hypotheses can be specified as

$$H_0 : \mu_{\text{Post}} - \mu_{\text{Pre}} = 0 \quad \text{versus}$$
$$H_A : \mu_{\text{Post}} - \mu_{\text{Pre}} \neq 0$$

In this case, the test is called a paired t test and the test is carried out by calculating the difference in paired observations (e.g., SBP post minus SBP pre) and forming the test statistic using the sample mean difference divided by the standard error of the difference in paired values:

$$t = \frac{\overline{x}_d}{s_d / \sqrt{n}}$$

If there is no difference between the paired observations, the test statistic will be close to zero. The rejection region is defined using a t distribution with $n-1$ degrees of freedom, where n is the number of subjects with paired observations.

When the independent groups t test cannot be used, such as when the distribution is not approximately normally distributed, a nonparametric test (which does not assume any shape to the underlying distribution) may be appropriate. A nonparametric analog to the independent groups t test is the Wilcoxon rank sum test which addresses the equality of mean ranks. The Wilcoxon rank sum test is carried out by ranking all individual observations across the two groups from lowest to highest, calculating the sum of ranks for one of the groups, and comparing this sum to tabled values (representing percentiles of the distribution) in order to reject or fail to reject the null hypothesis. The rejection region is defined according to tabled values of a distribution defined just for this particular test. When ranking the observations, ties are managed by assigning the mean of the ranks that would have been assigned if the observations had not been tied. For example, if the third, fourth, and fifth smallest observations are all tied, the assigned rank for each of these observations will be 4. The Wilcoxon rank sum test assumes that the two samples came from the same population and therefore have the same variance under the null hypothesis. If the null hypothesis of a common population distribution is rejected, the interpretation is that the distribution of one population is shifted away from the other. It is worth noting that the nonparametric analog to the paired t test is the Wilcoxon signed-rank test for pairs, although the details of this method are not discussed. Interested readers are referred to LaVange and Koch (2006) [9] for additional information on the Wilcoxon rank sum test and the Wilcoxon signed-rank test.

In studies involving comparisons of the population mean among more than two populations, an appropriate statistical method is called analysis of variance (ANOVA). If interest is in the equality of k population means, the null hypothesis tested in ANOVA is stated as

$$H_0 : \mu_1 = \mu_2 = \ldots = \mu_{k-1} = \mu_k$$

If the null hypothesis is rejected, the alternative hypothesis will be favored:

H_A: at least one pair of the population means is unequal. That is, at least one of the following inequalities is true: $\mu_1 \neq \mu_2, \ldots, \mu_1 \neq \mu_{k-1}$, and … $\mu_{k-1} \neq \mu_k$.

The assumptions required for use of ANOVA are that the samples represent simple random samples from the populations of interest, the random variable is normally (or approximately normally) distributed in the populations, and the population variance is equal among the populations. The overall variation of the individual

Table 11.1 ANOVA for mean VAS pain score from three dose groups

Source	Sum of squares	df	Mean square	F
Drug	99.89459	2	49.947295	6.28
Error	238.67896	30	7.955965	
Total	338.57355	32		

responses is partitioned into within-group variability (the inherent variability within each sample) and among-group variability (the variability of the sample means relative to the overall mean). The test statistic F is calculated as the ratio of the variability among samples (e.g., treatment groups) to the variability within samples:

$$F = \frac{V_{\text{Among}}}{V_{\text{Within}}}$$

That is, if the sample means vary more than the inherent variability, the ratio will be greater than one, and the evidence will suggest that the sample means did not arise from populations with a common population mean. Results from an analysis of variance are often displayed in an ANOVA table, such as the results displayed in Table 11.1 from an analysis of a clinical trial of three doses of an analgesic. The response of interest is the mean pain score recorded using a visual analog scale (VAS). The mean square for drug (49.95) represents the average variability of means relative to the grand mean response. The mean square error (7.96) represents the variability of responses within each treatment group. The ratio of these two is the test statistic and can be interpreted as the extent to which the variability in mean responses across groups exceeds the inherent variability in response.

The test statistic calculated in such a manner follows an F distribution, for which the shape (and therefore the critical region) is determined by two parameters: the "numerator degrees of freedom," defined as the number of degrees of freedom required to estimate the variability among sample means ($k-1$), and the "denominator degrees of freedom," defined as the number of degrees of freedom for estimating variability within samples ($N-k$), where N represents the total sample size across the k samples:

$$N = \sum_{i=1}^{k} n_i$$

If the null hypothesis of equal means is rejected, one would like to know which pairs of the population means are unequal.

Following a significant test result from the F test, one can compare the population means among samples (e.g., treatment groups in a clinical trial) using numerous methods that appropriately control the overall type I error rate. This is important since one could test each of $c=k(k-1)/2$ pairs of population means using an independent groups t test with $\alpha=0.05$, but the type I error rate is only controlled at $\alpha=0.05$ with this method when $k=3$. When $k>3$, the probability of incorrectly rejecting at least one hypothesis increases with the number of individual hypotheses tested. In general, if c null hypotheses each have independent tests at the α level, the probability of rejecting at least one by chance alone is

$$\begin{aligned} &= \text{P}(\text{rejecting at least one of } c \text{ hypotheses}) \\ &= 1-(1-\alpha)^c \end{aligned}$$

For example, if five such independent comparisons of treatment groups are tested at $\alpha=0.05$, the probability of rejecting at least one by chance alone could be as large as 0.226.

One appropriate method for controlling the experimentwise error rate is the Bonferroni test which involves testing each of the c pairs of means using a t test with $\alpha_B=\alpha/c$. For example, if a study with four groups was conducted and the F test was rejected ($\alpha=0.05$), then the six comparisons of means could subsequently be tested using $\alpha_B=0.05/6=0.0083$. This method controls the experimentwise error rate since the probability of incorrectly rejecting at least one null hypothesis is bounded by $6(0.05/6)=0.05$.

Another method which can be used to compare pairs of means is Tukey's Honestly Significant Difference test. This test requires the use of additional tabled values to determine the minimum absolute difference in means that would lead to rejection of the null hypothesis of the equality of two means. However, Tukey's method is more powerful than the Bonferroni test, meaning the absolute difference in means leading to rejection is smaller than that required for the Bonferroni test. Another method which may be used when comparing a number of group means to a common control is Dunnett's test. Additional details about methods used to control the experimentwise error rate in the setting of multiple tests can be found in Schork and Remington (2000) [5] and, on a more advanced level, in Westfall et al. (1999) [10].

If the shape of the underlying distribution cannot be assumed to be normal, a nonparametric approach may be used. The Kruskal-Wallis test is to the ANOVA as the Wilcoxon rank sum test is to the independent groups *t* test. That is, for the Kruskal-Wallis test, the original random variable is ranked across all *k* groups. The test statistic is the ratio of the variability in ranks among groups to the variability in ranks within groups. The null hypothesis for the Kruskal-Wallis test is that the groups have the same population distribution. If the null hypothesis is rejected, one would conclude the alternative hypothesis is true, that the population distributions are different, particularly for their location. The assumptions required for the use of the Kruskal-Wallis test are that the observations are independent, the samples are simple random samples from the populations of interest, and the variance is equal among the populations under the null hypothesis. The test statistic is evaluated using a chi-squared distribution, for which the shape (and therefore the critical region) is determined by the number of degrees of freedom $(k-1)$.

Many medical studies examine the proportion of subjects with a particular response, such as deaths, myocardial infarctions, or some risk factor for disease as the outcome of interest. The difference in proportions between two groups (e.g., represented by cases or controls in an observational study or treatment groups in a clinical trial) can be expressed as one proportion minus another, $p_1 - p_2$, or as a ratio of the two, $\frac{p_1}{p_2}$, a quantity called the relative risk. Data from studies with these kinds of outcomes are usually presented in the form of a table displaying the counts of subjects with and without the outcome of interest for each group.

Table 11.2 Number of events for subjects exposed and not exposed

		Exposed	Not exposed	
Workplace injury?	Yes	30	8	38
	No	70	132	202
		100	140	240

Data from a hypothetical cohort study are displayed in Table 11.2. In this study, patients with a confirmed diagnosis of a particular neurological condition ("exposed") and age- and sex-matched controls ("not exposed") were followed for a period of 1 year to ascertain the occurrence of workplace injuries.

Note that if the proportions of subjects between the groups were equal, the observed counts of subjects with each outcome (yes or no) would be distributed in equal proportion among the groups (exposed or not exposed). One method that can be used to test the hypothesis of equal proportions between two populations is the chi-squared test of homogeneity. The chi-squared test is an example of a goodness-of-fit test, for which the observed counts of subjects with and without the event are compared to the expected number of subjects with and without the event when no difference exists (or under the null hypothesis). For goodness-of-fit tests, the expected counts are obtained on the basis of an assumed model. In the case of the test of equal proportions, the expected counts would be obtained by applying the overall (across groups) proportion with response to each group's sample size. The test statistic for a chi-squared test is expressed as the ratio of the squared difference of the observed and expected counts (denoted by O and E, respectively) to the expected count for each cell and summed over all four cells (indexed below by j) of the table:

$$\chi^2 = \sum_{j=1}^{4} \frac{(O_j - E_j)^2}{E_j}$$

Squaring the deviations of observed counts from the expected ensures the difference is positive, which is required for a random variable from a chi-squared distribution. An alternative, mathematically equivalent, form of the test statistic is

$$\chi^2 = \frac{(\hat{p}_1 - \hat{p}_2)^2}{\left(\frac{1}{n_1} + \frac{1}{n_2}\right)\overline{p}(1-\overline{p})}$$

where $\hat{p}_1$ represents the sample proportion from group 1, $\hat{p}_2$ represents the sample proportion from group 2, and $\overline{p}$ is the overall proportion across the two groups.

In the case of a hypothesis test for two proportions, the null and alternative statistical hypotheses can be stated as follows:

$$H_0 : p_1 - p_2 = 0,\ H_A : p_1 - p_2 \neq 0$$

where the population proportions for each of two independent groups are represented by p_1 and p_2.

Under the null hypothesis, the test statistic has a chi-squared distribution with 1 degree of freedom. Therefore, the null hypothesis will be rejected if the test statistic is in the rejection region defined by $\chi^2 > \chi^2_{1-\alpha,1}$. Note that only large values of the test statistic contradict the null hypothesis. Therefore, the rejection region for the chi-squared test is represented by only the upper tail of the distribution. The chi-squared test is appropriate when the groups are independent, the outcomes are mutually exclusive, and most of the expected cell counts are at least five. The use of the chi-squared test is illustrated with the data from Table 11.2.

The null and alternative hypotheses concerning the proportion of subjects exposed and unexposed with workplace injuries are

$$H_0 : p_{\text{Exposed}} - p_{\text{Not Exposed}} = 0$$
$$H_A : p_{\text{Exposed}} - p_{\text{Not Exposed}} \neq 0$$

If the null hypothesis is true, the proportions of subjects with injuries would be equal. Therefore, the expected counts of subjects with events are calculated by applying the overall proportion of events to the sample size in each group. The expected number of events among exposed subjects is $\left(\frac{38}{240}\right)100 = 15.83$.

Similarly, the expected number of events among unexposed subjects is $\left(\frac{38}{240}\right)140 = 22.17$.

The expected numbers of subjects exposed and not exposed without the event is obtained by applying the overall proportion without event to the sample size in each group. The test statistic is then obtained as

$$\chi^2 = \frac{(30-15.83)^2}{15.83} + \frac{(8-22.17)^2}{22.17} + \frac{(70-84.17)^2}{84.17} + \frac{(132-117.83)^2}{117.83} = 25.817$$

For a test with α=0.05, the rejection region is defined as any value of the test statistic >3.84 (chi-squared distribution with 1 degree of freedom). Therefore, the null hypothesis is rejected with a conclusion that the proportion of exposed subjects with workplace injuries is greater than the proportion of age- and sex-matched unexposed subjects.

A confidence interval can also be constructed for the difference in two proportions. A two-sided $100(1-\alpha)\%$ confidence interval for the difference in sample proportions, $\hat{p}_1 - \hat{p}_2$, is given by

$$(\hat{p}_1 - \hat{p}_2) \pm z_{1-\alpha/2} SE(\hat{p}_1 - \hat{p}_2), \text{ where}$$

$$SE(\hat{p}_1 - \hat{p}_2) = \sqrt{\frac{\hat{p}_1(1-\hat{p}_1)}{n_1} + \frac{\hat{p}_2(1-\hat{p}_2)}{n_2}}$$

For this particular example, the corresponding 95% confidence interval is calculated as

$$(0.300 - 0.057) \pm 1.96\sqrt{\frac{(0.300)(0.700)}{100} + \frac{(0.057)(0.943)}{140}}$$
$$= 0.243 \pm 1.96(0.050) = (0.15, 0.34)$$

Since the hypothesized value of the difference in population proportions, zero, is outside of the calculated interval, this result is consistent with rejection of the null hypothesis.

The chi-squared test can be used in the instance when there are more than two groups (k>2) for

Table 11.3 Number of subjects with and without symptom pre- and postintervention

		Post		
		Yes	No	
Prior	Yes	a	b	$a+b$
	No	c	d	$c+d$
		$a+c$	$b+d$	n

which the proportions are compared. The test statistic is computed in the same manner as for the two groups case, except the test statistic is computed by summing over all $2k$ cells. In the more general case, under the null hypothesis of equal proportions across the k groups, the test statistic has a chi-squared distribution with $k-1$ degrees of freedom.

When the sample size requirements for the chi-squared test cannot be met due to small expected cell counts, an exact test is more appropriate. The fundamental concept of Fisher's exact test is that the margins of the table are considered fixed (e.g., count of subjects with and without events over all groups and the count of subjects in each group). Given the fixed margins, it is possible to specify all possible patterns of event counts. Then the exact probability of each pattern of counts of events is calculated using the hypergeometric distribution. The p value corresponding to the test is calculated exactly by summing the probabilities associated with all tables which have probabilities as small as, or smaller than, that for the observed table.

Medical studies involving assessment of the presence or absence of a characteristic in the same subjects before and after an intervention (e.g., negative or positive for a symptom before and after treatment) yield counts of paired observations, as shown in Table 11.3.

For assessment of whether the intervention had an effect on the response, McNemar's test can be used. The null and alternative hypotheses from such a study are

$$H_0 : p_{\text{Pre}} - p_{\text{Post}} = 0,\ H_A : p_{\text{Pre}} - p_{\text{Post}} \neq 0$$

If the intervention had no effect, the proportion with response would be the same prior to and postintervention, and therefore the marginal counts, (a+b) and (a+c), should be about equal. Therefore, the test statistic is calculated as

$$\chi^2 = \frac{(b-c)^2}{b+c}$$

and has a chi-squared distribution with 1 degree of freedom under the null hypothesis. A useful general reference that includes additional details about this test is Stokes, Davis, and Koch (2000) [11].

Statistical Issues in Diagnostic Testing and Screening

Tests which are used as an aid to diagnosing a disease are called diagnostic tests. An ideal diagnostic test would not identify a patient as positive for disease if she or he did not have it. Nor would an ideal diagnostic test fail to identify a patient as negative for disease if she or he did have it. The diagnostic accuracy of a new test is often compared to an existing gold standard test. For such studies, two samples of patients are selected: those who test positive for the disease using the gold standard test and those who test negative for the disease using the gold standard. All participants from both groups are subjected to the new test and the outcome, either test positive or test negative, is noted.

Two measures of diagnostic accuracy are sensitivity and specificity. Sensitivity is the probability that a subject who has the disease will test positive. Specificity is the probability that a subject who does not have the disease will test negative. If a diagnostic test does not have high sensitivity or specificity, it will be of limited use as important diagnoses will be missed in the former and unnecessary medical follow-up may result from the latter.

Many assays produce a quantitative result which must be interpreted as either negative or positive. Using different cutoff values for the result yields sensitivity and specificity for each one. Consider the use of the prostate-specific antigen (PSA) test as a diagnostic for prostate cancer. Higher values of PSA level (ng/mL) are more indicative of cancer. One may be interested in what specific value of PSA should be used to

Table 11.4 Sensitivity and specificity of PSA as a diagnostic for prostate cancer

PSA (ng/mL)	Sensitivity	Specificity
1.0	1.0	0.46
2.0	1.0	0.72
3.0	0.98	0.82
4.0	0.95	0.88
5.0	0.81	0.92
6.0	0.54	0.95
7.0	0.35	0.96
8.0	0.22	0.97
9.0	0.13	0.98
10.0	0.09	0.98
11.0	0.06	0.98
12.0	0.03	0.99
13.0	0.01	0.99
14.0	0.01	0.99
15.0	0.01	0.99

indicate a positive test result for cancer. To address this question, sensitivity and specificity are calculated for all possible cut points or thresholds. For example, a PSA≥2 can be interpreted as a positive test, and PSA<2 can be interpreted as a negative test. Using this criterion yields an estimate of sensitivity and specificity. When this is repeated for all possible cutoff values for PSA, it becomes evident that there is a tradeoff between sensitivity and specificity, as shown in Table 11.4. As seen in Table 11.4, nearly all patients with cancer have PSA≥2 (sensitivity of 1), but only three-fourths of patients without cancer have PSA<2 (specificity of 0.72).

The results obtained for multiple cutoff values can be plotted in a receiver operating characteristic (ROC) curve. For each cutoff, the value of sensitivity is plotted on the *y*-axis and the value of (1-specificity) is plotted on the *x*-axis. The value of the cutoff that is closest to the upper left quadrant (sensitivity of 1 and specificity of 1) is the cutoff that provides the greatest diagnostic accuracy. A ROC curve is displayed in Fig. 11.4 for the PSA data.

For this data set, a PSA value of 4.0 ng/mL is the cutoff that optimizes both sensitivity and specificity. Sensitivity and specificity can be interpreted as sample proportions for which confidence intervals can be constructed to estimate the precision of the sample estimate relative to the underlying population proportion. A two-sided $100(1-\alpha)\%$ confidence interval for a sample proportion $\hat{p}$ is

$$\hat{p} \pm z_{1-\alpha/2} SE(\hat{p}), \text{ where}$$

$$SE(\hat{p}) = \sqrt{\frac{\hat{p}(1-\hat{p})}{n}}$$

For example, an estimate of sensitivity of 0.95 among 100 study subjects would result in a 90% confidence interval for the population sensitivity of

$$0.95 \pm 1.64\sqrt{\frac{(0.95)(0.05)}{100}}$$
$$= 0.95 \pm 0.036 = (0.91, 0.99)$$

Apart from a test's accuracy relative to a gold standard diagnostic protocol, its ability to accurately screen for disease is of interest. The probability that a patient who tests positive for disease actually has the disease is called the positive predictive value. Similarly, the probability that a patient who tests negative for disease does not have disease is called the negative predictive value. Through the use of a mathematical expression called Bayes' theorem, it can be shown that the positive predictive value is a function of the sensitivity and specificity of the test and the underlying prevalence (expressed as a proportion) of disease in the population of interest:

$$\text{positive predictive value} = \frac{(\text{sensitivity})(\text{prevalence})}{(\text{sensitivity})(\text{prevalence}) + (1-\text{specificity})(1-\text{prevalence})}$$

The negative predictive value is also a function of these quantities. It is important to note that it is usually not appropriate to estimate the prevalence of disease from the same study used to define the diagnostic accuracy of the test since the two groups sampled (those who test positive and those who test negative) are typically not chosen at random from the population of interest. Estimates of

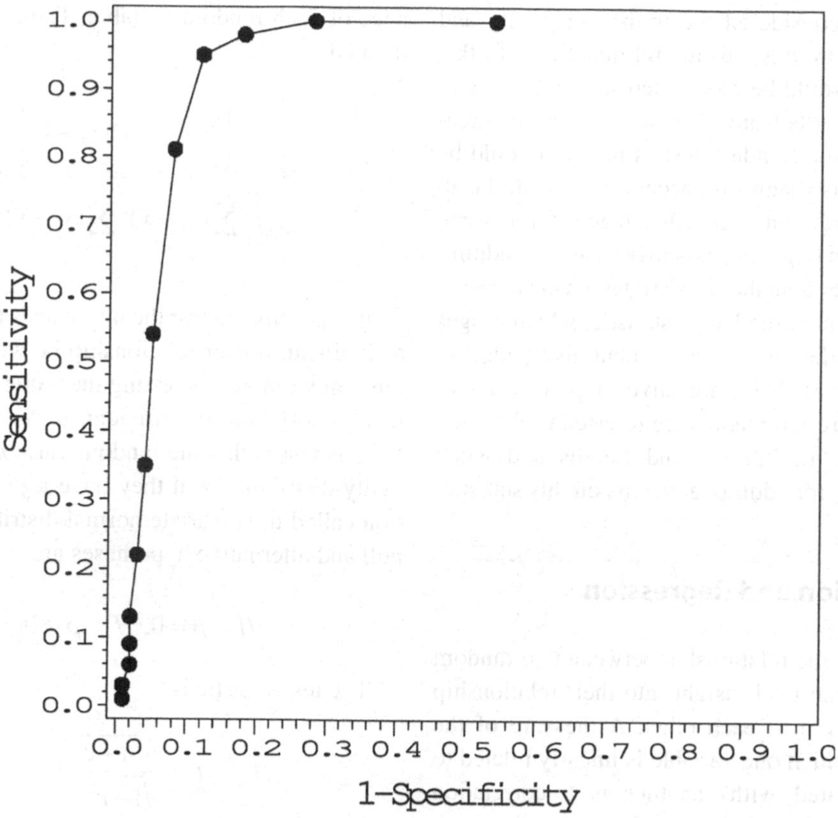

Fig. 11.4 Receiver operating characteristic curve for PSA levels

the prevalence of disease are more appropriately estimated from epidemiologic studies.

As an example, consider a test with sensitivity and specificity of 0.95 each. If the prevalence of the disease is 0.1 (a common disease), the positive predictive value is 0.68. However, if the prevalence of the disease is 0.05, 0.01, or 0.001, the positive predictive value is 0.5, 0.16, and 0.02, respectively. These results suggest that, despite high diagnostic accuracy, the use of a diagnostic test may not be informative. Secondly, this example is an illustration of how Bayes' theorem is used to combine prior information (in this case, the prevalence of disease) with newly collected data (a result from a diagnostic test with certain accuracy) to estimate the probability of disease given the test result. Confidence intervals about the positive predictive value and negative predictive value also can be calculated to assess the precision of the sample estimates.

Some methodological issues are worth mentioning for diagnostic studies. As described by Ransohoff and Feinstein (1978) [12], there are a number of biases that may be introduced that affect the results of assessments for sensitivity and specificity. When carrying out a study to assess the diagnostic accuracy of a test, it is important to select participants carefully, so they are similar to a population of patients for whom the test may ultimately be used. Failure to include an appropriately broad group of participants may lead to the so-called spectrum bias. Further, it is important to use the same gold standard diagnostic test among all participants. Lastly, carrying out the gold standard and test diagnoses separately can eliminate the possibility that one influences the other, thereby artificially inflating the estimates of diagnostic accuracy.

When the standard diagnostic test cannot be considered a gold standard (i.e., results from it cannot be considered the truth), sensitivity and specificity are not meaningful quantities. In this case, one would be more interested in the extent to which results from the new test were in agreement with the standard test. A new test could be helpful if its diagnostic accuracy was similar to the standard, but was advantageous for some other reason (e.g., less expensive, easier to administer, or safer than the standard test). One measure of agreement is the kappa statistic, which ranges from 0 (indicative of agreement likely due to chance alone) to 1 (indicative of perfect agreement). Interested readers are referred to Woolson and Clarke (2002) [6] and Landis and Koch (1977) [13] for additional details on this statistic.

Correlation and Regression

Describing the relationship between two random variables can lend insight into their relationship or association to each other. A measure of the extent to which one variable is linearly related to (or associated with) another is a correlation coefficient. Correlation coefficients can range from −1 to 1. Negative correlation coefficients imply that as values of one variable increase in value (e.g., displayed on the *x*-axis) values of the second variable (displayed on the *y*-axis) decrease in value. Similarly, positive correlation coefficients mean that as values of one variable increase in value, values of the second variable also increase in value. Correlations of −1 or 1 imply perfectly linear relationships. A correlation of 0 implies that there is no linear relationship between the two random variables. One significant limitation of correlation coefficients is that one random variable may be related mathematically to another, but has a small correlation coefficient because the relationship is not linear (e.g., as a quadratic function).

The Pearson correlation coefficient, for which the sample estimate is denoted by the symbol r, is appropriate when the random variables are continuous and approximately normally distributed. The Pearson correlation coefficient is a function of the extent to which the two random variables vary jointly (the covariance) as well as the variance of each random variable. The coefficient is defined as

$$r = \frac{\left\{\sum_{i=1}^{n}(x_i - \bar{x})(y_i - \bar{y})\right\}}{\sqrt{\left\{\sum_{i=1}^{n}(x_i - \bar{x})^2 \sum_{i=1}^{n}(y_i - \bar{y})^2\right\}}}$$

It is possible to test the hypothesis that there is a significant linear relationship between the two random variables by testing the value of the population correlation coefficient, ρ. An assumption for this test is that the random variables are normally distributed and they have a joint distribution called the bivariate normal distribution. The null and alternative hypotheses are

$$H_0 : \rho = 0,\ H_A : \rho \neq 0$$

The test statistic is

$$t = \frac{r\sqrt{n-2}}{\sqrt{1-r^2}}$$

which has a t distribution with $n-2$ degrees of freedom when the null hypothesis is true. If the null hypothesis is rejected, it is in favor of the alternative hypothesis that the correlation coefficient is not equal to zero, meaning there is a significant linear relationship between the two random variables. Confidence intervals for r are useful and can be obtained from statistical software. A note of caution is that cause and effect cannot be established solely on the basis of a statistical association.

When at least one of the random variables is not intervally scaled, but at least ordered (e.g., a rank or count variable), a nonparametric correlation coefficient is more appropriate. The Spearman rank correlation is computed by ranking both of the random variables and calculating the correlation coefficient on the ranks. For large sample sizes ($n > 30$), the hypothesis test of the Spearman rank correlation is based on a test statistic similar to that for the Pearson correlation coefficient.

A statistical method used to describe the relationship between an outcome (or dependent variable) and one or more independent or explanatory variables (considered fixed) is called regression. Regression techniques use observed data to estimate model coefficients for the explanatory variables that account for the variability in the response. The simplest example is linear regression for which the dependent variable, often denoted for regression as *Y*, is expressed as a linear function of one or more explanatory variables, denoted as *X* or X_1, X_2, etc.

A linear regression model with a single explanatory variable, called simple linear regression, is $y = \beta_0 + \beta_1 x + \varepsilon$. One can obtain estimates of the model parameters for the *y*-intercept (β_0) and the slope (β_1) by fitting a line to a set of observed data points (paired values of *x* and *y* for all subjects in the study). The assumptions required for the use of linear regression are that for fixed values of *X*, the distribution of *Y* is normal (with potentially different means across *X*) and the variance of *Y* is equal for all values of *X*. The estimates of the model parameters, $\hat{\beta}_0$ and $\hat{\beta}_1$, are used to predict values of *y* for given values of *x*. The resulting prediction equation is $\hat{y} = \hat{\beta}_0 + \hat{\beta}_1 x$. The interpretation of the slope coefficient is that for every unit change in *x*, the change in *y* is $\hat{\beta}_1$. For values of *x*, the difference between the actual and predicted values, $y - \hat{y}$, is called the residual because this difference represents the variability in the response that is remaining after fitting the model. The best fitting line is the one with the smallest sum of squared deviations between the observed and predicted values (i.e., smallest sum of squared residuals). Hence, the usual method to obtain the model estimates is called the method of least squares.

A hypothesis test may be used to test whether the value of the slope coefficient is different from zero. The corresponding hypotheses are

$$H_0 : \beta_1 = 0,\ H_A : \beta_1 \neq 0$$

If the null hypothesis is rejected, the appropriate conclusion is that there is a significant linear relationship between the independent variable and the dependent variable. The test statistic (and a corresponding confidence interval) for the slope coefficient use the standard error of the sample estimate, $se(\hat{\beta}_1)$. For the sake of brevity, the exact formulation of the standard error is not included in this chapter. The test statistic is defined as

$$t = \frac{\hat{\beta}_1}{se(\hat{\beta}_1)}$$

which follows a *t* distribution with $n-2$ degrees of freedom under the null hypothesis. Other references for this topic note that this *t*-statistic is identical to that used for testing the null hypothesis, $H_0 : \rho = 0$. Likewise, a $100(1-\alpha)\%$ confidence interval can be constructed as

$$\hat{\beta}_1 \pm t_{1-\alpha/2,n-2} se(\hat{\beta}_1)$$

Interested readers can find additional details in Schork and Remington (2000) [5].

In a prospective observational study of 202 adults between the ages of 20 and 60, triglycerides and other lipoproteins were tested over a period of several weeks. A linear regression model was fitted to the triglycerides levels as a function of age. The least squares estimates of the *y*-intercept and the slope yielded the following prediction equation:

$$triglycerides = 411.2 - 1.80\,age$$

So for every year increase in age, triglycerides were lower on average by 1.80 mg/dL. Likewise, for every 10-year increase in age, triglycerides were lower on average by 18 mg/dL. A test of the slope coefficient for age based on the *t* distribution is rejected at the α=0.05 level, indicating a significant linear relationship (negatively associated) between triglycerides and age. Kleinbaum et al. (1998) [14] have written a helpful reference for linear regression.

Survival Analysis and Logistic Regression

In many studies, subjects do not participate for the planned length of observation. When researchers are interested in the occurrence of a particular event or not (e.g., death, occurrence of a disease or condition, or onset of a symptom), the outcome

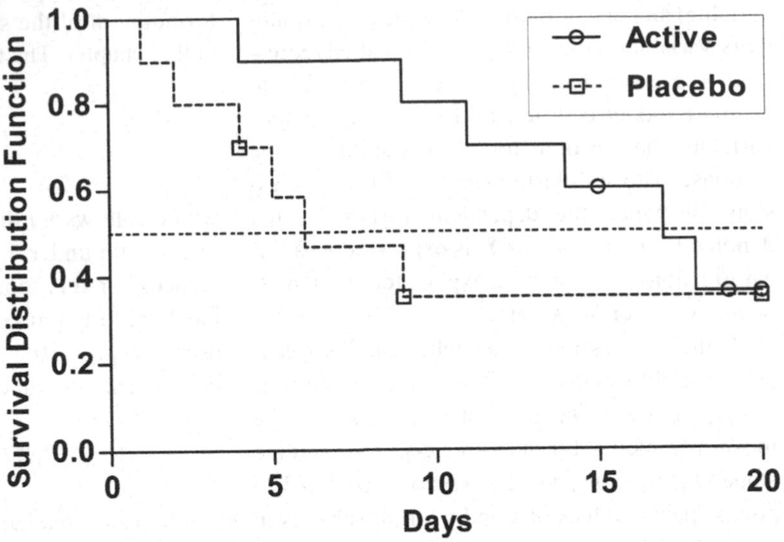

Fig. 11.5 Kaplan-Meier estimate of the survival distribution for unfavorable outcome from a clinical trial

may or may not occur during the period of observation. It is often desirable to utilize the experience of subjects for the time they were under investigation, whether or not they had the outcome of interest. Consider a study of subjects who were newly diagnosed with a fatal disease. One may be interested in the death rate for the 5 years following diagnosis. Some subjects who enter such a study will die while under observation, some will survive the 5-year observation period, and some will withdraw from the study during the middle of the observation period with a last known status of alive. Among subjects who will eventually have the outcome of interest, the occurrence may not be during the period of observation. These subjects are said to be censored at the last known observation time.

Survival analyses are used when the outcome of interest is a binary outcome (event or not), and it is desirable to account for the time subjects are at risk for the event. The survival function, denoted *S(t)*, describes the probability that a subject in the study will survive without having the event past a time, *t*. For example, *S*(1 year) is the probability subjects will survive past year 1 without the event. There are a number of statistical techniques used to describe and make inferences about the survival distribution.

One common method is Kaplan-Meier estimation of the survival function. The Kaplan-Meier estimate is constructed by calculating the conditional probability of subjects surviving a time interval (e.g., year 1–2) conditional on surviving all previous time intervals (e.g., year 0–1). Subjects who have the event or drop out prior to the time interval are not included in the risk set (i.e., they are no longer at risk) for that time interval and subsequent time intervals. The probability of surviving past a given time is calculated as the product of the probability of surviving the interval among those at risk and the probability of surviving all other previous time intervals. The survival function from the Kaplan-Meier estimate is often depicted graphically as shown in Fig. 11.5 for an unfavorable outcome.

The Kaplan-Meier estimate is a step function according to the shape of the distribution. One can read off values of the survival function for a value of *X*, as follows. In this figure, the survival distribution is plotted against time (days since start of treatment in a clinical trial). In the placebo group on Day 1, the estimate is 0.9, and then it drops down to 0.8 on Day 2. An important property of the step function defined using discrete event times is that it is a discontinuous function (i.e., not defined) between event times.

For example, the survival distribution function for the placebo group equals 0.46 on Days 6, 7, and 8 (no events occurred), and then at Day 9, the estimate is 0.35. Looking at the Kaplan-Meier curve for the placebo group, one could read Day 9 as having an estimate of 0.35 or 0.46, but it is appropriate to remember that the outside edge of the step (right at Day 9) is discontinuous, and thus the estimated probability of survival for Day 9 or later is 0.35.

A commonly cited measure of central tendency from the Kaplan-Meier estimate is the median survival time. The median survival time is the value of t beyond which approximately 50% of subjects survive without the event, i.e., $S(\text{median time } t)=0.5$. Using this guideline, one can read off the median survival times by drawing a reference line across the figure at $S(t)=0.50$ and finding the earliest value of time on the curve below the reference line. The median times are 6 and 16 days for the placebo and active groups, respectively.

Cohort studies or clinical trials may have the comparison of survival distributions between two or more groups as an objective. This can be accomplished through the use of the logrank test. The logrank test is carried out by treating each distinct event time as a stratum, calculating contributions to a chi-squared test statistic within each stratum, and combining over the strata. The null hypothesis is that the survival distributions are the same. Under the null hypothesis, the expected counts of events would be expected to be similar to observed counterparts across the groups being compared. Therefore, large deviations between the observed and expected counts at a number of event times will lead to a large value of the logrank test statistic. The resulting test statistic from the logrank test is distributed as a chi-squared statistic with 1 degree of freedom. If the null hypothesis is rejected, the conclusion is that the survival distributions did not arise from the same population.

A second analysis approach used with censored data is called Cox regression. For Cox regression, the outcome is not the probability of survival but the hazard, defined loosely as the risk of the event in a small interval of time. The hazard is modeled as a function of one or more explanatory variables (e.g., age, treatment in a clinical trial, baseline severity status). The contrast between the simple linear regression model and the Cox regression model is important to understand, as the model coefficients are interpreted differently in the two cases. The Cox regression models the hazard (y) as a function of a single explanatory variable x and is given by

$$y = \beta_0 e^{\beta_1 x}$$

The term β_0 can be thought of as the baseline hazard for a reference group represented by $X=0$. If the explanatory variable X is dichotomous (e.g., 1=hypertensive vs. 0=normotensive), the baseline hazard represents the hazard for normotensive patients. That is, $X=0$ implies $y = \beta_0$. Note that when $X=1$, $y = \beta_0 e^{\beta_1}$. The ratio of these two, e^{β_1}, is called the hazard ratio, which can be thought of as the relative risk of the event for hypertensive patients compared to normotensive patients. When the explanatory variable, X, is continuous, the hazard ratio corresponds to the multiplicative increase in hazard associated with a one-unit change in X. Since the hazard for many events does not change with small increments in the explanatory variable, it is often helpful to recode or rescale the explanatory variable. The Cox regression model can be extended to include multiple explanatory variables. An important assumption for the model is that the contribution of the explanatory variable(s) has a constant multiplicative effect on the hazard over time. This is often referred to as the proportional hazards assumption.

As with simple linear regression, fitting the model results in estimates of each of the coefficients and corresponding standard errors. Exponentiation of the coefficient estimates for an explanatory variable results in a hazard ratio expressing the increase in risk for one value of the explanatory variable compared to another while adjusting for other explanatory variables in the model. Confidence intervals and tests for the coefficients can be constructed which can be transformed to confidence intervals and tests for the hazard ratio. Care must be taken to code the model correctly so the interpretation can be made with respect to a meaningful reference group (or baseline hazard group) and not an arbitrary one. Cox models can be particularly helpful in observational studies since the primary interest is typically in one experimental factor (exposed or not) while controlling for other potential explanatory effects for the response. An introduction to this topic can be found in a text by Woolson and Clark (2002) [6]. A reference at a more advanced level has been written by Lee (1992) [15].

A technique called logistic regression is helpful when the outcome of interest is dichotomous (e.g., death, seroconversion), and the research objective is to describe how the probability of the outcome is related to one or more explanatory variables without accounting for the time at risk. Instead of modeling the probability of outcome as a linear function of explanatory variables, the log odds of the outcome is the dependent variable, where the odds is defined as $\frac{p}{1-p}$, the probability of outcome divided by the probability of no outcome. The reason for this choice is that a probability is bounded by 0 and 1, whereas the log odds or logit, $\ln\left(\frac{p}{1-p}\right)$, is continuous on the scale from negative to positive infinity. The logistic model with a single independent variable is specified as

$$\ln\left(\frac{p}{1-p}\right) \equiv y = \beta_0 + \beta_1 x$$

Model estimates can be interpreted in a manner similar to that described for the Cox regression model. If X is a dichotomous variable (e.g., gender), the predicted value $\hat{y} = \hat{\beta}_0$ is the log odds of the event for a reference group with $x=0$. When $x=1$, the predicted value $\hat{y} = \hat{\beta}_0 + \hat{\beta}_1$ is the log odds of the event for the group with $x=1$. The difference of these two is the log odds ratio, $\hat{\beta}_1$. Exponentiation of the log odds ratio results in the odds ratio, $e^{\hat{\beta}_1}$, which is an estimate of the relative risk of the event for subjects with $x=1$ compared to those with $x=0$. Logistic regression models can be extended to multiple explanatory variables (either categorical or continuous). When an explanatory variable is continuous, the odds ratio is interpreted relative to a unit change in x. For example, in a logistic model of coronary heart disease as a function of LDL cholesterol, an odds ratio of 1.02 means that a patient with LDL of 130 has greater risk of developing CHD in terms of a 1.02^{10} times greater odds and thereby greater risk of developing CHD than a patient with LDL of 120. Standard errors for the estimates may be used in the construction of confidence intervals for the odds ratio. Thus, the precision of the sample estimate can be evaluated, and tests of the hypotheses can be carried out to determine if an explanatory variable is significantly associated with increased risk of the outcome or event. Excellent references for logistic regression include Kleinbaum and Klein (2002) [16], Stokes et al. (2000) [11], and Hosmer and Lemeshow (2000) [17].

Summary

This chapter has served as an introduction to statistical methods in medical research. Descriptive statistics were discussed and are commonly used to characterize the experience of study subjects and their background characteristics. Inferential statistical methods, such as confidence intervals and hypothesis testing, are frequently used to evaluate observed associations relative to chance variation in the sampling process. The research process begins with a research question that motivates a study designed to answer the question for which relevant data are collected. The involvement of statistics ideally begins at the start of the research process and concludes with the final interpretation of the analyses. Further study of these topics is encouraged so that readers may enhance their abilities to interpret results of published medical literature.

Take-Home Points

- Descriptive statistics are used to summarize individual observations from a study and estimate a typical value (measures of central tendency) and the spread of values (measures of dispersion). Measures of central tendency include the mean and median. Measures of dispersion include the standard deviation and the range.
- Hypothesis tests and confidence intervals are two general forms of inferential statistical methods, for which the aim is to make an inference from a sample of subjects to a relevant population.
- Confidence intervals represent a plausible range of values of for a population parameter, such as the difference in mean response, the difference in proportions, or the relative risk.
- *p* values are reported from hypothesis tests. Small *p* values (e.g., <0.05) suggest that the observed result was unlikely to have occurred by chance alone.
- There are many statistical methods which may be appropriate for any given research study. The most appropriate statistical approaches must consider the research question and the study design.

References

1. Senn S. Dicing with death: chance, risk, and health. Cambridge: Cambridge University Press; 2003.
2. Campbell MJ, Machin D, Walters SJ. Medical statistics: a textbook for the health sciences. 4th ed. Chichester: Wiley; 2007.
3. Durham TA, Turner JR. Introduction to statistics in pharmaceutical clinical trials. London: Pharmaceutical Press; 2008.
4. Bowers D, House A, Owens D. Understanding clinical papers. 2nd ed. Chichester: Wiley; 2006.
5. Schork MA, Remington RD. Statistics with applications to the biological and health sciences. Upper Saddle River: Prentice-Hall; 2000.
6. Woolson RF, Clarke WR. Statistical methods for the analysis of biomedical data. 2nd ed. New York: Wiley; 2002.
7. Cohen J. A power primer. Psychological bulletin. 1992;112:155–9.
8. Chow S-C, Liu J-P. Design and analysis of clinical trials. 2nd ed. Hoboken: Wiley; 2004.
9. LaVange LM, Koch GG. Rank score tests. Circulation. 2006;114:2528–33.
10. Westfall PH, Tobias RD, Rom D, Wolfinger RD, Hochberg Y. Multiple comparisons and multiple tests using SAS®. Cary: SAS Institute, Inc.; 1999.
11. Stokes ME, Davis CS, Koch GG. Categorical data analysis using the SAS® system. 2nd ed. Cary: SAS Institute Inc.; 2009.
12. Ransohoff DF, Feinstein AR. Problems of spectrum and bias in evaluating the efficacy of diagnostic tests. N Engl J Med. 1978;299:926–30.
13. Landis JR, Koch GG. The measurement of observer agreement for categorical data. Biometrics. 1977; 33:159–74.
14. Kleinbaum DG, Kupper LL, Muller KE, Nizam A. Applied regression analysis and other multivariable methods. 3rd ed. Pacific Grove: Duxbury Press; 1998.
15. Lee ET. Statistical methods for survival data analysis. 2nd ed. New York: Wiley; 1992.
16. Kleinbaum DG, Klein M. Logistic regression: a self-learning text. 2nd ed. New York: Springer; 2002.
17. Hosmer DW, Lemeshow S. Applied logistic regression. 2nd ed. New York: Wiley; 2000.

Ethical Issues in Clinical Research 12

Eli A. Friedman

Introduction

For more than four millennia, professionals involved in human medical examination and research have pondered the boundaries for responsible patient care, and many have questioned the ethical limits of human subjects research. The goals of this chapter are to:

- Briefly review the historical background of contemporary research ethics
- Elucidate the ethical issues to be considered when constructing human research studies
- Provide workable definitions and guidelines governing benefits and risks involved in human subjects research.

A study "benefit" is a positive effect gained from participating in a research study that might accrue in an individual, such as obtaining a better therapeutic outcome (e.g., life extension, morbidity reduction) or a less tangible advantage such as learning that a medical treatment might reduce the need for a more invasive procedure or improve quality of life in a specific patient. The "risks" of a study, particularly one examining the impact of a purposively applied intervention, may range from a minor skin rash to a major complication such as liver failure, stroke, and even death. Even with purely observational studies, risks to patient privacy (especially the potential loss of that privacy) must always be carefully considered while preparing and subsequently performing an investigation. Risks to the subject are always weighed relative to the probability of benefit (both to the subject and to society in general).

For any research study, the benefits and risks can never be known ahead of time, nor can the effects be fully determined before investigation is finished. (Indeed, if they could be known beforehand, there would be no need for a study to take place.) While seemingly obvious, this precept should be a conscious pragmatic reality for all clinical researchers so that necessary discretion is followed prior to drawing important conclusions. Even when preliminary anecdotal information is suggestive or prior animal studies appear to support a hypothesis related to disease processes or treatment outcomes in humans, clinical circumstance or results obtained in an animal model of a disease may not translate into solid evidence for human clinical practice. As an illustration of the limits of preclinical investigation, in a study conducted by this author in the late 1990s [1], treatment with agents that block the enzyme aldose reductase effectively halted progression of diabetic retinopathy and nephropathy in induced diabetic rats but was of minimal to no value when tested in diabetic humans.

E.A. Friedman, MD (✉)
Department of Medicine, Sate University of New York, Downstate Medical Center, Brooklyn, NY 11203, USA
e-mail: elifriedmn@aol.com

P.G. Supino and J.S. Borer (eds.), *Principles of Research Methodology: A Guide for Clinical Investigators*, DOI 10.1007/978-1-4614-3360-6_12,

Background: Recognition and Introduction of an Ethics Base in Medicine

For the purposes of this chapter, the following discussion on medical ethics will focus primarily on clinical research involving human subjects. With that said, the contemporary notion that the "individual" is inherently valuable, and as such should be protected by policies that regulate human investigation, is derived from a sense of humanism evidently valued long before the enactment of twentieth century legislation. Thus, in order to provide context for the contemporary state of ethics in human investigation, this section will provide a brief introduction to some historical figures and influential schools of thought that helped to shape the vast field of modern-day health care. We find evidence of attention to medical ethics and the nature of the relationship between practitioner and patient in prominent ancient civilizations, such as early Chinese and Greek cultures.

Many of the principles of medical ethics that arose from these two cultures can be traced to the teachings of two renowned historical figures: Confucius and Hippocrates. Confucius was a Chinese thinker and educator of the fifth century B.C., while Hippocrates lived in ancient Greece in the fourth century B.C., practicing as a physician and providing instruction on "the art of medicine" [2].

Central to Confucianism, the ideology based on the teachings of Confucius, is the "*chun-tze*," the morally ideal person. Confucius' concept of persons, according to his theories of *chun-tze*, gives a two-dimensional approach to life: the "autonomous person" and the "relational person" [3]. Rather than promulgating a universal code of behavioral guidelines, Confucius proposed that each person subject himself to self-examination. Accordingly, physicians following Confucian teachings practiced self-cultivation through self-examination, self-criticism, and self-restriction. At the same time, a significant aspect of personhood is based on the individual's interpersonal relationships. This is the "relational" aspect of personhood, from which it follows that the "humaneness" (*jen*) one must attain in striving toward *chun-tze* can only be achieved through interaction with other individuals [3]. Thus, according to Confucianism, physicians are in the position of striving for *chun-tze* and humaneness on a personal level but, as doctors, they help others to maintain balance in the autonomous and relational aspects of their lives. Daniel Fu-Chang Tsai [4] evaluated the vast teachings of ancient Chinese medical ethics that Confucianism has engendered. The principles that he identified as common threads throughout the various teachings and texts from this school of thought are given in Table 12.1.

Table 12.1 Central principles of ancient Chinese medical ethics

"To appreciate the value of life and practise medicine with a heart of compassion and humaneness
To master Confucianism prior to learning medicine
To master medical knowledge by studying reliable sources diligently and extensively
To improve clinical skill and maintain a high professional standard
To be frugal, not to be greedy for wealth and fame
To treat patients equally, and as if they were your family
To be sincere, decorous, devoted, absorbed and selfless in treating patients
To treat female patients only in the presence of an attendant; respecting their confidentiality, and not being lustful
To be modest and prudent toward other physicians, not to belittle and criticize one's colleagues" [4]

Hippocrates (460 B.C.) became one of the most well-known ancient scientists for formally favoring constraints on physician behavior [5]. His credo for neophyte physicians, known as *The Hippocratic Oath*, requires practitioners to follow a system of guidelines that ultimately benefits patients while abstaining from any actions that are mischievous or would not be in the patient's best interest; various versions of this oath currently exist [6, 7], and to this day, one version or another is recited throughout the world by new physicians. Conflicting interpretations of this oath are evident when physicians defend their

Table 12.2 Early unregulated human research efforts: An incomplete chronology

1845–1949:	Dr. J. Marion Sims performs a series of experimental gynecological operations without anesthesia on enslaved African-American women [15]
1874:	Dr. Roberts Bartholow inserts needle electrodes into the exposed brain of a "feeble-minded" servant woman as part of a series of experiments in cerebral localization [16]
1895:	Dr. Henry Heiman infects two "idiot" boys with gonorrhea to investigate the causative agents of the disease [17]
1896:	Dr. Arthur Wentworth withdraws spinal fluid from 29 hospitalized children to determine the effectiveness of "spinal tapping" [18]
1906:	Dr. Richard P. Strong, researching vaccines for tropical diseases in the Philippines, injects inmates at a Manila prison with cholera, 13 of whom later die [19, 20]
1908:	Three Philadelphia physicians infect children at the St. Vincent's Home orphanage with tuberculin in order to compare the effectiveness of several diagnostic tests [18]
1918–1922:	Dr. Leo Stanley subcutaneously injects over 600 inmates at San Quentin prison with animal testicular tissue while researching a "cure" for criminality [19, 20]
1914:	Dr. Joseph Goldberger, in an effort to prove that pellagra is caused by nutritional deficiencies, induces the disease in a dozen Mississippi inmates, denying their requests to be removed from the study [19, 20]
1921:	Dr. Alfred F. Hess, studying the effect of varying dietary factors on the development of disease, withholds orange juice from infants until they show the characteristic hemorrhages of scurvy [18]
1931:	Dr. Cornelius Rhoads, studying hookworm and tropical sprue anemia in Puerto Rico, "transplants cancer" in several human subjects (killing eight) after writing in a confidential note to a colleague that the entire population should be "exterminated" [21]

treatment decisions on the basis of perceived ethical obligation to never cause the death of any patient. Contrary to this view is the belief that a physician holds an ethical obligation to relieve pain even if the patient dies as a consequence of the advocated treatment. (One of the most widely known modern examples includes the views of Dr. Jack Kevorkian [8–11]).

It was Celsus, a Roman encyclopedist, who is thought to have been the first to consider the rights of subjects under experimentation [12]. He spoke strongly against procedures such as vivisection on condemned criminals in Egypt, calling physicians who performed them "assassinating medical practitioners" [13]. Though it certainly is the case that both the ethics regarding human subjects research and regulations for such research have evolved substantially since the time of Celsus, his belief that medical practice should be a "work of mercy" as opposed to one of "dire cruelty" laid the ethical foundation for human subjects research long ago, eventually becoming the moral standard by which such research is judged today.

One would be hard-pressed to challenge the influence of Confucius and Hippocrates on modern-day medicine. More than 2,000 years have passed since their deaths, dynasties have risen and fallen, and religious figures, revolutions, and explorations have led to vast changes in virtually every aspect of civilization. Yet, as noted above, to this day, most graduating medical students in the United States of America (USA), Canada, and in certain other parts of the world recite some form of the Hippocratic Oath, and current US federal legislation incorporates principles identified by Confucianism as central to the practice of medicine. Thus, society continues to acknowledge the importance and relevance of the ancient Greek and ancient Chinese teachings on medical ethics, both of which championed one particular concept above all others: the veneration of human life, today termed "benevolence." From Hippocrates forward, all guides to the ethical practice of medicine included this concept [14]. Although benevolence in medicine implies that physicians should do everything in their power to ensure no harm is done to the patient, hundreds of incidents, as sampled in Table 12.2 [15–21], reflect efforts to exploit availability of prisoners, slaves, impoverished adults, and even children in sometimes lethal medical investigations prior to the establishment of regulatory boundaries for human subjects studies.

For the majority of cases referenced in Table 12.2, informed consent was obtained neither from the adult subjects nor the parents of the children. Furthermore, for the cases in which consent was obtained, the subjects were either mentally limited individuals without a proxy or prisoners promised pardon for participation in research. As reflected by the chronology of the table, abuses of "patients" by their "doctors" existed long before Germany invaded Poland, initiating World War II in 1939. In fact, it was German governmental regulations in 1931 that first promulgated a code for conducting human investigation in what was termed the *Reich Health Council Regulations of 1931* [22]. This document (obviously ignored by Adolph Hitler, throughout his 11-year Third Reich) consisted of 14 points demanding complete responsibility of the medical profession, including informed consent and risk-benefit analysis for human medical research experimentation. Included were technical and ethical standards for maintaining written records describing the justification for studying vulnerable populations.

The Post-WWII Evolution of Ethical Policies for Human Subjects Research

Many scholars trace modern concerns about the unethical treatment of "patients" to the findings of the Nuremberg Military Tribunal (also known as the "Doctors Trial"), which followed sadistic unscientific "research" involving forced human exposure to the effects of freezing, incendiary devices, mustard gas, and other experimental atrocities performed under Nazi Germany during World War II. Of 23 Nazi doctors and scientists tried for the murder of concentration camp inmates who were used as research subjects, 15 were convicted (7 were condemned to death by hanging, while 8 received prison sentences from 10 years to life [23]). An outgrowth of the judgment and sentences handed down at the trial was an outline of required elements for conducting research with humans, collectively known as the Nuremberg Code [24, 25] (Table 12.3) which currently is recognized as the most important document in contemporary human subjects research ethics. Table 12.3 lists the elements of the code.

As the eyes of the world focused on the activities in Nuremberg in the 1940s, events

Table 12.3 The Nuremberg Code of 1947

1. "The voluntary consent of the human subject is absolutely essential.
2. The experiment should be such as to yield fruitful results for the good of society, unprocurable by other methods or means of study, and not random and unnecessary in nature.
3. The experiments should be so designed and based on the results of animal experimentation and knowledge of the natural history of the disease or other problem under study that the anticipated results will justify the performance of the experiment.
4. The experiment should be so conducted as to avoid all unnecessary physical and mental suffering and injury.
5. No experiment should be conducted where there is a prior reason to believe that death or disabling injury will occur, except perhaps, in those experiments where the experimental physicians also serve as subject.
6. The degree of risk to be taken should never exceed that determined by the humanitarian importance of the problem to be solved by the experiment.
7. Proper preparations should be made and adequate facilities provided to protect the experimental subject against even remote possibilities of injury, disability or death.
8. The experiment should be conducted only by scientifically qualified persons. The highest degree of skill and care should be required through all stages of the experiment of those who conduct or engage in the experiment.
9. During the course of the experiment the human subject should be at liberty to bring the experiment to an end if he has reached the physical or mental state where continuation of the experiment seems to him to be impossible.
10. During the course of the experiment the scientist in charge must be prepared to terminate the experiment at any stage, if he has probable cause to believe, in the exercise of the good faith, superior skill, and careful judgment required of him, that a continuation of the experiment is likely to result in injury, disability, or death to the experimental subject" [25].

concurrently unfolding and earning publicity in the USA were slowly beginning to draw audible concern from the American public, government officials, and professionals in various fields regarding the ethical nature of human subjects research being conducted domestically. Criticism followed a paper published in 1936 on the "Tuskegee Study of Untreated Syphilis in the Negro Male," a research project initiated by the US Public Health Service in conjunction with the Tuskegee Institute in 1932. The purpose of the study was to investigate the effects of untreated syphilis [26]. Six hundred black males in Macon County, Al., approximately two thirds with syphilis, were enrolled in the program under the premise that they were to be treated for what was at the time colloquially termed "bad blood" [27]. This vague term was used to refer to a number of ailments, including syphilis. As critics charged, treatment was withheld from the men in the study even after treatment with penicillin was accepted as the standard of care for syphilis in 1945; unwitting subjects were led to believe they were being treated. Despite eliciting concern as early as 1936, the study remained in progress until 1972. In fact, it took 30 years from that first Tuskegee publication for the movement toward evaluating ethical practices in human subjects research to gain any truly sustained momentum on a national level.

Internationally, discussions on the ethics of human experimentation continued following the Nuremberg proceedings. The World Medical Association (WMA) prominently adopted the Declaration of Helsinki in 1964 to serve as a guide for regulating human subjects research. Though ratified by multiple WMA General Assemblies, most recently in October 2008, the wide-ranging principles and policies of the Declaration of Helsinki (spanning fundamentals of ethical recruitment of study subjects, to principles of good study design, to essential elements of a research protocol, to ethical considerations in publication of the results of the research) remain active to this day [28].

The worldwide presentation of these principles may have helped prominent Harvard-trained anesthesiologist Henry K. Beecher, M.D., to capture the attention of members of the medical and science communities in the USA to whom he had attempted to voice his concerns about the ethical nature of human subjects research since the late 1950s. Beecher, at one point the anesthesiologist-in-chief at Massachusetts General Hospital, was a renowned researcher in his own right, a significant factor contributing to his concern about the ethical quality of research practices [29]. As David J. Rothman described, "Beecher's sharpest fear was that research of dubious ethicality might impugn the legitimacy of experimentation, discrediting the prime force bringing progress to medicine" [30].

Though Beecher's 1959 *JAMA* publication, "Experimentation in Man," did not achieve the reverberating impact for which he had hoped, a 1965 speech that he gave to an audience of journalists invited by the Upjohn Pharmaceutical Company had a far more tangible influence on ethical human subjects research discourse in the USA. Beecher's revelations of ethical misconduct and his assertion that such questionable activities were being conducted at leading medical schools, medical centers, even in the military, caused enough of a stir among his audience to spark dramatic headlines throughout the nation, such as the Boston Globe's "Are humans used as guinea pigs not told?" As one might expect, Beecher faced a strong backlash from colleagues who felt as though he had "violated professional etiquette" [29] by discussing his concerns and in such a public manner. Despite the hostile response, Beecher continued to push the issue.

In 1966, the *New England Journal of Medicine* published a paper, "Ethics and Clinical Research," by Beecher in which he reported his survey of 22 published medical studies documenting exposure of subjects to substantive risks without their knowledge or approval [31]. Of note, these studies were conducted at some of this country's most prestigious institutions, gaining publication in highly prestigious journals. Examples of investigator misdirection and/or abuse of their study patients included:

- Performing heart catheterizations in patients who believed that they were to have bronchoscopy
- Assigning patients with life-threatening diseases to placebo control groups, where effective treatments were known to be available
- Randomizing US soldiers suffering from streptococcal pharyngitis to penicillin versus treatments known to be ineffective.

While Beecher's article drew attention in its own right, his crusade gained remarkable steam through the publicity generated by a 1972 *New York Times* article. Whistleblower Peter Buxton revealed the shocking truths behind the Tuskegee study to the paper, which subsequently published "Syphilis Victims in US Study Went Untreated for 40 Years" as its front-page headline on July 26, 1972 [32]. When the study was terminated in 1972, congressional hearings were held to address the matter of ethical conduct in human investigation.

The National Research Act of 1974 was passed in the USA as a direct response to these above-mentioned ethical abuses (especially the revelation of the Tuskegee experiment) [33]. Through the act, congress called for the establishment of the *National Commission for the Protection of Human Subjects of Biomedical and Behavioral Research* [34], which was charged with the tasks of identifying key ethical issues to be addressed by researchers and injecting clear ethical practices into human subjects research that would help assure the public of the safety of medical research and avoid future atrocities. Following Beecher's disturbing portrayal of extreme overriding of patient rights in medical investigation by US investigators and the rules established by the 1974 Research Act, additional reports were published that recounted instances of exposing subjects, without their consent, to radiation, infectious agents, or injection of cancer cells. Of the responses generated, perhaps the single most important resource used as a basis for governing both the practice of medicine and conduct of research involving human subjects was *The Belmont Report* [35], released by the commission in 1979, which established:

- Boundaries between clinical practice and otherwise unneeded research
- Basic ethical principles to be preserved during all research studies (respect for persons, beneficence, and justice)
- Fundamental applications (guidelines for informed consent, assessment of risk and benefits, and selection of subjects).

Notably, we find that *The Belmont Report* [35]—a document created late in the twentieth century in a highly developed Western nation—presents morality-driven guidelines similar to those of ancient Confucian ideology and Hippocrates. In "Part B: Basic Ethical Principles" of the report, "respect for persons" asserts the importance of respecting an individual's autonomy and protecting those persons with diminished autonomy, "beneficence" requires that actions do not cause harm and that treatments aim to maximize potential benefit while minimizing risks, and "justice" entails considering various factors in determining the "fairness in distribution" with regard to the benefits and risks of human subjects research.

In the decades both leading up to and following the release of the *Belmont Report,* the USA undertook a substantial review and overhaul of federal regulations in human subjects research. A chronology of key events is provided in Table 12.4.

The Genesis of Institutional Review Boards in the USA and Their Regulatory Role

With the guidance of *The Belmont Report*, the US Department of Health, Education, and Welfare (now the Department of Health and Human Services [HHS]) established requirements for the development of Institutional Review Boards or IRBs [36]. ("IRB" is a generic term used by governmental agencies, but each institution that establishes an IRB may maintain any name to describe such a board.) As a general rule, the role of the IRB is to regulate human subjects research by advocating, upholding, and maintaining the

Table 12.4 Post-World War II developments aimed at protecting human subjects in research

1947:	*Nuremberg Code* defines subject-centered principles for ethical human subjects research in response to unethical medical experimentation by the Nazi's during WWII [25].
1964:	World Medical Association adopts the *Declaration of Helsinki,* defining new guidelines for human subjects was an outline of required research (last revised in October 2008) [28].
1965:	A speech addressing problems in clinical research is given by *Henry Beecher, M.D.,* to journalists assembled by the Upjohn Pharmaceutical Company and draws attention nationwide through prominent media outlets [29].
1966:	*Henry Beecher M.D.* publishes "Ethics and clinical research" in The New England Journal of Medicine, expressing concern over the potentially vast impact of unethical procedures in clinical research, and referencing 22 studies without explicitly identifying the studies or investigators [30].
1972:	Tuskegee whistleblower Peter Buxtin contacts the Associated Press with information on the study, leading to *The New York Times* July 26, 1972, article, "Syphilis Victims in U.S. Study Went Untreated for 40 years; Syphilis Victims Got No Therapy"; the study is terminated that same year [32].
1973:	Congressional hearings are held to address human experimentation primarily in response to the Tuskegee revelations [33].
1974:	The *National Research Act* is created, establishing the *National Commission for the Protection of Human Subjects of Biomedical and Behavioral Research* [34].
1979:	The Commission releases *The Belmont Report,* identifying relevant ethical principles and guidelines for human subjects research [35].
1981:	Human subject regulations are amended to provide a common framework within which Institutional Review Boards (IRBs) can review human subjects research [36].
1991:	Regulations for the protection of human subjects are codified under Title 45, Part 46 of the Code of Federal Regulations; Subpart A is accepted by 17 US Federal Agencies as "*the Common Rule*" [38].

rights and welfare of humans participating in research. IRBs are universally engaged in all health and social science studies funded by the National Institutes of Health (NIH) and HHS. Such studies include, but are not limited to, clinical trials of new, novel, or repurposed devices or drugs regulated by the Food and Drug Administration (FDA); investigations of behavior, opinions, and attitudes; or studies on health-care management.

In 1991, the US Federal Policy for the Protection of Human Subjects was published in the Federal Register (56 FR 28003) and incorporated into the regulating codes of 17 Federal departments [37]. The policy, known as the "Common Rule," provides specific direction for the operations and regulation of IRBs, outlines requirements for obtaining informed consent, and requires written assurance of institutional compliance with federal research regulations. The policy was codified by HHS as Title 45 Code of Federal Regulations [CFR] Part 46 Subpart A, "Basic HHS Policy for Protection of Human Research Subjects" [38]. It later was codified by the FDA in 21 CFR §56.107, which covers FDA oversight of drugs and medical devices.

The Common Rule requires that IRBs approve and oversee all human research supported directly or indirectly by, what is today known as, HHS. It is within the purview of the Office for Human Research Protections (OHRP) within HHS to regulate all IRBs, but today, all IRBs also are subject to additional governmental organization (e.g., FDA) regulations. Similar regulatory boards have been in place for animal research since the enactment of the Laboratory Animal Welfare Act of 1966, like the Institutional Animal Care and Use Committees, which may be considered IRBs for nonhuman research subjects. For a broader discussion of ethical issues considered in preclinical research which is beyond the scope of this chapter, the reader is referred to *Animal Experimentation. The Moral Issues* (Baird and Rosenbaum, 1991) [39] or *Animal Experimentation: A Guide to the Issues* (Monamy 2000) [40].

Historically, academic institutions and medical facilities created their own IRBs to oversee human subjects research, specifically to avoid or limit ethical problems in such research. In this era, there are additional for-profit *independent* or *commercial* IRBs that institutions may choose to contract out to monitor their research; their role, accountability, and composition are no different than that of traditional IRBs. In brief, all IRBs must contain at least five members, chosen in a nondiscriminatory fashion, with sufficient expertise to judge the scientific merit of each proposed protocol and to assess whether the rights of the subjects are properly safeguarded. In its early days, concerns were raised over the relatively homogeneous composition of IRB membership. In response, the HHS Common Rule provided regulations in 45 CFR §46.107 designed to ensure satisfactory and unbiased review of clinical research projects by requiring diversity of IRB members with regard to their field of expertise, affiliations, experience, gender, race, and cultural background [38]. A majority of the members must be present for voting to take place, at least one of whom is a nonscientist, and IRB members may not vote on their own projects [38, 41]. As necessary, IRBs can invite nonvoting content experts to assist in the review process [38].

IRBs must review all research protocols and related materials (e.g., informed consent documents and promotional fliers) to ensure that proposed investigations are ethically conducted. For example, they must determine that patients are properly selected, that the proposed protocol is designed so that valid inferences can be drawn, that subjects are fully informed about the risks and benefits of the study, and that their participation is entirely voluntary (or, for special patient populations [e.g., those with dementia, mental retardation, severe neuropsychiatric disorders] that informed permission is appropriately obtained by proxy). Their role is to maximize safety in the delicate balance between risk and benefit for subjects once they are enrolled in research.

Each IRB must advocate and uphold the interests of all research subjects. Such advocacy includes protection of the future interests of subjects, especially in situations involving tissue storage. Clearly, future technologies may arise that can yield potentially valuable new data. However, these findings may pose considerable unexpected risk to subjects, especially if that information was later revealed and linked back to the subject.

The underlying concern for governing bodies regulating clinical research is the level of risk posed to human subjects. As such, the cornerstone for virtually all IRB operations is the evaluation of risks to study subjects. Beginning at the earliest stages of application for study approval, the nature of identified risks to human subjects in a research study directs the procedures for IRB review and approval. For example, the "level of risk" (a concept to be further described momentarily) is a significant factor in determining whether a research study qualifies for exempt status or expedited review or requires full-committee review. It should be noted that certain types of research protocols (as mentioned below) may qualify for "exempt" status with regard to IRB review. Clinical research studies considered "exempt" by the IRB are additionally absolved from standard informed consent requirements *unless* the research involves protected health information, in which case patient authorization or IRB waivers of authorization must be obtained for each subject [42].

For the purposes of IRB review, there are three "levels of risk" to which subjects can be exposed in any given research study: *less than minimal risk, minimal risk,* and *greater than minimal risk* [43]. Studies that involve "less than minimal risk" include those that pose no known physical, emotional, psychological, or economic risk to subjects. Such studies may be deemed "exempt" from IRB review and, therefore, would not require review by an IRB committee member.

As stipulated in 45 CFR § 46.101(b), a proposed investigation may be classified as "exempt" (unless otherwise mandated by a department or agency head) if it limits involvement of human subjects to one or more of the following categories: (1) educational practices and assessments (e.g., comparing two or more teaching methods), (2) interviews or observations of public behavior, and (3) studies of public data or specimens without accompanying information that might permit subject identification [38]. Also exempt is research examining public benefit or service programs, procedures for obtaining benefits or services under those programs, possible changes in (or alternatives to) those programs or procedures, or modification of payment for benefits or services in these programs. Other exemptions include dietary studies of nontoxic food deemed to be safe for human consumption by the FDA, Environmental Protection Agency, or the Food Safety and Inspection Service of the US Department of Agriculture [38]. The participation of certain populations (e.g., minors, prisoners, pregnant women) generally excludes studies that otherwise may be viewed as posing "less than minimal risk" from qualifying for exempt status.

Studies that involve "minimal risk," as defined by 45 CFR §46.102(i) [38], are those in which "the probability and magnitude of harm or discomfort anticipated in the research are not greater in and of themselves than those ordinarily encountered in daily life or during the performance of routine physical or psychological examinations or tests." Minimal risk studies include, but are not limited to, observational investigations which involve the collection of medical test data that are ordered for routine clinical purposes. Studies that involve medical chart review would be considered to pose no more than minimal risk, provided that no unique identifiers are included in the records. Often subsumed in the category of "minimal risk" are studies that use questionnaires or surveys, provided that no unique identifiers are included and that it is unlikely that the questions would cause emotional distress to the participant. Thus, "minimal risk" studies frequently are eligible for "expedited" review by select members (e.g., the IRB chair or a designated board member) [43].

Studies are considered to pose "greater than minimal risk" to subjects if they "include risk beyond that ordinarily encountered by subjects" [43]. Research procedures that require subjects to take experimental drugs, mandate implantation of medical devices, or involve surgical procedures are among the more obvious types of such studies [43]; however, there are less evident factors that can elevate the level of risk.

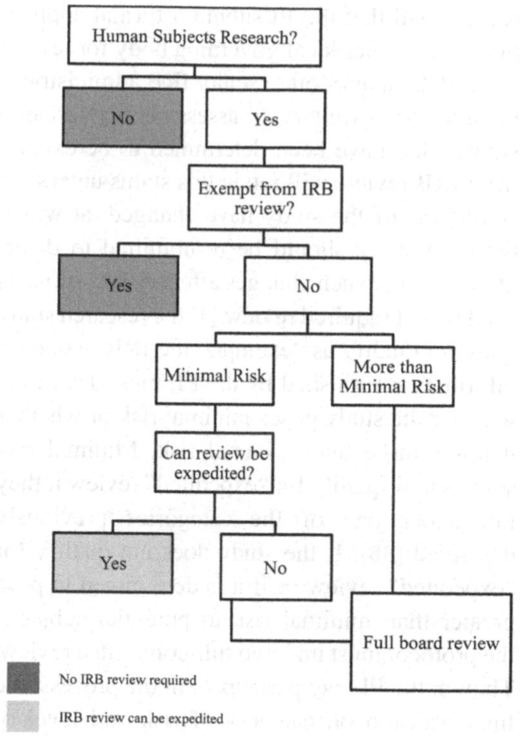

Fig. 12.1 Regulatory questions to be considered prior to study initiation

For example, an activity such as walking, which is considered to be a normal daily activity for the majority of the population, may pose a greater than minimal risk to certain subjects (e.g., individuals suffering from moderate to severe angina). Thus, a crucial factor to consider is how the subject interprets or responds to the "perceived risk" and what the individual considers "minimal risk" to be in the context of his or her life [44]. All research studies posing "greater than minimal risk" require a full-committee review by the IRB.

Figure 12.1 provides a summary of the regulatory questions that must be considered before initiating a clinical research study. In brief, the Principal Investigator (PI) should first determine whether the proposed project qualifies as human subjects research (as defined by 45 CFR §46.101 and 45 CFR § 46.102). Even if the criteria for IRB-exempt status appear to have been satisfied under 45 CFR § 46.101(b), most institutions recommend that the PI submit a formal application to his or her local governing body for review by an IRB chair or other senior IRB administrator in order to permit *their* assessment. (Research studies that have been determined to be exempt from IRB review will retain this status unless the conditions of the study have changed, at which time the study should be resubmitted to determine whether such changes affect risk to subjects and level of required review.) If the research study does *not* qualify as "exempt," the IRB, based on information furnished by the PI, must determine whether the study poses minimal risk or whether it poses more than minimal risk. Minimal risk studies may qualify for "expedited" review if they fall under one of the categories previously described [38]. If the study does not qualify for "expedited" review or if it is determined to pose greater than minimal risk to potential subjects, the protocol must undergo full-committee review. Though the PI may participate in the process, the final decision on category of risk and level of review ultimately is governed by the IRB chair or his or her designee(s).

The IRB considers a number of complex issues in its review of proposed protocols. The impact of the *study design* on human subjects is evaluated with careful attention paid to any protocol implementing *deception or withholding of information.* Deception is a particularly complex issue in human subjects research due to the extensive federal regulations regarding informed consent and disclosure of information. The IRB conducts an extensive assessment of *risks and benefits* and may require additional safeguards to be implemented. It also may examine the *selection of subjects,* evaluating both inclusion and exclusion criteria and ensuring that the process is free of coercion. The IRB considers the planned methods for *identification of research participants* and associated procedures in place to *protect the privacy* of study subjects. Its members evaluate the *process for obtaining informed consent* and thoroughly review the *informed consent forms* as well as any *other documents* or *devices* that will be introduced to study subjects or will be used in recruitment. The qualifications of all *investigators* on the protocol are to be considered, as are potential *conflicts of interest.* Finally, the IRB will determine if the study warrants additional reviews during a one year period. The protocols for all ongoing research studies are considered to be undergoing "continuing review" and are required to be reviewed at least annually [45].

In addition to previously cited requirements, all IRBs must review any amendments, including updates to any research-related forms, along with any other documents that the IRB deems necessary to protect potential human study subjects. (There may be local variation in the order in which an IRB verifies the propriety of proposed and/or ongoing research of human subjects.)

In 1996, the International Conference on Harmonisation of Technical Requirements for Registration of Pharmaceuticals for Human Use Guideline for Good Clinical Practice (ICH-GCP) [46] established additional guidelines for IRB oversight of clinical trials, which later were adopted by the FDA [47]. In this context, "clinical trials" are defined as studies that involve investigational products. In addition to the general procedures discussed previously for human subjects research studies, the requirements set forth in the Guideline for Good Clinical Practice mandate that ongoing IRB reviews of clinical trials must include proposed drug and device safety documentation.

The role of the IRB comprises far more than extensive document review. The *Belmont Report* cited above states that research on human subjects must ethically address "beneficence," "respect for persons," and "justice" [35]. This edict can be fulfilled only when the IRB approves research that fully informs subjects (or when necessary, their proxies) about the risks of the study before they provide consent for participation in the research.

IRBs are required to provide special attention to proposed studies of persons with diminished comprehension, pregnant women, prisoners, the elderly, or children. In his well-focused Lancet review of David Wendler's book on *The Ethics of Pediatric Research* [48] (provoked by intended use of children as the subjects of investigation), Peter Singer poses the daunting question: "Is it ever ethical to do research on human subjects without their consent?" [49]. Arguing that research with children is justifiable with parental consent, Singer bases this inference on his belief in the subject's inherent altruistic desire to benefit others—an objective that, in the broadest interpretation, infers that contributing to a significant research project is an accomplishment of ultimate value to the contributor. While the question remains hotly debated, Singer suggests that parents should be able to give consent for their child to enroll in a "well-designed study of an important question … despite the fact that doing so involves momentary pain and, in good medical practice, a risk … that is greater than zero, but still extremely small" [49]. In sum, current ethical standards in the USA permit parent-approved research on children when the risk of harm to the child is minor and potential benefit to others is likely or in situations when no alternative mechanism exists to attain those benefits.

IRBs have not been free of criticism, even in this new millennium. As late as 2010, Hall, Friedman, King et al. noted that academic medical center IRBs and conflict of interest committees "usually are *not* involved in reviewing research budgets to determine whether per capita payments are excessive" [50] (italics added); in certain circumstances (to be described later), excessive payments may be seen as undue inducement for participation in the study. In addition, due to what is perceived to be misunderstanding of specific social science research methods (e.g., ethnography, oral histories) by many IRB members, some social scientists have argued that current regulation of social science research is insufficiently flexible; they believe that current regulatory requirements (e.g., lengthy and/or complicated consent forms) are overly burdensome in light of the fact that social science studies generally pose only limited risk to subjects. In an attempt to address these concerns, the OHRP, in conjunction with the Oral History Association (OHA) and the American Historical Association (AHA), stated in 2003 that investigative procedures (e.g., oral histories, collection of anecdotes, unstructured interviews, and other related methods) often do not constitute human subjects research as commonly defined [51]. A year later, problems persisted, causing the representatives from the OHA and AHA to issue a reaffirmation of their 2003 statement [52].

HIPAA, the Privacy Rule, and "Preparatory to Research" Activities

In the US, IRBs took on additional tasks following the enactment of the Health Insurance Portability and Accountability Act (HIPAA) of 1996 [53], passed by Congress "to improve portability and continuity of health insurance coverage in the group and individual markets, to combat waste, fraud, and abuse in health insurance and health care delivery, to promote the use of medical savings accounts, to improve access to long-term care services and coverage, to simplify the administration of health insurance, and for other purposes" [53]. To accomplish these tasks, the act called for a vast overhaul of the methods used to transmit medical information, including a shift toward standardized electronic transmissions. HIPAA has been modified a number of times since its enactment in 1996 [54–56], and though initially the act most evidently applied to health-care providers and health-care plan providers, extensions of the act have had a significant impact on clinical research. Most notably, a provision was made requiring compliance with the HSS-issued *Standards for Privacy of Individually Identifiable Health Information*, known as the HIPAA Privacy Rule, by most covered entities as of April 2003. HSS provides the following statement on "covered entities" with regard to research:

> Covered entities are health plans, health care clearinghouses, and health care providers that transmit health information electronically in connection with certain defined HIPAA transactions, such as claims or eligibility inquiries. Researchers are not themselves covered entities, unless they are also health care providers and engage in any of the covered electronic transactions. If, however, researchers are employees or other workforce members of a covered entity (e.g., a hospital or health insurer), they may have to comply with that entity's HIPAA privacy policies and procedures. [57]

Table 12.5 Information that must be removed for deidentification

1. Names
2. Contact information (e.g., phone or fax #, website or internet protocol [IP] or electronic mail addresses, geographic address smaller than State, except first three digits of zip code)
3. Identifying dates (more detailed than year, e.g., birth, death, admission, discharge)
4. Age over 89 years (unless listed as 90 or older)
5. Social security, medical record, insurance identification number
6. Vehicle identification numbers (e.g., serial numbers, license plate numbers)
7. Device identification or serial numbers
8. Certificate or license numbers
9. Biometric identity (e.g., voice or retinal print, fingerprint, full face image)
10. Any other unique account numbers or material [58]

The purpose of the HIPAA Privacy Rule is to regulate the use and disclosure of certain "individually identifiable health information," termed protected health information (PHI). An individual's PHI includes information pertaining to (1) his or her past, present, or future physical or mental health or condition, (2) the provision of health care to the individual, and (3) the past, present, or future payment for the provision of health care to the individual [58]. An individual's genetic information also is considered to be PHI. PHI is protected under the Privacy Rule when it contains information that possibly could be used to determine the identity of the individual. It is possible to deidentify PHI by removing certain information pertaining to the individual. The information that must be removed in order to deidentify an individual's PHI is listed in Table 12.5.

Just as medical professionals must maintain the security and privacy of their patients' PHI, so too must clinical researchers who are covered entities, work for covered entities, or who obtain data from covered entities (as defined above). The legislation established to regulate the transmission of PHI significantly impacts the clinical researcher in two specific ways: (1) a subject's PHI must be obtained and used in a manner deemed permissible by the Privacy Rule, and (2) activities that are considered to be "preparatory to research" and that involve the review of PHI must be carried out in accordance with specific guidelines [57]. The ways by which a covered entity may use or disclose an individual's PHI for research purposes are outlined in Table 12.6.

Table 12.6 Conditions permitting the use or disclose of PHI for research by covered entities

• "If the subject of the PHI has granted specific written permission through an Authorization that satisfies section 164.508
• For reviews preparatory to research with representations obtained from the researcher that satisfy section 164.512(i)(1)(iii) of the Privacy Rule
• For research solely on decedents' information with certain representations and, if requested, documentation obtained from the researcher that satisfies section 164.512(i)(1)(iii) of the Privacy Rule
• If the covered entity receives appropriate documentation that an IRB or Privacy Board has granted a waiver of the Authorization requirement that satisfies section 164.512(i)
• If the covered entity obtains documentation of an IRB or Privacy Board's alteration of the Authorization requirement as well as the altered Authorization from the individual
• If the PHI has been de-identified in accordance with the standards set by the Privacy Rule at section 164.514(a)–(c) (in which case, the health information is no longer PHI)
• If the information is released in the form of a limited data set, with certain identifiers removed and with a data use agreement between the researcher and the covered entity, as specified under section 164.514(e)
• Under a 'grandfathered' informed consent of the individual to participate in the research, an IRB waiver of such informed consent, or Authorization or other express legal permission to use or disclose the information for research as specified under the transition provisions of the Privacy Rule at section 164.532(c)" [57]

As mentioned, the Privacy Rule has had a substantial impact on "activities preparatory to research." Activities preparatory to research include reviews of data that enable researchers to determine whether or not it would be purposeful or reasonable to pursue a particular research study. This may include reviewing medical records to determine whether or not there are enough potential subjects to be able to carry out the study. Such activities also may be used to allow the researcher to identify potential research participants for recruitment purposes and to contact potential study participants. Each of these activities must be carried out in accordance with particular requirements. For example, a covered entity may allow a researcher to review PHI, but they may not permit the researcher to remove any PHI from the covered entity. Additionally, the researcher would not be permitted to contact a potential study participant based on the PHI reviewed without the researcher being a workforce member of the covered entity or without the researcher securing proper documentation of a "waiver of authorization" from the IRB or Privacy Board [59].

The regulations previously discussed specifically address the researcher's ability to obtain and utilize a subject's PHI; however, there are additional directives under the Privacy Rule that stipulate the handling of PHI beyond the permissibility of transmission. The rules for maintaining privacy and security include written privacy procedures in which a privacy officer, who is responsible for upholding such procedures, is designated. It must be clearly stated who has access to specific private health information and how to modify levels of accessibility. Appropriate training must occur on a scheduled and ongoing basis for all persons with access to PHI. Research information must be securely backed up in case the original information is lost or corrupted in an emergency.

A key guideline for ensuring the privacy of PHI is to transmit only the minimal amount of information necessary. Any equipment used for research or patient management that contains PHI must be monitored and protected from unauthorized access. With the growth of digital information systems, any PHI that is sent over an open network must have adequate encryption, but there is some leeway with regard to PHI sent via closed networks. In the case of closed networks, encryption is optional and the existing network access controls are considered sufficient. Safeguards must be in place for any third parties to uphold the same level of security and privacy with regard to PHI. Plans for audits of these procedures to make sure problems are clearly identified and rectified are required.

Additionally, plans must be in place for responding to breaches of private information. Breaches of PHI generally are defined as "the unauthorized acquisition, access, use, or disclosure of protected health information which compromises the security or privacy of such information …" [56]. In the event that a breach occurs, all individuals whose PHI may have been inappropriately disclosed (or their next of kin, if the individual is deceased) must be informed. Furthermore, a notice of breach is to be listed on the affiliated institution's website or disseminated through a major media outlet. Cases in which a large number of individuals (500 or more) have been affected require that the secretary of HHS also be notified. Affected parties should be informed as to what they can do to further protect themselves after a breach occurs [56].

Human Research Requires Informed Consent

As mentioned previously, the informed consent process for human subjects is a cornerstone of ethical standards in human research. It is important to note the distinction between "authorization," as discussed in relation to the HIPAA Privacy Rule, and "informed consent." Authorization is written permission from an individual permitting the disclosure and/or use of his or her PHI for research. Informed consent is an individual's permission to participate in research.

To the extent possible, one must receive clearly stated information explaining the study's "purpose, methods, risks, benefits, and alternatives to research" in order to be considered an "informed" subject [60]. However, violations of this precept occasionally occur even in developed societies. A particularly horrific example was given in a 2005 paper [61] that described how a mother learned, after the death of her baby, that the child had been buried without its heart by the staff of the Bristol Royal Infirmary in the United Kingdom (UK). This was done without her knowledge and consent so that tissue samples could be used for future research by investigators.

After the subject has been adequately informed, it is up to him or her to decide whether to participate in the study. If the research undertaken is to be considered ethical, it is imperative that this decision be completely voluntary. The subject must be able to freely decide not only whether to begin participation at the outset but also whether to *continue* participation after the study has commenced. An important point often overlooked during this process is that the subject must fully understand the conveyed information. Otherwise, the decision made may not reflect the true wishes or interests of the individual. However, in cases where the potential subject is a child, an unconscious adult, or an individual of otherwise limited mental capacity, informed consent from the individual is not required. In these instances, consent is obtained instead through a proxy (a decision maker who is empowered to ensure that the subject's involvement in the study is consistent with his or her values, beliefs, and interests). In this way, the decision that is ultimately made will most closely represent what the subject would have willfully done if he or she had been able to render a decision [60].

Fundamental to the process of informed consent is the concept of respect for potential and enrolled subjects. It is important that enrolled subjects be treated with respect from the time they are approached to be in the study to the time their participation has ended. Likewise, individuals who decline to participate nevertheless should be treated with respect throughout the entire recruitment process. Respect for subjects entails not only respecting their decisions and keeping private information confidential but also disclosing new information (e.g., novel risks and benefits that might emerge during the course of the study and affect their willingness to participate), monitoring their well-being to prevent and treat adverse effects, and informing them about what was learned from the research [60].

The responsibility to maintain the integrity of the processes of communicating details of a study to participants rests with the PI and all associate investigators who personally interact with the subject. This is to ensure that the subject (or his or her proxy) understands what is being proposed and comprehends any and all known potential adverse consequences that could arise from his or her participation. In other words, responsibility for obtaining consent should not be delegated to subordinates.

Consent must be obtained in a noncoercive and fully voluntary manner, avoiding the fraud of Tuskegee (cited previously) and the horrors of Nazi experimentation as a prelude to murder. As it is always the ultimate responsibility of the investigators to ensure that their research is properly conducted, they must remain alert (even if, as noted above, IRBs are not) to the reality that excessive payment to research subjects might be coercive. While compensation to subjects is generally viewed as an acceptable way of covering their expenses and rewarding them for their time and effort related to the study, the use of relatively large incentives to facilitate recruitment may comprise, in certain circumstances, a form of undue influence by inducing the individual to accept seemingly irresistible offers against his or her better judgment. [62]

A striking example is the series of experiments conducted at the Willowbrook State School, in which parents were asked to enlist their retarded children in a research project that required them to be infected with hepatitis [62]. As incentive, the child was offered a place in a residential treatment facility that otherwise would have been difficult to secure. It is not hard to see that such an incentive, as an attempt to induce parents to overcome their hesitation about the study by appealing to their concern for their child's treatment, is ethically unsound.

Those in favor of subject compensation argue that compensating subjects for participating in research is no different than paying people for working. As McNeill has noted, however, unlike work, experimentation on human subjects inherently exposes people to unnecessary risks of harm—"risks that cannot be known in advance" [63]. Therefore, while a completion bonus for a relatively harmless research study usually poses no ethical problems and is, in fact, a commonly employed method for emphasizing the importance of full commitment to the study, caution should be exercised when the research might be painful or distressing for the subject; in cases such as these, compensation may be seen as undue influence, seductively pressuring the subject to accept conditions they would otherwise deem unreasonable or aversive.

Investigators should always bear in mind that inequalities in authority between investigator and subject persist even after informed consent is given, creating potential threats to autonomy [64]. Certain strategies customarily are employed to minimize the impact of such potential vulnerability. For example, while consent for participation in a clinical research study may include agreement to certain pre- or postintervention procedures, subjects still retain the right to discontinue their participation at any time, even when their treating physician or a consulting physician for the study believes it may be life threatening for the subject to withdraw from the study [65].

Self-Experimentation Guidelines

Defined as the special case of single-subject scientific experimentation in which the experimenter conducts experiments on himself or herself, self-experimentation usually means that the designer, operator, subject, analyst, and ultimate user of resulting information are all the same person. Lawrence K. Altman has catalogued numerous instances of physician investigators who opted to first expose themselves to the risks of a new technique or therapy. [66]. Included is Karl Landsteiner's pursuit of what would be named the ABO blood groups repeatedly depended on blood samples drawn from himself and five members of his staff. Similarly, invasive cardiology was pioneered in Germany by Werner Forssmann, who would eventually receive the Nobel Prize in Physiology or Medicine following years of self-experimentation he performed by catheterizing his heart numerous times [66]. Another significant example of self-experimentation was an experiment conducted by Barry J. Marshall [67]. In order to confirm that Helicobacter pylori (H. pylori) caused gastritis and predisposed peptic ulceration even in patients with a healthy mucus lining, Marshall volunteered to ingest a sample of H. pylori. After he developed the characteristic symptoms of gastritis, it was shown that ingested H. pylori is able to colonize completely normal gastric mucosa and lead to the acute inflammatory changes collectively referred to as acute H. pylori gastritis [67].

Current federal regulations, however, do not distinguish between self-experimentation and experimentation on subjects recruited for a specific project. Clinicians may feel that if they are experimenting with their own bodies, then as doctors, they are cognizant of all the risks and may consider circumventing the IRB approval process altogether. However, as a general rule, IRBs require prior submission and approval of an application detailing all aspects of any study incorporating self-experimentation before it starts. The rationale for IRB approval is the concern that overly zealous investigators may subject themselves to inappropriate, unnecessary, and unforeseen risk without the IRB's oversight. As an example, proper IRB oversight would protect an investigator, with early signs of Huntington's disease, from self-experimenting with a "promising" drug undergoing early animal trials for safety and efficacy that ultimately may cause more deaths than standard-of-care treatment. Control of self-experimentation is a delicate issue since respect for each individual's right of autonomy is a key feature of federal governance via IRBs.

Scientific research is, of course, not the only context in which people are likely to expose themselves to potentially harmful situations. In a free society, individuals can daily engage in a wide range of risky behaviors at their own discretion. For example, individuals may willingly have unprotected sex, maintain an unhealthy diet, consume alcohol in excessive amounts, or ride a motorcycle without wearing a helmet for protection. However, if a research study requires the individual to engage in a risky activity *due* to the research, it obligates the investigators (with IRB oversight) to, truthfully and without restriction, fully inform each potential research subject of all aspects of an intended study, including risks, which the candidate would not have assumed had the research not been performed.

This task is especially daunting in the setting of self-experimentation because investigators may not be objective about risks to their own health and safety, especially (as noted above) when the likelihood of risk for potential major adverse effects may not already be known.

Evaluating a New Human Research Study: Scientific Value of Research Methods and Reporting

As best elucidated by Emanuel, Wendler, and Grady [68] and summarized by the NIH for their own recommendations [60], the seven main principles presently guiding the conduct of ethical research are social and clinical value, scientific validity, fair subject selection, favorable risk-benefit ratio, independent review, informed consent, and respect for potential and enrolled subjects [68]. Fellows and junior faculty preparing to initiate or join ongoing human research involving possible injury to the subject (as may follow organ or tissue biopsy or penetration for measurement of fluid pressures in pulmonary, renal, or cardiac vasculature) can test whether their protocol addresses, and is responsive to, all seven principles. Below is a brief explanation of how the first five principles help guide the ethical review process. Informed consent and respect for potential and enrolled subjects have been described in detail previously (see "*Human Research Requires Informed Consent*").

Clinical and Social Value

An overriding concern in research is the question of whether the proposed study explores questions that, if answered, will provide new information of significant value for present or future patients with a specified illness or for society in general: If the new information pursued is deemed to be important, are the risks inherent in the study sufficiently reasonable to justify exposure and inconvenience of the research subjects? Is it anticipated that answers to the research question will contribute to scientific understanding of health or improve our disease management?

Scientific Validity

Research that leads to invalid conclusions is unethical because it wastes time and resources while needlessly exposing subjects to risk. For this reason, IRBs consider the scientific credibility of the study to be an important ethical consideration. For example, are the questions addressed by the study likely to be answered by the techniques and methods to be utilized? Are the questions investigators are asking answerable and are the research methods valid and feasible for this purpose? Has the study been designed with a clear scientific objective using accepted principles, methods, and reliable practices? Does the sample size detailed in the statistical plan provide good precision for estimation of population parameters or sufficient power to adequately test the research hypothesis?

Fair Subject Selection

According to the NIH, those accepting the risks and burdens of the research also should "be in a position to enjoy its benefits, and those who may benefit should share some of the risks and burdens" [60]. Therefore, researchers should carefully assess who is to be included in the study such that the issues being investigated may be addressed appropriately. In other words, has study recruitment been based on the weighing of scientific goals against subject vulnerability, privilege, or other factors unrelated to the purposes of the study? For the purposes of fairness, specific subgroups (e.g., minorities, women, children, and the elderly) cannot be excluded from research unless a good scientific reason or a particular susceptibility to risk exists [60].

Favorable Risk-Benefit Ratio

A fundamental principle that was stressed at the beginning of this chapter was that the risks and benefits associated with a given research project or experiment can never be determined before the actual study has been conducted. In fact, the very definition of research implies uncertainty regarding the effects of whatever drug, device, or therapy is being tested. Because it is impossible to predict if a given risk (whether physical, psychological, economic, or social) will be trivial or serious, transient or long term, it is of the utmost importance that clinical researchers strive to achieve a favorable risk-benefit ratio by minimizing all potential risks to subjects while maximizing all potential benefits. Furthermore, it must be ascertained that the study's potential benefits to other individuals outweigh the risks to its subjects. Only with these measures can the uncertainty inherent in every research pursuit be approached safely and sensibly.

Independent Review

The ultimate question to be asked, of course, is whether local IRBs have reviewed the study and deemed it to be ethically acceptable before it starts. As is inferable from the preceding discussion, the IRB is usually the main body in the USA that will determine whether the investigators conducting the trial are sufficiently free of bias, whether adequate protection has been afforded to research volunteers, and whether the trial has been ethically designed with an acceptable risk-benefit ratio.

Ethically sensitive issues (often relating to the seven above-mentioned guiding principles) also can arise in disciplines such as interventional nephrology or cardiology, especially when proposing invasive bodily research. Local circumstances predominantly take precedence over a simple resolution based on what appears ethically correct. For example, some institutions will not perform a kidney transplant for patients older than age 70; thus, consideration of this procedure for an intensive care unit patient above this age at one of these facilities is moot and such a patient could not be eligible for a kidney transplant research projects even if, as may be the case in multicenter studies, the overarching protocol would allow inclusion of such a patient. Similarly, criteria for acceptability of HIV-positive patients may have been established by a hospital IRB.

Ethical Misconduct and Consequences

With potentially decades of work, reputations, and financial and professional interests at stake, clinical research certainly is vulnerable to ethical misconduct. The Office of Research Integrity, maintained by HHS, provides the following definition of research misconduct:

> Research misconduct means fabrication, falsification, or plagiarism in proposing, performing, or reviewing research, or in reporting research results.
>
> (a) Fabrication is making up data or results and recording or reporting them.
> (b) Falsification is manipulating research materials, equipment, or processes, or changing or omitting data or results such that the research is not accurately represented in the research record.
> (c) Plagiarism is the appropriation of another person's ideas, processes, results, or words without giving appropriate credit.
> (d) Research misconduct does not include honest error or differences of opinion. [69]

Ethical misconduct relating to data tampering and related abuses is well documented, and penalties for such misconduct can be quite severe. In a notable example of research fraud, a 1998 publication in the *Lancet* alleged the identification of a new "brain-bowel" syndrome and a link between that syndrome and the measles, mumps, and rubella (MMR) vaccine, based on a research study conducted in the UK in the 1990s by Andrew Wakefield, M.D., and colleagues [70]. Wakefield et al. claimed that the onset of behavioral symptoms in eight of the 12 children involved in the study was directly associated with receiving the MMR vaccine. Their paper also cited a high correlation between "regressive" autism and "nonspecific colitis" to lend support to the claims of a new "brain-bowel" syndrome. These reported findings had a substantial adverse impact on adherence to recommended vaccination regimens here in the USA, leading to a rise in previously controlled childhood diseases such as measles, mumps, and rubella.

Following more than a decade of contentious debate over the validity of the study (during which countless parents considered the much discussed "link" between the MMR vaccine and autism when deciding whether or not to vaccinate their children), the paper was retracted in February 2010. Revelations of ethical misconduct in Wakefield's study included (1) nine of the children were reported as having regressive autism, but a third lacked any autism diagnosis, and only one child actually showed clear signs of the condition; (2) five of the 12 children described as being "previously normal" actually had documented preexisting developmental concerns; (3) the immediacy of the onset of symptoms following MMR vaccination was greatly exaggerated in some instances; (4) following a medical school "research review," the diagnosis for nine of the children was changed from "unremarkable" to "nonspecific colitis"; (5) while 11 families actually alleged the MMR vaccine caused their children's' symptoms, three late cases were intentionally omitted in order to create the false impression of a 14-day window between vaccine exposure and symptom onset and (6) recruitment and funding aspects of the study correlated closely to anti-MMR programs, accounting for substantial grounds for conflict of interest claims [71]. It also was revealed that Wakefield profited from a future lawsuit against the patent holders of current vaccines. Wakefield and John Walker-Smith, the senior clinician involved in the study, were subjected to the UK's longest *General Medical Council Fitness to Practice Hearing* and were eventually "struck off the medical register" [71].

In 2009, Scott Reuben, M.D., previously a renowned anesthesiologist and pain management investigator, published flagrantly fraudulent findings from studies that he performed without the approval of his own institution's IRB, going so far as to fabricate patient data and to forge the name of a colleague in order to list him as a coauthor on a publication [72–74]. In the aftermath of that scandal, Dr. Reuben lost all credibility in his field, has served jail time for health-care fraud, and a large fine was levied against him by a US federal court [75].

In his article published in the Cleveland Clinic Journal of Medicine, James G. Sheehan cited four additional cases of ethical misconduct in research throughout the past decade [76]. Included was the case of Dr. Eric Poehlman who was sentenced to one year in prison in 2006 for falsifying and fabricating research data for a study on menopause and metabolism. Also in 2006, Elizabeth Goodwin, a University of Wisconsin professor, resigned following the revelation that she made false statements in her genetics research. Dr. Gary Kammer resigned from Wake Forest University in 2005 when it was discovered that he had fabricated families in his NIH grant application, this a year after Harvard professor Ali Sultan resigned due to false information in his own grant application [76].

The previous examples are just a few selected cases of misconduct, with many more cases reported in the literature about falsification of data, plagiarism, research conducted without proper consent, undisclosed conflicts of interest, and much more [77]. It is difficult to calculate how much research funding has been squandered and how much harm has been caused to the public health by generating and advancing fraudulent findings.

Final Thoughts and Closing Unanswered Moral Research Dilemmas

The vast regulations, protocols, and governing bodies developed over the course of history to protect the ethical integrity of clinical research are evidence that the issue is a cornerstone of human subjects investigation. While current legislation provides answers to many of the questions that may be posed today regarding the ethicality of research activities, it is important to keep two considerations in mind: (1) It is often the case that as societies evolve, so too do the standards of "appropriateness" governing the nature of principles, and (2) the passage of time will inevitably force workers in the field of clinical investigation to take into consideration issues or concerns that simply could not be projected as possibilities at an earlier time. Mentioned below are some questions that can, and should, be asked by clinical researchers in this era. Is investigation of one's self ethically appropriate? Is any age "too old" for subjects in an invasive biopsy study such as kidney, lung, or major vessel transplantation or replaceable device? For an organ transplant study, should young candidates be selected before geriatric candidates? In studies allocating an expensive and limited therapy (e.g., bone marrow, heart, or kidney transplant) should individuals in advantaged positions be accepted into a research protocol ahead of people not so advantaged? Must undocumented noncitizens be excluded from innovative, experimental, or potentially life-sustaining therapy that may be scarce or expensive? Are women to be approached for research on an equal basis with men? Is it reasonable to include race and religion as inclusion/exclusion criteria for study candidates? Is HIV infection a reasonable exclusion criterion for a study of an experimental surgical procedure? Should absence of insurance coverage or being impoverished (and thus, in both cases, inability to pay for standard care that may not be covered by a research grant) dictate exclusion from a research protocol that might provide beneficial therapy? Should prisoners be excluded from recruitment? In an experimental life-sustaining device (e.g., aortic balloon pump or a hypothermia catheter) study of coma patients after resuscitated cardiac arrest, if the study subject fails to respond to the experimental device, who decides to discontinue use of the device (e.g., the patient, family/proxy decision maker) and when should that decision be made? How should a subject's nonadherence to a protocol [78], hostility to staff, or criminality [79] be managed? (e.g., is it ethical to withdraw therapy or to consult with psychiatry, social services, administration, lawyers, clergy, family members or friends, or members of the Ethics Committee under these circumstances?) Sensitivity to the need for respect, autonomy, and dignity of individuals subjected to investigation in these types of situations allows researchers to detect and correct deviations from appropriate conduct in modern human research.

Take-Home Points

- From the earliest prebiblical writings to modern day, concern for and debate on the appropriate conduct by caregivers toward patients has been a central theme of appropriate ("ethical") medical practice.
- Resulting from awareness of World War II German atrocities performed on prisoners, the mentally deficient, and defenseless civilians, the Nuremberg Code and Belmont Report were devised to protect patients and society from inappropriate assault on their body and psyche, later to be followed by regulations regarding the importance of patient privacy.
- Central to acceptable ethical behavior in human research are three main principles: respect for persons, beneficence, and justice.
- When possible, a fully informed written consent based on protocol comprehension must be obtained and preserved from each subject.
- With reservation and caution, parental consent may be sufficient for child participation in a study of low risk but potential importance to society.
- Currently, international guidelines for ethical human research require prior approval of research protocols by an Institutional Review Board (IRB). The IRB must document its views in writing, clearly identifying the trial being assessed, which documents were reviewed, and the dates of its reaching decisions for approval, disapproval, or need for restructuring.
- The US National Institutes of Health (NIH) names the principles governing acceptable human research: social and clinical value, scientific validity, fair subject selection, favorable risk-benefit ratio, independent review, informed consent, and respect for potential and enrolled subjects.

References

1. Friedman EA. Diabetic nephropathy: fresh perspectives. Facta Univ. 1999;6:31–47.
2. Carrick P. Medical ethics in the ancient world. Washington, DC: Georgetown University Press; 2001.
3. Tsai DF. How should doctors approach patients? A Confucian reflection on personhood. J Med Ethics. 2001;27:44–50.
4. Tsai DF. Ancient Chinese medical ethics and the four principles of biomedical ethics. J Med Ethics. 1999; 25:315–21.
5. Chadwick J, Mann WN. Hippocratic writings. London: Penguin; 1950.
6. Owsei T, Temkin C. Ancient medicine. Selected papers of Ludwig Edelstein Johns. Baltimore: Hopkins University Press; 1987.
7. "The Hippocratic Oath: Today". Doctors' Diaries. WGBH Educational Foundation. 1964. http://www.pbs.org/wgbh/nova/body/hippocratic-oath-today.html. Accessed 15 Sept 2011.
8. Betzold M. Appointment with doctor death. Troy: Momentum Books; 1993.
9. Kevorkian J. Medicine, ethics, and execution by lethal injection. Med Law. 1985;4:307–13.
10. Kevorkian J. A comprehensive bioethical code for medical exploitation of humans facing imminent and unavoidable death. Med Law. 1986;5:81–197.
11. Kevorkian J. The long overdue medical specialty: bioethiatrics. J Natl Med Assoc. 1986;78:1057–60.
12. Jonsen AR. The birth of bioethics. Experiments perilous: the ethics of research with human subjects. New York: Oxford University Press; 1998.
13. Spencer WG. Celsus' De Medicina— a learned and experienced practitioner upon what the art of medicine could then accomplish. Proc R Soc Med. 1926;19(Sect Hist Med):129–39.
14. Friedman EA. Stressful ethical issues in uremia therapy. Kidney Int. 2010;78(Suppl 117):S22–32.
15. Ojanuga D. The medical ethics of the 'father of gynaecology', Dr J Marion Sims. J Med Ethics. 1993; 19:28–31.
16. Lederer SE. Subjected to science: human experimentation in America before the Second World War. Baltimore: John Hopkins University Press; 1997.
17. Grodin MA. Children as research subjects: science ethics and law. New York: Oxford University Press; 1994.
18. Lederer SE. Orphans as guinea pigs: American children and medical experimenters, 1890–1930. In: Cooter R, editor. The name of the child: health and welfare, 1880–1940. New York: Routledge; 1992.
19. Caelleigh AS. Prisoners. Acad Med. 2000;75:999.
20. Hornblum AM. They were cheap and available: prisoners as research subjects in twentieth century America. BMJ. 1997;315:1437–41.
21. Rosenthal ET. The Rhoads not given: the tainting of the Cornelius P. Rhoads Memorial Award. Oncol Times. 2003;25:19–20.
22. Sass HM. Reichsrundschreiben 1931: pre-Nuremberg regulations concerning new therapy and human experimentation. J Med Philos. 1983;8:99–111, (reprint of German original and English translation).
23. Mitscherlich A, Mielke F. Epilogue: seven were hanged. In: Annas GJ, Grodin MA, editors. The Nazi doctors and the Nuremberg Code – human rights in human experimentation. New York: Oxford University Press; 1992.
24. Nuremberg Code [from Trials of War Criminals before the Nuremberg Military Tribunals under Control Council Law No. 10. Nuremberg, October 1946–April 1949. Washington, DC: U.S. G.P.O, 1949–1953].
25. Shuster E. Fifty years later: the significance of the Nuremberg Code. N Engl J Med. 1997;337:1436–40.
26. Jones JH. Bad blood: the Tuskegee Syphilis Experiment. New York: The Free Press; 1993.
27. Shamoo AE, Resnick DB. The use of human subjects in research. Responsible conduct of research. New York: Oxford University Press; 2003.
28. Declaration of Helsinki: Ethical Principles for Medical Research Involving Human Subjects. Adopted by the 18th WMA General Assembly Helsinki, Finland, June 1964, and amended by the 29th WMA General Assembly, Tokyo, Japan, October 1975; 35th WMA General Assembly, Venice, Italy, October 1983; 41st WMA General Assembly, Hong Kong, September 1989; 48th WMA General Assembly, Somerset West, Republic of South Africa, October 1996; and the 52nd WMA General Assembly, Edinburgh, Scotland, October 2000. http://www.wma.net/en/30publications/10policies/b3/. ccessed 15 Sept 2011.
29. Harkness J, Lederer SE, Wikler D. Laying ethical foundations for clinical research. Bull World Health Organ. 2001;79:365–6. Epub 2 Jul 2003.
30. Rothman DJ. The doctor as whistle-blower. Strangers at the bedside. New York: Basic Books; 1991.
31. Beecher HK. Ethics and clinical research. N Engl J Med. 1966;274:1354–60.
32. Heller J. Syphilis victims in U.S. study went untreated for 40 years. New York Times (New York) 26 July 1972;1,8.
33. Cobb WM. The Tuskagee Syphilis Study. J Natl Med Assoc. 1973;65:345–8.
34. Brody B. The ethics of biomedical research. New York: Oxford University Press; 1998.
35. The Belmont Report. Ethical principles and guidelines for the protection of human subjects of research. The National Commission for the Protection of Human Subjects of Biomedical and Behavioral Research. 18 Apr 1979. http://ohsr.od.nih.gov/guidelines/belmont.html. Accessed 13 May 2011.
36. US Food and Drug Administration. The genesis of human subjects protections regulations and biomedical research in the 21st century. CDER small business assistance training clinical trial workshop, September 2011. http://www.fda.gov/downloads/

Drugs/NewsEvents/UCM275441.pdf. Accessed 20 Nov 2011.
37. Federal Policy for the Protection of Human Subjects; Notices and Rules. Federal Register. 1991;56(117). http://www.hhs.gov/ohrp/policy/frcomrul.pdf. Accessed 15 Sept 2011
38. Public Welfare, Protection of Human Subjects, Basic HHS Policy for Protection of Human Research Subjects, Title 45 CFR Part 46, Subpart A. 2005. http://ohsr.od.nih.gov/guidelines/45cfr46.html. Accessed 15 Sept 2011.
39. Baird RM, Rosenbaum SE. Animal experimentation. The moral issues. Buffalo: Prometheus Books; 1991.
40. Monamy V. Animal experimentation. A guide to the issues. Cambridge, UK: Cambridge University Press; 2000.
41. Brown, JG. Department of Health and Human Services. Office of Inspector General. Institutional review boards: their role in reviewing approved research. Office of Evaluations and Inspections, June 1998.
42. UVA IRB-HSR Research Guidance. Informed consent. University of Virginia, 2010. http://www.virginia.edu/vpr/irb/HSR_docs/Guidance/UVA InvestigatorGuide5-1-08.doc. Accessed 15 Sept 2011.
43. Assessing Level of Risk and Type of IRB Review. Research compliance news. University of South Alabama. 2008. www.southalabama.edu/research-compliance/pdf/compliancenews0908.pdf. Accessed 15 Sept 2011.
44. Mazur DJ. Evaluating the science and ethics of research on humans: a guide for IRB members. Baltimore: The Johns Hopkins University Press; 2007.
45. Protocol Review Process. Institutional review board for health sciences research. University of Virginia IRB-HSR. 2008. http://www.virginia.edu/vpr/irb/hsr/reviewprocess_background.html#issues. Accessed 10 Sept 2011.
46. Guideline for Good Clinical Practice E6 Harmonisation of Technical Requirements for Registration of Pharmaceuticals for Human Use. 1996. http://www.ich.org/fileadmin/Public_Web_Site/ICH_Products/Guidelines/Efficacy/E6_R1/Step4/E6_R1__Guideline.pdf p10. Accessed 5 Apr 2011.
47. Guidance for Industry E6 Good Clinical Practice: Consolidated Guidance. U.S. Department of Health and Human Services. 1996. http://www.fda.gov/downloads/Drugs/GuidanceCompliance RegulatoryInformation/Guidances/ucm073122.pdf p10. Accessed 5 Apr 2011.
48. Wendler D. The ethics of pediatric research. New York: Oxford University Press; 2010.
49. Singer P. When is research on children ethical? Lancet. 2011;377:115–6.
50. Hall MA, Friedman JY, King NM, Weinfurt KP, Schulman KA, Sugarman J. Commentary: per capita payments in clinical trials: reasonable costs versus bounty hunting. Acad Med. 2010;85:1554–6.
51. Ritchie D, Shopes L. Oral history excluded from IRB review: application of the Department of Health and Human Services regulations for the protection of human subjects at 45 CFR part 46, subpart A to oral history interviewing. Oral History Association. 2003.
52. Shopes L, Ritchie D. An update on the exclusion of oral history from IRB review. Oral history association. 2004. http://classicweb.archive.org/web/20080115224655/alpha.dickinson.edu/oha/org_irbupdate.html. Accessed 6 Apr 2011.
53. Health Insurance Portability and Accountability Act of 1996. Public Law 104-191. 104th Congress. 1996. http://www.gpo.gov/fdsys/pkg/PLAW-104publ191/pdf/PLAW-104publ191.pdf. Accessed 15 Sept 2011.
54. HHS, Health Insurance Reform: Security Standards; Final Rule. 45 CFR parts 160, 162 and 164. 2003. Federal register. http://aspe.hhs.gov/admnsimp/final/fr03-8334.pdf. Accessed 12 May 2011.
55. HHS Strengthens HIPAA Enforcement. 2009. http://www.hhs.gov/news/press/2009pres/10/20091030a.html. Accessed 12 May 2011.
56. Guidance for Securing Protected Health Information. 2009. http://www.hhs.gov/ocr/privacy/hipaa/understanding/coveredentities/hitechrfi.pdf. Accessed 12 May 2011.
57. Clinical Research and the HIPAA Privacy Rule. NIH Publication Number 04-5495. 2004. http://privacyruleandresearch.nih.gov/clin_research.asp. Accessed 15 Sept 2011.
58. HSS, Summary of the HIPAA Privacy Rule. http://www.hhs.gov/ocr/privacy/hipaa/understanding/summary/privacysummary.pdf. Accessed 5 Sept 2011.
59. Institutional Review Boards and the HIPAA Privacy Rule. NIH Publication Number 03-5428. 2003. http://privacyruleandresearch.nih.gov/irbandprivacyrule. Accessed 15 Sept 2011.
60. NIH & clinical research. Ethics in clinical research. http://clinicalresearch.nih.gov/ethics_guides.html. Accessed 5 Apr 2011.
61. Diamond B. Removal, retention and storage of organ and tissue in the UK. Br J Nurs. 2005;14:107–8.
62. Grant RW, Sugarman J. Ethics in human subjects research: do incentives matter? J Med Philos. 2004; 29:717–38.
63. McNeill P. A response to Wilkinson and Moore. Paying people to participate in research: why not? Bioethics. 1997;11:390–6.
64. Litton P, Miller FG. What physician-investigators owe patients who participate in research. JAMA. 2010; 304:1491–2.
65. Schwarze ML, Bradley CT, Brasel KJ. Surgical "buy-in": the contractual relationship between surgeons and patients that influences decisions regarding life-supporting therapy. Crit Care Med. 2010;38:843–8.
66. Altman Lawrence K. Who goes first? The story of self-experimentation in medicine. New York: Random House; 1998.
67. Marshall BJ, Armstrong JA, McGechie DB, Glancy RJ. Attempt to fulfil Koch's postulates for pyloric campylobacter. Med J Aust. 1985;142:436–9.
68. Emanuel EJ, Wendler D, Grady C. What makes clinical research ethical? JAMA. 2000;283:2701–11.

69. Definition of Research Misconduct. HHS, Office of Research Integrity. http://ori.hhs.gov/misconduct/definition_misconduct.shtml. Accessed 15 Sept 2011.
70. Wakefield AJ, Murch SH, Anthony A, Linnell J, Casson DM, Malik M, Berelowitz M, Dhillon AP, Thomson MA, Harvey P, Valentine A, Davies SE, Walker-Smith JA. Ileal lymphoid nodular hyperplasia, non-specific colitis, and pervasive developmental disorder in children [retracted]. Lancet. 1998;351:637–41.
71. Deer B. How the case against the MMR vaccine was fixed. BMJ. 2011;342(C5347):77–82.
72. Borrell BA. Medical Madoff: anesthesiologist faked data in 21 studies. Scientific American, 10 Mar 2009.
73. Harris G. Doctor admits pain studies were frauds, hospital says. New York Times, 11 Mar 2009.
74. Marret E, Elia N, Dahl JB, McQuay HJ, Møiniche S, Moore RA, Straube S, Tramèr MR. Susceptibility to fraud in systematic reviews: lessons from the Reuben case. Anesthesiology. 2009;111:1279–89.
75. Johnson P. Scott Reuben, a former Baystate doctor who faked research, sentenced to 6 months for health care fraud. MassLive.Com, 24 June 2010.
76. Sheehan JG. Fraud, conflict of interest, and other enforcement issues in clinical research. Cleve Clin J Med. 2007;74(Suppl 2):S63–7. discussion S68–S9.
77. Wells JA. Final report: observing and reporting suspected misconduct in biomedical research. 2008. http://ori.dhhs.gov/research/intra/documents/gallup_finalreport.pdf. Accessed 13 May 2011.
78. Stewart DO, DeMarco JP. Rational noncompliance with prescribed medical treatment. Kennedy Inst Ethics J. 2010;20:277–90.
79. Cleaveland C. "We are not criminals": social work advocacy and unauthorized migrants. Soc Work. 2010;55:74–81.

How to Prepare a Scientific Paper

13

Jeffrey S. Borer

The Purpose of the Research Paper

It has long been a commonly accepted precept that the process of research is complete only when the research has been reported in appropriate form to the scientific community. Currently, that form is the scientific "paper." Without the scientific paper, the research cannot be replicated, clinicians and researchers cannot evaluate it and act upon it, and society cannot benefit from it.

To best understand the purpose and scope of the scientific paper, one must understand the purpose and scope of research. These characteristics, considered in the opening chapter, are also clearly delineated in a monograph, entitled "Clinical Judgment," by the late Alvan Feinstein, which provides illuminating insight into the relation of science and medicine [1]. Dr. Feinstein's thesis was that clinical judgment must be based on application of the scientific method. As indicated earlier in this book, the scientific method is an intellectual concept referring to the development of a hypothesis, testing of the hypothesis by observations employing relevant methodology, appraisal and analysis of the resulting data, and the development of conclusions by interpretation of these data. In Feinstein's words, the goal of this process is to "answer the original questions [on which the research was based], and to establish knowledge that may clarify the past, illuminate the present, and anticipate the future" [1]. Thus, the fundamental goal of medical research is the creation of new knowledge.

Dr. Feinstein argued that the same method, the scientific method, underlies the reasoning of a physician in selecting a management strategy for a single patient, the work of a clinical researcher studying large groups of patients, and the efforts of the laboratory scientist observing and experimenting with animals, cells, or molecules. These activities differ only in the procedures employed for making observations and the precision and representativeness of the resulting data. All these activities can create new knowledge which, either directly or ultimately, may carry forth the goals of the physician-scientist: relief of suffering and improvement in quality and, perhaps, length of life. Thus, Feinstein suggests that all activities of the physician, both in the laboratory and at the bedside, are the product of the same problem-solving methods, including application of Boolean algebra and its associated logic.

The scientific paper reports and describes the problem that was studied, the methods employed, the results of the research, and the interpretation drawn from these results by the investigator. Consistent with the possible scope of the research, discussed above, in medicine the scientific paper

J.S. Borer, MD (✉)
Department of Medicine, Division of Cardiovascular Diseases, Howard Gilman Institute for Valvular Heart Diseases, and Cardiovascular Translational Research Institute, State University of New York (SUNY) Downstate Medical Center, 450 Clarkson Avenue, 50, Brooklyn, NY 11203, USA
e-mail: canadad45@aol.com

P.G. Supino and J.S. Borer (eds.), *Principles of Research Methodology: A Guide for Clinical Investigators*, DOI 10.1007/978-1-4614-3360-6_13, © Phyllis G. Supino and Jeffrey S. Borer 2012

can range from a report of a well-studied single clinical experience (case report) to a highly complex, controlled, and carefully blinded study of the impact of a transfected gene on myocardial protein degradation in tissue culture. The term "scientific paper" may seem relatively nonspecific. However, given the explosion of biomedical literature during the past generation, the concomitant recruitment of highly talented and experienced journal editors, and the relative paucity of costly journal publication space, it is not surprising that a fairly rigorous definition for the term can be found.

The definition of a scientific paper is comprehensively developed and discussed by Robert A. Day, professor emeritus of English at the University of Delaware and past president of the Society for Scholarly Publishing and of the Council of Biology Editors, in his definitive book, "How to Write and Publish a Scientific Paper" [2]. As stated by Professor Day, "a scientific paper is a written and published report describing original research results." However, it must be written and published "as defined by [three centuries of developing] tradition, editorial practice, scientific ethics, and the interplay of printing and publishing procedures." Professor Day quotes the definition of an acceptable primary scientific publication developed by the Council of Biology Editors: it "must be the first disclosure containing sufficient information to enable peers (1) to assess observations, (2) to repeat experiments and (3) to evaluate intellectual processes; moreover, it must be susceptible to sensory perception, essentially permanent, available to the scientific community without restriction, and available for regular screening by one or more of the major recognized services (e.g., currently, Biological Abstracts, Chemical Abstracts, Index Medicus, Excerpta Medica, Bibliography of Agriculture, etc., in the United States and similar services in other countries") [2].

Today, considerable publication is performed via electronic media and the Internet, and may never appear in an edition printed on paper. The definition of the scientific paper is not altered by the use of electronic media. As indicated by the American Association for the Advancement of Science (AAAS), the essential elements of the electronically published scientific paper are that the final published version of an article after peer review (or any future peer-review equivalent), which AAAS denotes as "the *Definitive Publication*," needs to be clearly identified as such and "must be publicly available, the relevant community must be made aware of its existence, a system for long-term access and retrieval must be in place…it must not be changed (technical protection and/or certification are desirable), it must not be removed (unless legally unavoidable), it must be unambiguously identified…it must have a bibliographic record…containing certain minimal information, [and] archiving and long-term preservation must be provided for" [3].

As indicated by the AAAS criteria, the definition of the scientific paper, either printed on paper or in electronic media, encompasses the concept of prepublication peer review. Peer review is the process by which other professionals, understood on the basis of their own publications or other credentials to have expertise in paper's area of focus, evaluate the paper and grade it as to priority for publication. Most journals employ a system of peer review to select manuscripts to be published from within the larger pool of those submitted. The number of peer reviewers for most publications usually is two, though more or fewer may be employed in any instance. The criteria for judgment generally include the intrinsic importance of the subject about which the paper is written (hypothesis to be tested, research problem, etc.), the adequacy of the methodology for the stated purpose, the credibility of the results and the adequacy of the data analysis, the reasonableness and fairness of the conclusions/interpretations, the adequacy of the bibliography, and the adequacy of the formal presentation (i.e., is the reader likely to be able to understand the material as it is presented). In addition, it is hoped that peer reviewers will help to identify submissions that already are in review by more than one venue or that present data already published (both findings indicate transgression of copyright laws and general standards for publication). Peer reviewers also are expected to have some sense of the likelihood that the data are real and not fraudulent, though the latter is largely impossible for a reviewer to verify. It is essential for authors to recognize the characteristics by which peer reviewers will judge a manuscript (and, subsequently, to respond courteously and appropriately to suggestions for additions, clarification, or other alterations to the manuscript) if the work is to be accepted for publication.

The definition of the scientific paper also implies a certain amount of detail in reporting methodology and results; the degree of such detail ultimately is the product of a complex interplay of intellectual and moral/ethical considerations and may vary with the mores of the era and the context within which the publication is conceived and written. Centuries ago, a scientific treatise did not necessarily conform to the rigorous research standards that prevail today, with the necessity for substantiating data. The concept was paramount; data reporting was less rigorous and often relatively inaccurate. Scientific thought was evolving, but scientists did not have the luxury of the technological resources available today that mark the often exquisite details of current research.

The degree of detail that is required depends in part on the familiarity of the intended audience with the methods employed. In many instances, techniques that are widely used and generally accepted as "standard" (e.g., electrocardiography) require no more than recitation, with no supporting bibliographic reference. On the other hand, other aspects of methodology, and particularly elements of study design, may be so critical to interpretation of the results by the reader that considerable descriptive detail may be necessary.

The need for a scientific paper to enable the reader to "evaluate the intellectual process" requires either direct discussion of that process in the manuscript or, more commonly, organization of the manuscript such that relevant inferences can be drawn. As noted by Feinstein, the latter has resulted in the complaint by Peter Medawar in the Saturday Review that "scientific writing is often intellectually 'fraudulent' because the careful organization given to the published material do[es] not reflect the way things happened. After conquering his ignorance, the scientist presenting his 'new' ideas in print may be reluctant to discuss how much ignorance he had to overcome" [4]. Fortunately, however, given the limited journal publication space available, the capacity to evaluate the logic underlying a given piece of research far outweighs the need to scrutinize the specific and often circuitous path by which that logic was revealed, Dr. Medawar and the Saturday Review notwithstanding!

Since a scientific paper must communicate several aspects of a research project, a logical, standardized reporting format is preferred. Currently, the most commonly used format is known by the acronym, IMRAD: introduction, methods, results, and discussion. This probably should be changed to AIMRAD to reflect the almost universal placement of an abstract at the head of the scientific paper, a relatively recent development. The abstract is important since it may alter the information content required of the introduction. The IMRAD format (or AIMRAD, or TAAIMRAD, if the title and authors are considered, since they, too, can convey important information) indicates sequentially what problem was studied, why it was studied, what was found, and how these findings should be interpreted, particularly within the context of related work in the field.

The best aid to crafting a useful scientific paper is a well-organized, well-planned, and clearly written research proposal or protocol. The well-crafted proposal will (1) clearly state the specific aims of the research, including hypotheses to be tested (if any); (2) provide a context and justification for the study with reference to the literature; and (3) define precisely the methods to be employed, including the research design, measurement techniques and approach to statistical analysis, the principal results expected, and the conclusions that might be suggested by them. In other words, the protocol provides the basis for the introduction and methods sections of the paper. However, since the best laid plans often go somewhat astray, the proposal must be supplemented by consideration of the procedures actually employed and data truly collected before the scientific paper can be written. As Turato et al. have noted, "Investigative studies without explicit hypotheses give rise to the supposition that these enterprises have a merely mechanical course. That is, they uncritically repeat the dominant group's methodological models in the world of academic medicine. Failure to present hypotheses, before enumerating the objectives, usually represented a failure to respect the *logical sequence of stages*, which are understood as occurring naturally in the mind of the thinker" [5]. As Knottnerus also has observed, "We should not forget that mathematical indices are just ways to summarise collected research data. For the quality of research, defining the research question, and methodological challenges in study design, are far more important" [6].

A summary of some specific characteristics of the components of the scientific paper follows, organized as per the TAAIMRAD format. This summary owes a considerable debt to the published comments of Professor Day, as well as to personal experiences in applying the generally accepted precepts.

The Title

The title is the first and, often, only contact of the reader with the paper. Therefore, it must convey considerable information with an economy of words. The primary consideration in crafting a title is clarity. Jargon should be avoided, and the relevant rules of grammar should be followed.

Equally importantly, a title should be specific and focused. Thus, the title must refer specifically to the subject of the research, rather than merely to the field within which the research is undertaken. (Of course, the operating definition of "subject" and "field" can vary with the research.) For example, in a prospective study employing radionuclide cineangiography and echocardiography to develop prognostic indices for survival in patients with mitral regurgitation who had not undergone valve replacement or repair, the title "Prediction of Survival in Patients with Mitral Regurgitation by Use of Noninvasively Defined Indices of Left and Right Ventricular Performance" would be preferable to, for example, "Prediction of Survival in Mitral Regurgitation." While the latter indicates the general subject of the study, the former also indicates the methodological approach, including the variables measured. Although more verbose, the longer title helps to define the scope of the study and to distinguish it from others in the field. If no study of prognostication in mitral regurgitation had been performed previously, the lengthier title would be less essential. However, since other studies have been performed, the additional verbiage is useful, providing the knowledgeable reader with some indication of the uniqueness of the paper and its relevance for his or her work.

Other important considerations, suggested above, include the desirability of conveying more of the IMRAD information than merely the subject of the study and the desirability of brevity. The criterion for acceptable brevity varies with fashion (e.g., Darwin's title for his account of his voyages on the Beagle, "On The Origin of Species by Means of Natural Selection, or The Preservation of Favoured Races in the Struggle for Life" [7], acceptable in 1859 but not in a medical journal in 2010!).

In summary, in crafting a title, effort is well spent attempting to minimize words while maximizing clarity, focus, and information content.

Authorship

Different criteria exist for inclusion in an authors list and for the order of listing. When this author worked at the National Institutes of Health (NIH), a simple rule of thumb was proposed: listed authors should have made an important contribution to the research and should be able to present and defend the paper at a scientific meeting. This definition implies that an author has acquired a body of knowledge which can serve as a context for the reported research and that he or she is intimately familiar with the intricacies of the methodology employed in the research as well as with the results. However, with the rapid increase in technological and biological information in recent years, it has become increasingly necessary for projects to be carried out by teams comprising collaborators with different, and often widely disparate, areas of expertise. For example, in the randomized Collaborative Study of Coronary Artery Surgery (CASS) [8], a trial designed to assess the effects of coronary artery bypass grafting plus standard (ad hoc) pharmacological/dietary therapy compared with standard (ad hoc) pharmacological/dietary approaches alone on natural history of patients with coronary artery occlusive disease, public health specialists/epidemiologists and statisticians were critical to the study design and analysis. In fact, an epidemiologist and a statistician were the first and second authors of one of the most important papers resulting from the trial.

However, surgeons and cardiologists participated in the trial, and the cardiologists included those who performed catheterizations and those who did not. It is likely that representatives of all these groups, and more, participated in the conceptualization of the study, that all but the statistician participated in primary data collection, and that many participated in interpretation of the results. However, it would be excessive to expect the epidemiologist or statistician to understand the methodological pitfalls of the catheterization (much less to identify them when they occurred), or to expect the cardiologist, the epidemiologist, or the statistician to fully understand and identify methodological problems associated with surgical procedures, or for the cardiologist or the surgeon to understand fully or to be able to defend the procedures employed by the statistician. Therefore, Day's definition is now most appropriate: "an author of a paper should be defined as one who takes intellectual responsibility for the research results being reported" [2]. Thus, authors should include those who actively or substantially contributed to the conceptualization, design, and performance of the research. It is sometimes true that individuals intimately involved in conceptualization and design of research and in analysis and/or interpretation of results have little or no responsibility for primary data collection and that individuals involved in primary data collection have little or no involvement in the other processes. The latter is particularly true of technicians or research assistants, who in most circumstances do not provide intellectual input into the process (though many exceptions exist). Problems can also arise regarding the inclusion of senior scientists in whose area of responsibility the research occured but who may have had little direct input into the specific project. Clearly, the distinction between those whose intellectual responsibility is sufficient to warrant authorship and those whose responsibility is not is difficult to make with precision. Ultimately, this determination probably depends on a consensus of the involved investigators. However, those who allow their names to be listed as authors incur another responsibility, specifically for the veracity of the reported data. In several celebrated cases of research fraud three decades ago, some renowned senior scientists, not associated with collecting or analyzing data but involved (sometimes distantly) in project conceptualization, were listed among the authors of papers found to be fraudulent; though none of them was aware of the fraudulence of the reported data, they were perceived as irresponsible in allowing their names to be used without adequately assessing the reported projects.

Regarding the order of authorship, again per Day, "authors should normally be listed in order of importance to the experiments" [2]. Sometimes a senior investigator or group leader chooses to move out of such ordering into the last position on the list, from which his or her senior status can be inferred and which provides added recognition to junior authors by moving them up the list. In some cultures, authors are listed alphabetically. No universally accepted rules exist for ordering the authors list; the ultimate test of the appropriateness of the list is consensus of the individuals involved.

The Abstract

The Abstract represents a brief summary of the paper. As such, it should contain a concise statement of the research problem, sufficient methodological information to orient the reader, a summary of the results of primary importance, and the authors' principal conclusions.

The length of the Abstract and, often, its format are governed by the policy of the publication to which the paper is submitted.

Important considerations in Abstract writing include (1) avoidance of abbreviations whenever possible and, when they are needed, limitation to those which are generally recognized; (2) minimization of words without disregard for grammar and syntax; and (3) avoidance of reference to data or methods not reported in the paper. The latter requires careful final editing since substudies or subanalyses sometimes are eliminated from the final edition of a paper because of considerations of relevance or space, but still may appear in the previously written Abstract.

Introduction

The Introduction is a tool for communication and is critical to the success of the paper. It serves several functions. These include, but are not limited to, engaging the reader's interest sufficiently to justify proceeding into the details of methodology and results, suggesting the logic of the methods, and providing a framework for assimilating and interpreting the results.

To serve these purposes, the Introduction must (1) clearly state the problem or problems (hypotheses, research questions, specific aims) under study; if more than one problem has been studied, the relation of the problems, and the reason for studying them together, should be elucidated; (2) provide a basis, usually from the literature, for choosing to study the problem(s); (3) outline the approach to the problem indicating, when appropriate, why this approach, rather than others, was chosen; and (4) indicate the importance or uniqueness of the paper, i.e., justify the performance of this particular study. Though some writers choose to briefly describe results and conclusions in the Introduction, most do not. These are available in the Abstract and are redundant when more complete exposition of these aspects of the research will follow. In stating the problem, the writer should avoid distracting irrelevancies. For example, if one has studied the effect of alcohol consumption on left ventricular ejection fraction, it would be inappropriate to include in the Introduction a paean to the value of ejection fraction as an index of prognosis in heart disease. Though ejection fraction is a useful prognostic index, the problem under study has nothing to do with the use of ejection fraction for prognosis. The mention of this property of ejection fraction may suggest to the reader that prognostication strategies have been studied. The resulting confusion may preclude clear assimilation of the data actually presented. If the reader is performing prepublication peer review for a journal, this confusion may be translated into rejection for an otherwise worthy effort.

As we have emphasized in Chap. 2 of this book, the statement of the problem must be sharply focused. Many authors have documented a relation between alcohol consumption, acute or chronic, and deterioration of left ventricular performance. Few have defined the quantitative relation between alcohol consumption and ejection fraction change. If the study in question was designed to provide such information, and the relevant data were collected, then the statement of the problem should focus on the effort to quantify the relation between the intervention and the parameter employed.

The author should not promise something, directly or by implication, that he or she does not deliver. Thus, for example, in justifying the study of the effect of alcohol consumption on ejection fraction, it would be best to avoid suggesting that the study was performed because it might help to guide therapy unless (a) the results include data on the effects of therapy in this condition and (b) the relationship of the effects of therapy to ejection fraction is described. (In certain situations, this speculation might be appropriate in the Discussion.)

It is important to inform the reader if multiple problems have been assessed. All but the most compulsive readers generally will remember no more than one fact or concept after reading a paper. If multiple concepts or types of results have been generated in a study, a well-constructed Introduction may improve the likelihood of their recognition and retention. A negative example may illustrate the point. In 1979, this author and colleagues assessed response of left ventricular volume and function to exercise in patients with aortic regurgitation [9]. In a brief, two-paragraph Introduction, only the study of "function" (measured as ejection fraction) was mentioned. The assessment of volume change received no comment. In the many subsequent references to this frequently cited paper, the citation invariably has been to the effect of exercise on ejection fraction. To this author's knowledge, no one ever has mentioned our finding of marked reduction in left ventricular end diastolic filling during exercise, which was reported in this paper. Other authors subsequently reported studies of volume changes during exercise in aortic regurgitation, without reference to these data. This oversight is likely related in large part to an incomplete Introduction to the paper. As a result, other investigators could not benefit from these findings in designing their studies.

A brief description of the methodological approach employed in the study will permit the knowledgeable reader to place the study in an appropriate context for interpretation while other sections of the paper are being read. If methodology somehow was unique, this should be indicated, together with the reason for use of the new method. For example, in 1977, this author and colleagues reported a study of the effect of exercise on regional and global left ventricular function/performance in 11 patients with coronary disease who had normal performance descriptors at rest [10]. In this instance, the method employed to study performance during exercise was of greater interest than the effect of exercise itself. Application of radionuclide cineangiography during exercise had not been previously reported in a scientific paper. Therefore, the Introduction included a paragraph explaining the theoretical importance of studying the effect of exercise in coronary disease and another paragraph describing the relevance of radionuclide cineangiography in permitting such study.

The introduction should be organized according to journalistic precepts: the most important concept should be presented first, and subsidiary concepts should be presented thereafter. Neither the Introduction nor the scientific paper as a whole should be treated as a guessing game or as a finely wrought mystery-drama. The busy reader should be engaged early by references to material which the author considers most important.

Finally, the Introduction should be brief. Detailed review of collateral or supporting literature is appropriate for the Discussion, but not for the Introduction. Generally, the Introduction should be limited to one double-spaced typed page (approximately 250 words). If the Introduction substantially exceeds this limit, the author must consider the possibility that he or she has not clearly identified the key concepts in his or her own mind.

Methods

As Day has noted, the primary purpose of this section "is to describe and (if necessary) defend the experimental design and then provide enough detail that a competent worker can repeat the experiments" [2].

Clear and accurate description of methods is critically important. The careful reader cannot properly interpret the results or evaluate the conclusions without a fundamental understanding of the methods employed in making the observations. As a corollary, the limitations of the methods should be understood. This may require a specific statement by the author if he or she believes that the interpretation or generalizability of results is importantly mitigated by some aspect of the methodology or, conversely, if the author believes that an apparent methodological limitation can be explained in a manner that minimizes circumscription of conclusions.

In general, the Methods section should begin with a detailed statement of the subjects employed (physical models or devices, cells, tissues, or animals if the study is nonclinical) or humans studied (if the study is clinical). This statement should include generally accepted group descriptors (i.e., demographic data in clinical studies), criteria for acceptance and/or exclusion of subjects from the study population, and a description of any special procedures employed to determine fitness for acceptance. If rabbit hearts have been homogenized for analysis of protein content, the weight, age, and breed of rabbit should be noted, as well as the total number of rabbits instrumented for study and reasons for any discrepancy between this number and the number whose hearts actually were homogenized and analyzed. This information helps the reader to evaluate possible interactive effects of selection bias, albeit unintentional, that might alter extrapolability of results. Similarly, in the previously noted example of the study to develop prognostic strategies in mitral regurgitation, in addition to age, sex, and, perhaps, other demographic descriptors if deemed relevant to interpretation of results, the author should define the basis for determining the diagnosis of mitral regurgitation and its severity (physical examination, echocardiography, catheterization, etc.), including the specific criteria employed for classification with the method[s] chosen. If the study were designed to develop prognostic strategies in systemic arterial hypertension, rather than in mitral regurgitation, then, in addition to age and sex, race, weight, and height might be important demographic descriptors since the pathophysiology of hypertension is known to vary with race and, to a lesser extent, with obesity.

Special note should be made of sample size estimates (see detailed discussion in Chap. 11). Sample size should be planned in the study protocol. It may be appropriate to relate the protocol-mandated plan in the Methods and the reasoning on which the plan was based. This is particularly true when the primary results, or some important secondaries, are "negative," i.e., the expected relationships are not found. Lack of statistical significance is not equivalent to true lack of relationships. Sample size estimates are based on the expected outcome, the expected variability of the measurement methods, the likelihood that the result is not due to chance alone (the alpha level, selected before the study by the investigators), and the likelihood of finding the expected outcome *if it really exists* (also chosen before the study by the investigators). The latter is known as the "power" to find the expected results and is expressed as a percentage. The hazards involved in not reporting the basis of sample size selection are best illustrated with reference to studies of therapeutic interventions, usually evaluated by comparing a new treatment modality with an established therapy. For such studies, the expected outcome event rate with the established therapy may be estimated from earlier studies; the difference to be sought between the new therapy and the comparator may be selected by the investigators based on their judgment of the magnitude of difference that may be clinically useful. However, if the event rate with established therapy is found to differ importantly from historical standards (particularly if it is lower), the calculated sample size may provide far less than the anticipated power to detect superiority of the new therapy, even if it exists. Presentation of the basis for selection of the sample size in the methods may help the reader to avoid erroneous ("negative") interpretation of the data.

As these examples suggest, the specific parameters described in a methods section will vary from study to study. Nonetheless, each aspect of the methodology must be defined rigorously and precisely. On the other hand, excessive detail which does not affect data interpretation (e.g., hair color, shoe size, and telephone numbers of the patients with mitral regurgitation) can be confusing, misleading, and inappropriate. One caveat: some journals may have specific requirements regarding identification of materials or methods. These will be related in *Instructions to Authors* in the journal and must be followed.

After describing the subjects/items on which studies were performed and, if appropriate, explaining the basis of sample size selection, the author should detail the materials employed in processing and testing the subjects, as well as the procedures used to make observations. Again, detail should be sufficient to permit interpretation and/or replication of results. If procedures have been well described in the literature and were performed without substantial change from those published, a general statement with a literary citation may suffice. As a hypothetical example, assume that the authors of a study state that "equilibrium radionuclide cineangiography was performed at rest and during symptom-limited supine bicycle ergometry according to methods analogous to those we have previously described and employing in vivo labeling of red cells with Tc^{99m}." If substantial changes have occurred since the previous publication of the method, these should be described and, if necessary, justified or defended (e.g., "radionuclide cineangiography was performed using a recently developed image rendering method to precisely define left ventricular borders. This method involves…. It was employed because cardiac function indices were significantly better correlated with independent standards than were older methods"). Appropriate references also should be supplied.

The research design also should be specified. If interventions are employed in some study subjects but not in others, the basis for allocation of subjects to treatment groups should be defined (e.g., randomization, stratification) as should other design elements that reduce bias (e.g., blinding in processing/evaluating primary data). The temporal sequencing of the observations relative to the intervention should be described.

Statistical methods employed to analyze data must be presented, including criteria for accepting or rejecting the null hypothesis (i.e., the p value below which result will be declared statistically significant). Most physicians are relatively unfamiliar with the details of statistics and with the criteria for selecting specific tests of significance in certain situations. However, the ready availability of statistical computer packages has led to widespread performance of statistical tests by nonstatisticians. While many of these procedures undoubtedly are correctly selected and performed, some probably are not. The best remedy for this problem is to consult a statistician in the design of the research protocol and in statistical analysis of results and to ask the statistician to write the appropriate portion of the methods section, explaining it conceptually to the other authors. However, if this is not done, the statistical methods employed should be carefully cited so that the statistically literate reader (and the peer reviewers) can evaluate the appropriateness of the analysis and resulting conclusions. During a study performed some years ago by this author's group, one nonstatistician spent considerable time familiarizing himself with statistical methodology and performed a multiple logistic regression analysis with some of the data. An astute peer reviewer noted that, given the size of the patient population, an excessive number of parameters had been tested for independent significance in the regression model. The description of the statistical methodology permitted detection and correction of this error.

In summary, description of methods requires judgment as to the appropriate degree of detail. When in doubt, it is usually better to include more rather than less, though much detail may be removed by editorial suggestion after peer review and before publication. The guiding principle should be that sufficient information is transmitted so that, in the view of the authors and journal editor, the results can be accurately interpreted.

Results

In the Results section, the author presents the observations which will permit assessment of his or her original hypotheses and specific aims. In a sense, the results represent the new knowledge which has been created by the research.

Narrative

In general, and particularly when complex mathematical analyses and subanalyses have been performed, it is useful to present the results in narrative form, supplemented by tables and figures. The narrative should indicate as clearly as possible the flow and thrust of the data, i.e., the overall sense of the findings. Interpolation of numbers into this narrative should be done with care and caution, preferably when they do not impede the flow. However, the narrative may be strengthened by judicious interpolation of evidence of the statistical significance of the findings ("p values"). This latter approach necessitates clarity and comprehensiveness in the design of tables and figures in which the data are presented quantitatively, since the narrative must be consistent with the numbers. Moreover, the narrative should present only the results and not the conclusions. A well-designed narrative plus graphics may lead obviously to certain conclusions, but statement of these should await the next section.

As with the methods, some judgment must be employed in deciding which results require presentation. Intensive analysis may reveal many relationships unsuspected in the planning of the study. Concern about the chance finding of a "statistically significant" relationship on the basis of overanalysis of data probably is well-founded. Therefore, unexpected relationships, particularly those derived from post hoc analyses, should be evaluated with caution. Nonetheless, some of these may be important in drawing conclusions from the research and certainly can be hypothesis-generating for future studies. Some may be irrelevant. The latter generally do not require presentation. Negative results often are important though these, too, must not be overinterpreted. A negative finding may have resulted from measurement error or from sample size that is inadequate to properly assess the relationship under study. In these instances, a positive, i.e., statistically significant, result would have been unlikely even if, in fact, the sought-after relationship actually exists. Such limitations in the extrapolability of the data generally should be noted in the discussion section.

Tables and figures need not be limited to the Results, but this is the section in which they are generally most appropriate and useful. Tables and figures can be employed in the Introduction or Discussion to summarize work done by others into which context the newly reported results must be integrated, or to diagram relationships (often pathophysiological relationships) believed to underlie the results that are being reported. In general, these strategies are best reserved for review articles and should be avoided in scientific papers (original research reports) because the use of space for this purpose is seldom justified by any gain in comprehension by the reader. Indeed, in order to make such tables comprehensible, an expanded explanatory text often is required (frequently drawing upon data not generated within the report being presented by the author), potentially increasing the size of the printed article beyond the limit allowed by the journal and diminishing space needed to present the new knowledge. In the current era in which Internet publication, with supplements and appendices, often is undertaken or accompanies printed versions of scientific papers, the space limitation may be overcome by adding tables (and figures) in electronic appendices, surmounting the proscription on such additions. However, the author must always remember that the primary purpose of publication is communication and that the accretion of additional material may obscure rather than clarify the focus and conclusions of the research. In the Results, however, tables and figures are invaluable and space-saving devices that often help to clarify complex results by removing them from the narrative, enabling comprehensible summary presentations supplemented by the data from which they are derived. In the following summary of considerations in the use and configuration of tables and figures, much has been gained from review of the chapters on these subjects in the monograph by Edward J. Huth ("How to Write and Publish Papers in the Medical Sciences") to which the reader is referred for greater detail [11].

Tables

Multiple well-focused tables are preferable to one massive compendium of all relevant data. However, the number of tables that can be employed often is defined or limited by the editorial policy of the individual journal and must be known when planning use of these devices. More importantly, the author must consider which tables would best further the communication at which the paper is aimed. Information involving few data that might be effectively displayed in tabular form for an oral presentation probably can be communicated more appropriately by narrative summary in a paper. If tables are employed, however, they must be cited and sequenced within the text so that their relation to the narrative results is easily discernable [11]. In any table, the title should clearly define the focus and nature of the data or relationships to be presented, and column and row headings should be simple and easily understood. If abbreviations or technical terms are employed for the sake of the esthetic/clarity of the layout, these should be precisely defined in a legend. The legend also may include a summary statement amplifying or totally replacing the table title to clarify the specific purpose of the table. It is critically important to define the units of measurement for any numerical data in the table [11]. In some tables, absolute numerical results are followed by parenthetical presentations of percentages of the data set represented by these absolute values. Unless the antecedent data set is precisely defined and obviously visible, such formats can lead to reader confusion and deterioration of communication. If statistical comparisons among elements of the table are presented, it must be made absolutely clear which elements are being compared and what type of comparison has been performed. For example, a "p value" for noninferiority between two data sets may indicate the high likelihood that one set is noninferior to the other, but unless the type of comparison has been explicitly stated and there is a numerical difference between the sets, the reader may assume the "p value" refers to superiority, an erroneous conclusion that could preclude comprehension and subsequent application of the results.

Figures

To be optimally effective, figures should be relatively uncluttered. In general, one fact or relationship should be illustrated by each figure, though many observations in the narrative may be supported by figures. It can be very confusing to decipher "three-dimensional" plots, or single figures with two or three different ordinate or abscissa scales, each referring to a different line identifiable with reference to black or white polygons, all within the same coordinate axes. Examples of figures that can be very useful in clarifying or amplifying (or replacing) text include graphic presentations of complex study designs, flow charts indicating reductions in population size as exclusions or other factors impact on the population studied, quantitative relations between important independent (input) variables and primary dependent (outcome) variables (particularly when the relation follows a clear pattern), etc. However, the latter figures only should be employed when they provide clear support for an author's subsequent conclusions [11]. It is not necessary, and, in my view, it is inappropriate to provide examples of individual data (e.g., a photograph of a histological sample of a degenerated myocyte from an organism with heart failure) unless some unique characteristic of the photograph supports the existence of a previously unsuspected process. It is not necessary to present illustrations to prove that certain analyses were performed: there is general agreement among researchers that statements of fact presented in the Results are true—it is the interpretations that may differ; figures are most useful when they support interpretations.

It should be intuitively obvious that any figure employed in a publication must be clean, technically well reproduced, and easy to read. In addition, however, considerable attention should be paid to labeling. In displays of coordinate axes, the ordinate and abscissa must be clearly labeled with units of measurement, amplified if necessary by statements in the legend. Similarly, interventions, time intervals, etc., must be precisely laid out in flow charts and study design diagrams. Idiosyncratic abbreviations in labels should be avoided when possible. Ultimately, as for tables, the use of figures should be undertaken only when they are clearly useful in potentiating comprehension of results and conclusions presented in the Discussion. It is an error, likely to be cited and extirpated by peer reviewers and editors, to present the same data both in tabular and graphic format—if the data require amplification beyond the narrative, select one format or the other, not both. Remember that the goal of the presentation is clear communication.

Discussion

The purpose of the Discussion is to present conclusions based on the results of the research. Thus, the Discussion is the authors' opportunity to interpret and identify the importance of their work and, as Day has noted, "to present the principles, relationships, and generalizations shown by the Results" [2]. Certain principles should be observed in writing a Discussion. If they are not, most editors and many reviewers will call the author to task and may even reject an otherwise laudable report.

Less generally is more. Lengthy discussions, extrapolating from every conceivable aspect of the data, often are not well received. Moreover, they can detract from the importance and originality of the primary observations by overwhelming and distracting the reader. As a corollary, summarization of the results is redundant and inappropriate in the Discussion and usually is not tolerated by editors jealous of their limited publication space.

Conclusions should be clearly and closely related to the data obtained in the study. Far-reaching speculations generally should be avoided. Fairness and balance are necessary in interpreting results. Excessive emphasis on a pet theory should be avoided, particularly if alternatives exist that may be credible. Therefore, the relation of the results to those of other parallel or similar studies should be discussed. If possible, some explanation should be provided for apparent differences. Often, these may be ascribable to differences in methodology, so that careful review of the methodology of collateral references can be very helpful. Claims of priority are appropriate if correct (e.g., "This study represents the first demonstration of parthenogenesis in the Syrian hamster"), but check the literature carefully to be certain of the claim (see below).

Support for or refutation of conclusions should be cited from the published literature and may require additional discussion. It is the responsibility of the authors to undertake a reasonable literature search to find appropriate references. As discussed in Chaps. 2 and 9, the explosion of scientific literature has made this a difficult and time-consuming undertaking. However, several computer-based literature search services can be helpful, including those readily available via the National Library of Medicine. It is true that the scientific paper reports the findings of the authors' project and that lack of placement of these findings in the appropriate literary context does not alter their intrinsic validity or value; nonetheless, lack of adequate literary references may lead a reader to under- or overvalue or otherwise misunderstand the importance and implications of the reported research. Also, lack of appropriate referencing is unfair to the work and workers thus disregarded. Even if the intrinsic moral issue here is uninteresting to an author, its practical consequences often are not. It is almost a truism that the author of a study you neglect will be a prepublication peer reviewer and may resent what is perceived as an inappropriate claim of priority.

Limitations of the work, in terms of methodology employed, inconsistencies in results, etc., should be discussed. Interpretation in light of these limitations should be defended when necessary. Readers and reviewers will be aware of these limitations, and failure to deal with them in the Discussion may detract from the credibility of otherwise excellent work.

Theoretical or abstract conclusions are appropriate when logically drawn from data, circumscribed in their scope, and supported by appropriate references to parallel work in the field. As stated by Howard Haggard in *The Doctor in History*, "…a theory affords an explanation for known facts. Theories, when correct … serve as guides in the search for new facts. But when incorrect, they obscure the truth" [12]. Whether or not truth is obscured, wide-ranging theorizing, only tenuously related to the data, often raises the ire of peer reviewers, with unfortunate consequences for the scientific paper.

Finally, as in the Introduction, the journalistic approach is useful: discuss primary conclusions first and secondary or subsidiary extrapolations later. Thus, in the study of prognostic strategies in mitral regurgitation, suppose that right ventricular ejection fraction less than 30% at study entry was associated with poor two-year survival and that, as an unexpected ancillary finding, an association exists between prior rheumatic fever and left ventricular ejection fraction less than 50% at rest. The Discussion might begin,

"These data indicate that right ventricular ejection fraction at rest is closely related to survival in the absence of valve replacement." While the author alternatively might choose to highlight the rheumatic fever association first ("These data indicate a significant association between a history of rheumatic fever and chronic depression of left ventricular performance"), this point is not germane to the primary focus of the study or the paper. Beginning the Discussion in this way probably would confuse the reader and detract from the impact of the study. It is useful to outline a Discussion prior to writing it. This approach permits a review of the logic and flow of the discussion and of the appropriateness of placement of collateral or supporting references from the literature. The need to check the logic of the conclusions cannot be overstressed. The basis for each conclusion must be clearly presented. If a Discussion is logically deficient, then the Results, and the relevant literature, should be searched for the missing puzzle piece. If the link remains unapparent, then the authors' conclusions require reappraisal.

Afterthoughts

The foregoing represents some considerations regarding the author's personal approach to scientific paper writing, supplemented by the published views of a professional who has devoted much of his professional life specifically to this area (Robert Day) and other authors who have presented ideas that have been influential. Many subjects (acknowledgements, concerns regarding grammar and usage, how to respond to reviewers, etc.) have not been covered and can be sought in texts devoted to medical writing, which also may provide more comprehensive comments regarding the areas discussed. Ultimately, however, the decision on how to write a scientific paper rests with the author, modified by the policies of the editor and prepublication reviewers. If the author remains always cognizant that the scientific paper is a tool for communication, a critical part of the research process by which new knowledge is made available for the benefit of others, then he or she will successfully accomplish the task.

Take-Home Points

- The scientific paper is the vehicle that reports what research problem was studied, why it was studied, what was found, and how these findings should be interpreted, particularly within the context of related work in the field. Its publication, making the data available to the scientific community, is the final step in the research process.
- The scientific paper is a communications tool. Clarity and precision of expression are critically important.
- The best aid to crafting a useful scientific paper is a well-organized, well-planned, and clearly written research proposal or protocol.
- The results (not the discussion or authors' interpretation) are the new knowledge; their evaluation by the reader requires clear exposition of the methods. The discussion is not a mystery novel—state the conclusions in order of their importance. Remember that less usually is more.

References

1. Feinstein AR. Clinical judgment. Baltimore: Williams and Wilkins; 1967.
2. Day RA, Gastel B. How to write and publish a scientific paper. 6th ed. Westport: Greenwood; 2006.
3. American Association for the Advancement of Science (AAAS), Science & Policy, Electronic Publishing in Science, *Defining and Certifying Electronic Publication in Science,* A Proposal to the International Association of STM Publishers Originally Drafted October 1999; Revised March and June/July 2000. Learned Publishing. 2000;13:251–258.
4. Medawar PB**.** Is the scientific paper fraudulent? Yes; it misrepresents scientific thought. Saturday Review, 1 Aug 1964; 42–43.
5. Turato ER, Machado AC, Silva DF, de Carvalho GM, Verderosi NR, de Souza TF. Research publications in the field of health: omission of hypotheses and presentation of common-sense conclusions. Sao Paulo Med J. 2006;124:228–33.
6. Knottnerus JA. Challenges in dia-prognostic research. J Epidemiol Community Health. 2002;56:340–1.
7. Darwin C. On the origin of species by means of natural selection, or the preservation of favoured races in the struggle for life. 1st ed. London: John Murray; 1859.
8. Alderman EL, Fisher LD, Litwin P, Kaiser GC, Myers WO, Maynard C, Levine F, Schloss M. Results of coronary artery surgery in patients with poor left ventricular function (CASS). Circulation. 1983;68:785–95.
9. Borer JS, Bacharach SL, Green MV, Kent KM, Henry WL, Rosing DR, Seides SF, Johnston GS, Epstein SE. Exercise-induced left ventricular dysfunction in symptomatic and asymptomatic patients with aortic regurgitation: assessment by radionuclide cineangiography. Am J Cardiol. 1978;42:351–7.
10. Borer JS, Bacharach SL, Green MV, Kent KM, Epstein SE, Johnston GS. Real-time radionuclide cineangiography in the noninvasive evaluation of global and regional left ventricular function at rest and during exercise in patients with coronary-artery disease. N Engl J Med. 1977;296:839–44.
11. Huth EJ. How to write and publish papers in the medical sciences. 2nd ed. Baltimore: Williams & Wilkins; 1990.
12. Haggard HW. The doctor in history. New Haven: Yale University Press; 1934.

About the Editors

Phyllis G. Supino, EdD
Dr. Supino is an internationally recognized expert in research methodology, cardiovascular epidemiology, and medical education who has spearheaded multiple innovative educational programs on research methods for clinical audiences, upon which this book is largely based. She has authored more than 140 publications on research training, program evaluation, psychometrics, evidence-based medicine, and various topics in clinical medicine including valvular and coronary heart diseases, geriatric screening and death and dying. She is Professor of Medicine at the State University of New York (SUNY) Downstate Medical College, Professor of Public Health at the SUNY Downstate School of Public Health, Adjunct Research Professor of Public Health at Weill Medical College of Cornell University, and Director of Clinical Epidemiology and Clinical Research in the SUNY Downstate Division of Cardiovascular Medicine. She has primary responsibility for leading and mentoring clinical and epidemiological research in cardiovascular medicine, and for teaching principles of clinical research methodology to medical students, postgraduate medical trainees, attending physicians, and other health professionals at SUNY Downstate. Formerly, Dr. Supino served as a full-time faculty member at Weill Cornell Medical College and at other academic medical institutions in the greater New York area, where she directed clinical research and designed, introduced, and taught new courses on research methodology and hypothesis and protocol design for clinicians and allied health professionals. Several of these courses have been published as curriculum models in the international medical literature. She has taught biostatistics, epidemiology, and evidence-based medicine to medical undergraduates, mentored hundreds of medical students and physicians on clinical research and epidemiological methods, and created novel programs to introduce area college students to clinical investigation. Dr. Supino received her BA in biological sciences from the City College of the City University of New York. She holds an earned doctorate, with research distinction, in science education from Rutgers—the State University of New Jersey, and has conducted seminal postdoctoral research on learning theory and teaching

P.G. Supino and J.S. Borer (eds.), *Principles of Research Methodology: A Guide for Clinical Investigators*,
DOI 10.1007/978-1-4614-3360-6, © Phyllis G. Supino and Jeffrey S. Borer 2012

methods at Princeton University, where she served as a member of faculty, and at the Personality and Social Behavior Research Group of the Educational Testing Service, both in Princeton, New Jersey. She has won numerous awards for excellence in research, teaching, and mentoring, chaired several committees on research education in medicine, served on a variety of editorial boards and scientific advisory committees, and has chaired various scientific sessions in cardiovascular medicine. Dr. Supino is a Fellow of the New York Academy of Medicine and has been included in Who's Who in America, Who's Who in the World, Who's Who in Medicine in Healthcare, Who's Who in Science and Engineering, and Who's Who among American Women.

Jeffrey S. Borer, MD

Jeffrey S. Borer, MD is Professor of Medicine, Cell Biology, Radiology, and Surgery at SUNY Downstate Medical Center and College of Medicine in New York City. He is Chairman, Department of Medicine and Chief, Division of Cardiovascular Medicine, and Director of the Howard Gilman Institute for Heart Valve Disease and of the Cardiovascular Translational Research Institute at SUNY Downstate. Dr. Borer received his BA from Harvard, his MD from Cornell and trained at the Massachusetts General Hospital. He spent 7 years in the Cardiology Branch of the NHLBI at the NIH and a year at Guy's Hospital in London as a Senior Fullbright Hays Scholar, where he completed the first clinical demonstration of the utility of nitroglycerin in acute myocardial infarction. Upon returning to the NIH, he developed stress radionuclide cineangiography, for the first time allowing non-invasive assessment of cardiac function with exercise. He then returned to Cornell for 30 years, where he was the Gladys and Roland Harriman Professor of Cardiovascular Medicine and Chief of the Division of Cardiovascular Pathophysiology. At Cornell, his primary research involved developing prognostic standards for regurgitant valve diseases and exploring the cellular and molecular biology of myocardial dysfunction in valve diseases, now continued at SUNY Downstate. He has been an Advisor to the USFDA for 33 years, chairing the CardioRenal Advisory Committee for three terms and the Cardiovascular Devices Advisory Committee for one, and Advisor to NASA for 24 years. He has served as President of the American College of Cardiology (ACC), New York State Chapter, and member of the Board of Governors of the national ACC, as well as on the Boards of Governors or Trustees of multiple other national professional societies. Currently, he is President of the Heart Valve Society of America and a member of the ISO US Valve Experts Committee. Dr. Borer has published 400 scientific papers and four books, edits the journal, *Cardiology*, and has received several awards and other recognitions, including the Public Service Medal of NASA. He has been extensively involved in the training of medical students, residents, fellows, and translational scientists. Since 1990, he has closely collaborated with Dr. Supino on a variety didactic teaching programs on research methodology for clinicians and other members of the academic communities of Weill Medical College and SUNY Downstate Medical Center.

Index

P.G. Supino and J.S. Borer (eds.), *Principles of Research Methodology: A Guide for Clinical Investigators*, DOI 10.1007/978-1-4614-3360-6, © Phyllis G. Supino and Jeffrey S. Borer 2012

Printed in the United States
By Bookmasters